The Nutrition for Fitness Answer Book

A COMPANION FOR YOUR ACTIVE LIFESTYLE

MELVIN H. WILLIAMS
Old Dominion University

wcb
Wm. C. Brown Publishers
Dubuque, Iowa

Cover Photo by Guido A. Rossi/The Image Bank

Copyright © 1983, 1985 by Wm. C. Brown Publishers. All rights reserved

Library of Congress Catalog Card Number: 85-71682

ISBN 0-697-00753-7

No part of this publication may be reproduced, stored in a
retrieval system, or transmitted, in any form or by any means,
electronic, mechanical, photocopying, recording, or otherwise,
without the prior written permission of the publisher.

Printed in the United States of America
10 9 8 7 6 5 4 3 2 1

Dedicated to
my brothers and sisters
Betty Jean
Bud
Gail
and
Georgia

Contents

To the Reader ix

1 The Essential Dietary Nutrients 1
Essential Nutrients and the RDA 1
Basic Four Food Groups and a Balanced Diet 6
Dietary Goals for Americans 14

2 Carbohydrates—The Main Energy Food 19
Types and Sources 19
Metabolism and Function 21
Carbohydrates and Your Health 24
Carbohydrates for Exercise 27
Carbohydrate Loading 31

3 Fat—An Additional Energy Source During Exercise 39
Types and Sources 39
Cholesterol 43
Metabolism and Function 44
Fats, Exercise, and Your Health 48

4 Proteins—The Tissue Builder 55
Types and Sources 55
Metabolism and Function 60
Proteins and Your Health 63
Proteins and Exercise 64

5 Vitamins—The Organic Regulators 69
Basic Facts 69
Supplements and Megadoses 72
The Individual Vitamins 75
Vitamins for Athletes 83

6 Minerals—The Inorganic Regulators 85
Basic Facts 85
The Individual Minerals 86
Dietary Recommendations 96

7 Water—The Medium 97
Metabolism and Function 97
Water and Exercise 102

8 Human Energy Sources and Human Energy Systems 103
Measures of Energy 103
The Caloric Concept of Energy 106
Human Energy Systems 110
Energy Utilization during Rest and Exercise 114

9 Energy Requirements of Physical Exercise 121
Basal and Resting Metabolism 121
Exercise and the Metabolic Rate 126

10 Body Weight and Composition 133
Ideal Body Weight 133
Body Composition and Physical Performance 136
Calories and Weight Control 140

11 Gaining Body Weight—Diet and Exercise 143
Basic Considerations 143
Exercise Principles 145
Nutritional Principles 149

12 Losing Body Weight—Dieting 153
Predicting Body Weight Loss 154
Rapid and Slow Weight Losses 158
Strategies to Lose Body Weight 159
Dietary Modifications 163

13 Losing Body Weight—Exercise 171
The Role of Exercise 171
Designing Your Own Exercise Program 175
Body Weight Losses 183
Diet versus Exercise 185

14 Exercise in the Heat 187
Body Temperature Regulation 187
Exercise Effects on the Body Temperature 189
Preventing Heat Illnesses 193
Fluid and Electrolyte Losses 198
Fluid and Electrolyte Replacement 200

15 The Drug Foods—Alcohol and Caffeine 205
Alcohol Nutrition and Metabolism 206
Alcohol and Physical Performance 209
Alcohol and Your Health 212
Caffeine and Physical Performance 213
Caffeine and Your Health 216

16 The Consumer Athlete 219
Nutritional Value of American Foods 220
Nutrient Density 225
Nutritional Quackery in Athletics 229

17 Special Considerations for Active People 235
Exercise and Nutritional Requirements 235
Eating for Physical Performance 241
Diet, Exercise, and Your Health 245
Nutrition for Athletes 248

Appendixes 249
Glossary 293

Index 309

To the reader

For the average American, there are two basic changes in life-style that may have a significant impact upon their health. Initiation of a sound exercise program and modification of current dietary patterns may be significant factors in reducing the incidence of obesity, high blood pressure, coronary heart disease, and other degenerative diseases seen in our society.

The past decade has witnessed a tremendous increase in physical fitness awareness among the American populace, with more people than ever becoming participants in action sports such as running, swimming, bicycling, tennis, and racketball. It is estimated there are now over 25 million people regularly jogging or running in order to maintain adequate physical fitness levels to help optimize their overall health.

Research has shown that adults who become physically active also become more interested in other aspects of their life-style—particularly nutrition—that may affect their health in a positive way. However, nowhere in the area of nutrition is there more quackery and fraud than is found in organized athletics, and the myths and misconceptions of athletic nutrition are now influencing the dietary behavior of many physically active individuals such as your daily jogger or average road runner. For example, perusal of a popular magazine for runners over the past year revealed a number of articles or advertisements extolling the virtues of such diverse alleged nutrients as caffeine, bee pollen, vitamins B_{15}, C, and E, wheat germ oil, mineral supplements, and beer. One purpose of this book is to help dispel the myths and misconceptions associated with nutrition for physically active individuals.

This book is designed to provide nutritional information to the individual who is physically active or to those who desire to initiate or are just initiating a personalized exercise program. Although nutrition for active individuals is not essentially different from that for the nonactive person, there are special nutritional considerations of importance to help insure optimal physical performance under certain conditions. The topics covered will be of interest to all individuals concerned about sound nutritional practices, but special attention is devoted to nutritional aspects of physical performance.

Topics discussed include basic nutritional principles; the role of carbohydrates, fats, protein, vitamins, minerals, and water in physical performance; the energy aspects of exercise; the determination of body composition; weight gaining and weight loss programs by diet and exercise; guidelines for initiating exercise programs; special concerns during exercise in the heat; vegetarianism and physical performance; alcohol and caffeine effects on physical performance; consumer awareness for the active person; and special dietary considerations relative to performance.

The book uses a question-answer format, thus presenting meaningful content in small segments. This is a convenient approach for the individual who may have occasional short periods of time to read such as riding a bus or during a lunch break. In addition, the questions are arranged in a logical sequence, the answer to one question often leading into the question that follows. Where appropriate, cross-referencing within the text is used to expand the discussion. No deep scientific background is needed for the chemical aspects of nutrition and energy expenditure as these have been simplified.

The essential dietary nutrients

This chapter is intended to be a brief overview relative to the nutritional needs of most healthy individuals and a general plan of how you may achieve adequate nutrition. The concepts of the Recommended Dietary Allowances (RDA), the Basic Four Food Groups, the balanced diet, dietary goals, and nutrient density are discussed. The scope of this text prevents a detailed discussion of each of these concepts in this chapter, but several will be expanded in later chapters.

What nutrients are essential to humans?

There are six general classes of nutrients considered necessary in human nutrition. They are carbohydrates, fats, protein, vitamins, minerals, and water. Some nutritionists also consider fiber, a form of carbohydrate, a specific necessity in the diet. Within several of these general classes, notably protein, vitamins, and minerals, there are a number of specific nutrients necessary for life. For example, over a dozen vitamins are needed for optimal physiological functioning. Table 1.1 represents the specific nutrients known to be or are probably essential to humans.

Essential nutrients and the RDA

Some foods, such as whole wheat bread, may contain all six general classes of nutrients, while others, such as table sugar, contain only one nutrient. However, whole wheat bread is not a complete food since it does not contain all the essential specific nutrients.

Essential nutrients are necessary for human life. An inadequate intake may result in disturbed body metabolism, certain disease states, or death.

Some of the nutrients listed in Table 1.1 have been shown to be essential for various animals and are probably essential for humans. Essential nutrients, or nutrients from which they may be formed, must be obtained from the foods we eat.

What is the key nutrient concept?

There are eight nutrients that are central to human nutrition and found naturally in plant and animal sources usually accompanied by other essential nutrients. If these eight **key nutrients** are adequate in the diet, you will probably receive an ample supply of all nutrients essential to humans. Table 1.2 presents the eight key nutrients and some significant plant and

Table 1.1 Nutrients essential or probably essential to humans

Protein (essential amino acids)

Isoleucine	Threonine
Leucine	Tryptophan
Lysine	Valine
Methionine	Histidine (for children, but not adults)
Phenylalanine	

Fats (essential fatty acids)

Linoleic

Carbohydrates

Fiber

Vitamins

Water soluble	Fat soluble
B_1 (thiamin)	A (retinol)
B_2 (riboflavin)	D
Niacin	E (tocopherol)
B_6 (pyridoxine)	K
Pantothenic acid	
Folacin	
B_{12} (cyanocobalamin)	
Biotin	
C (ascorbic acid)	

Minerals

Calcium	Iron	Selenium
Chloride	Magnesium	Silicon
Chromium	Manganese	Sodium
Cobalt	Molybdenum	Sulfur
Copper	Nickel	Tin
Fluorine	Phosphorus	Vanadium
Iodine	Potassium	Zinc

Water

Table 1.2 Eight key nutrients and significant food sources from plants and animals

Nutrient	Plant source	Animal source
Protein	Dried beans and peas Nuts	Meat Poultry Fish Cheese Milk
Vitamin A	Dark green leafy vegetables Yellow vegetables Margarine	Butter Fortified milk Liver
Vitamin C	Citrus fruits Broccoli, potatoes Strawberries, tomatoes Cabbage, dark green leafy vegetables	Liver
Vitamin B_1 (thiamin)	Breads Cereals Nuts	Pork Ham
Vitamin B_2 (riboflavin)	Breads Cereals	Milk Cheese Liver
Niacin	Breads Cereals Nuts	Meat Fish Poultry
Iron	Dried peas and beans Spinach, asparagus Prune juice	Meat Liver
Calcium	Turnip greens, okra Broccoli, spinach	Milk Cheese Mackerel Salmon

animal sources. As can be noted, the four food groups approach would be a useful guide to securing these eight key nutrients. In Chapter 16, we will discuss the concept of the eight indicator nutrients in relation to nutritional labeling.

What does the term nutrient density mean?

As mentioned before, the nutrient content of foods varies considerably, the difference between food groups being more distinct than the differences between foods in the same group. **Nutrient density** is an important concept relative to the proportions of essential nutrients such as protein, vitamins, and minerals, which are found in specific foods. This concept will be stressed throughout the text and be explored further in Chapter 16; but, to cite an extreme example, consider the nutrient differences between a seven-ounce can of tuna fish packed in water and a piece of Boston cream pie. The tuna fish would provide you with over 100 percent of your RDA for protein, niacin, and vitamin B_{12} along with substantial amounts of vitamin B_6 and phosphorus, and very little fat. The caloric content would only be 220. For 210 Calories of Boston cream pie, you would receive little protein, few vitamins, or few minerals with greater amounts of fat and refined carbohydrates. Hence, the tuna fish has greater nutrient density and considerably greater nutritional value.

Another term related to nutrient density is the **Index of Nutritional Quality (INQ)** of a given food. The INQ is a comparison of the nutrient content of a food to the RDA for that nutrient in relation to the caloric content of the food and the caloric RDA for an average individual. As an example, look at the INQ for vitamin C in a glass of orange juice for an average adult female:

Orange juice (6-oz glass)
    92 Calories
    90 mg vitamin C
RDA for average adult woman
    2,100 Calories
    60 mg vitamin C

$$INQ = \frac{90/60}{92/2100} = 34.23$$

The higher the INQ, the better. The lowest recommended INQ for the various nutrients varies in the range of 1–2. Thus, orange juice is an exceptionally nutritious food in relationship to vitamin C.

What are the functions of food?

There are three major functions of food. First, foods provide energy for human metabolism. Carbohydrates and fats are the prime sources of energy and, although protein may also provide energy, this is not its major function. Vitamins, minerals, and water are not energy sources. Second, foods are used to build and repair body tissues. Protein is the major building material for muscles and other soft tissues, while certain minerals such as calcium and phosphorus make up the skeletal framework. Third, foods are used to help regulate body processes. Vitamins, minerals, and proteins work closely together in order to maintain the diverse physiological processes of human metabolism. For example, hemoglobin in the red blood cell (RBC) is essential for the transportation of oxygen to the muscle tissue via the blood. Hemoglobin is a complex combination of protein and iron, and the RBC also requires vitamin B_{12} and folic acid for full development.

Although these functions of food are important to the sedentary individual, they become increasingly important to the physically active person who may increase metabolic activities more than ten-fold through exercise and maintain that high rate for an hour or more. A number of studies have shown that physical performance may be hampered seriously by inadequate nutrition. On the other hand, as will be seen generally throughout this book, supplemental feeding of nutrients beyond adequate dietary intake has not been shown to increase physical performance capacity. The key point is to insure that you are receiving the optimal amount of specific nutrients as recommended by current knowledge of nutritional requirements. Hence, proper nutrition is essential to optimize energy sources, tissue building and repair, and regulation of body processes during and following periods of increased physical activity levels.

What are the RDA?

As noted in Table 1.1, humans have an essential requirement for a variety of nutrients, including organic compounds, inorganic ions, and water. In the United States, the amounts of certain of these nutrients have been established by the Food and Nutrition Board, National Academy of Sciences—National Research Council. The **Recommended Dietary Allowances (RDA)** represent the levels of intake of essential nutrients considered in the judgment of the Food and Nutrition Board on the basis of available scientific knowledge to be adequate to meet the known nutritional needs of practically all healthy persons in the United States. The current RDA are found in Appendix A, the ninth revision since they were initiated in 1943.

It should be noted that the RDA are based on the median heights and weights for specific age groups. The average adult male weights 154 pounds or in metric terms, 70 kilograms (kg). One kilogram equals 2.2 pounds. Hence, an adult male who weighs 80 kg will need proportionately more of the RDA while a 60 kg male will need proportionately less. The values for women and children also need to be adjusted accordingly.

The RDA should not be construed to be the recommended ideal diet. They are not guaranteed to represent total nutritional needs, for there is insufficient evidence relative to some essential trace elements. Moreover, they are designed for healthy persons, not those needing dietary modifications on account of illness. The RDA have not been designed to be used as individual requirements, but they can be an effective guide for this purpose.

Although related, the RDA should not be confused with the **United States Recommended Daily Allowances (U.S. RDA).** The U.S. RDA are a simplified RDA. They appear on the labels of food products and simply represent the percentage of the RDA provided by a serving of the food product. They may serve as a useful guide in planning meals that will contain the daily RDA.

Again, one must interpret the U.S. RDA with care. They are based on the RDA, which have been established for the average sized male or female at a given age. Hence, a U.S. RDA for protein of 50 percent for a given food product may be 70 percent for one person and 30 percent for another if they weigh considerably less or more, respectively, than the average person for their age group. The U.S. RDA is discussed further in Chapter 16.

An individual does not necessarily have a deficient diet if the full RDA is not received daily. The daily RDA should average over a five-to-eight day period, so that one may be deficient in iron consumption one day but compensate for this one-day deficiency during the remainder of the week. A general recommendation to help meet the daily RDA requirements is to select as wide a variety of foods as possible when planning the diet.

The RDA provide sound information relative to nutritional needs. However, they are a rather cumbersome tool to use for the purpose of educating the public about sound nutrition. Hence, the food group approach, based upon the RDA, was developed as a practical method for nutrition education in the United States. A recent report from California showed significant improvement in the eating habits of teenagers following an innovative teaching program based on the four food groups.

What are the basic four food groups?

Basic four food groups and a balanced diet

The nutritional composition of foods varies tremendously. Perusal of the Food Composition Table of the United States Department of Agriculture reveals that no two foods are exactly alike in nutrient composition. However, certain foods are similar enough in nutrient content that they may be grouped accordingly. For educational purposes, foods have been grouped according to nutrients in which they are rich. A commonly used system in the United States is the **Basic Four Food Groups.** Foods of similar nutrient value are placed in groups such as the Meat Group, the Milk Group, the Bread-Cereal Group, or the Fruit-Vegetable Group. Some publications list a fifth group, the Fats, Sweets, and Alcohol Group. The meat group may also be described as the meat, poultry, fish, and beans group, while the milk group is also known as the milk and cheese group.

Table 1.3 lists some common foods found in each of the four groups. A more detailed list patterned after the Exchange Food Model is presented later in this book.

Table 1.3. Common foods found in the four major food groups

Meat group: two or more servings daily		Fruit-vegetable group: four or more servings daily		Bread-cereal group (whole grain or enriched): four or more servings daily	
Beef	Ground beef	Asparagus	Apple	Biscuits	Corn grits
Lamb	Stewing lamb	Beets	Apple juice	Boston brown bread	Hominy
Pork	Pork chops	Broccoli	Apricots	Cornbread	Macaroni
Veal	Veal chops	Brussels sprouts	Banana	Muffins	Noodles
Fish	Salmon	Cabbage	Blueberries	Pancakes	Oatmeal
Chicken	Tuna	Carrots	Cantaloupe	Raisin bread	Ready-to-eat cereal
Duck	Shrimp	Celery	Cherries	Rolls	Rice
Turkey	Oysters	Collard greens	Dates	Rye bread	Rolled oats
Ham	Lobster	Cauliflower	Figs	Waffles	Rolled wheat
Liver	Kidney	Corn	Grapefruit	White bread	Spaghetti
Frankfurter	Sausage	Cress	Grapefruit juice	Whole wheat bread	Crackers
Goose	Salami	Eggplant	Grapes		
Liverwurst	Bologna	Green beans	Honeydew melon		
Dry beans	Sardines	Green peas	Lemon juice		
Peanut butter	Dry peas	Green pepper	Lemons		
	Eggs	Kale	Limes		
Milk group: two or more servings daily		Lettuce	Mangos		
Whole milk	Dry milk	Lima beans	Nectarines		
Cheddar cheese	Cream cheese	Mushrooms	Orange juice		
Swiss cheese	Blue cheese	Onions	Oranges		
Buttermilk	Ice milk	Parsley	Papaya		
Ice cream	Coffee cream	Potatoes	Peaches		
Other foods		Pumpkin	Pears		
Beer	Margarine	Rutabaga	Persimmons		
Cake	Marmalade	Sauerkraut	Pineapple		
Candy	Mayonnaise	Spinach	Pineapple juice		
Cookies	Molasses	Sweet potatoes	Plums		
Honey	Olive oil	Swiss Chard	Prune juice		
Jam	Pickle	Tomato juice	Prunes		
Jelly	Preserves	Tomatoes	Raisins		
Syrup	Soda	Turnip greens	Raspberries		
Wine		Turnips	Rhubarb		
		Watercress	Strawberries		
		Wax beans	Tangelo		
		Zucchini squash	Tangerines		
			Watermelon		

Foods in the Basic Four Food Groups.
(Bob Coyle)

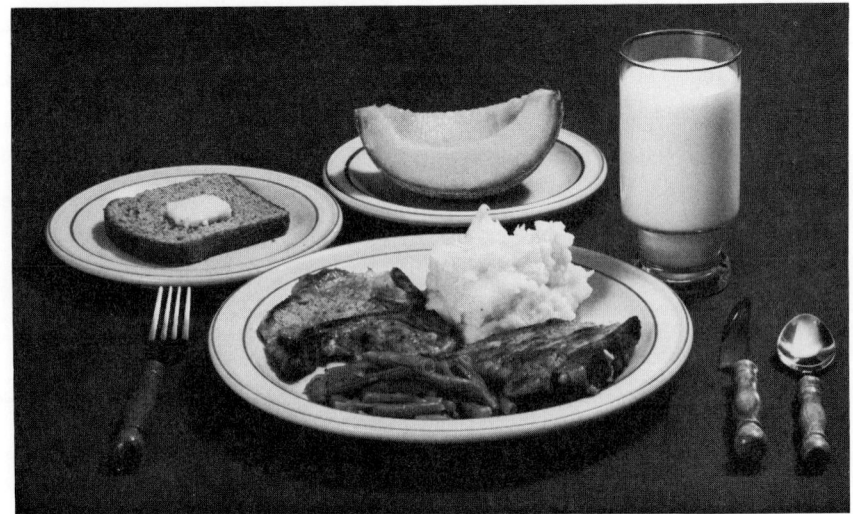

The value of the Basic Four Food Group approach is in its simplicity. Different patterns of nutrients are found in the four food groups, and since the American population has a tremendous variety of foods from which to select, it should not be difficult to get the necessary amount of nutrients if foods are selected from across the four groups. Admittedly, there are variations in the nutrient concentrations of different foods within each group (a peach and a pear are both fruits, but the peach has a considerably higher content of vitamin A), but if the individual selects foods widely throughout each group, the nutrient intake should be balanced over a period of time.

What major nutrients are found in the basic four food groups?

As noted previously, humans have a requirement for many diverse nutrients, including eight amino acids, three fatty acids, fourteen vitamins, and twenty-one minerals. Some of these requirements are only for trace amounts and can be met easily because several of the trace nutrients are distributed widely throughout the four food groups. On the other hand, substantial amounts of several major nutrients are needed and also can be obtained easily if foods are selected from the group that is rich in those nutrients. The following represents a listing of the major nutrients found in each of the four food groups. More specific information relative to vitamins and minerals may be found in Chapters 5 and 6.

Meat group	Milk group	Bread-cereal group	Fruit-vegetable group
protein	calcium	thiamin	vitamin A
thiamin	protein	niacin	vitamin C
niacin	riboflavin	riboflavin	vitamin E
vitamin B_6	vitamin A	iron	folacin
vitamin B_{12}	vitamin D	protein	biotin
iron	vitamin B_{12}		
	phosphorus		

It should be noted that this listing represents the major nutrient content of each food group, but that there is some variation in the proportion of the nutrients found between food groups as well as in different foods within each group. For example, the Bread-Cereal Group may be a good source of protein, but not as good as the Meat or Milk Group. Within the Fruit-Vegetable Group, oranges are an excellent source of vitamin C, but peaches are not.

There are also some foods that do not fall naturally into one of the four groups and are usually listed as *others* or *miscellaneous*. They usually supply very little nutritional value other than the calories of fat and simple carbohydrates. Fats, sweets, nonmilk and nonjuice beverages, and condiments are included in this listing.

What is a balanced diet?

Although everyone's diet requires the essential nutrients, the proportions differ at varying stages of the life cycle. The infant has needs differing from his grandfather, and the pregnant or lactating woman has needs differing from her adolescent daughter. There are also different needs between the sexes, particularly in the iron content of the diet. Moreover, individual variations in life-style may impose different nutrient requirements. A long distance runner in training for a marathon has some distinct nutritional needs compared to a sedentary colleague. The individual trying to lose weight needs to balance calorie losses with nutrient adequacy. The diabetic needs strict nutritional counseling for a balanced diet. Thus, there are a number of different conditions that may influence nutrient needs and the concept of a balanced diet.

It should be noted that the food supply in the United States is extremely varied, and most individuals who consume a wide variety of foods throughout the four food groups do receive an adequate supply of nutrients on a balanced diet.

Table 1.4. Recommended minimum number of servings from the basic four food groups with serving sizes

Food group	Recommended minimum number of servings				
	Child	Teenager	Adult	Pregnant woman	Lactating woman
Meat	2	2	2	3	2
Milk	3	4	2	4	4
Fruit-Vegetable	4	4	4	4	4
Bread-Cereal	4	4	4	4	4

Serving sizes

Meat: one serving is

2 ounces cooked, lean, boneless meat, fish, poultry or protein equivalent

2 eggs

2 slices (2 oz) cheddar cheese*

½ cup cottage cheese*

1 cup cooked dry beans, peas, lentils or soybeans

1 cup nuts

4 tablespoons peanut butter

Milk: one serving is

1 cup milk, yogurt or calcium equivalent

1½ slices (1½ oz) cheddar cheese*

2 ounces processed cheese food*

1½ cups ice cream or ice milk

2 cups cottage cheese*

Fruit-vegetable: one serving is

½ cup cooked or juice

1 small salad

1 orange

½ cantaloupe

1 medium potato

Bread-cereal: one serving is

1 slice bread

1 cup (1 oz) ready-to-eat cereal

½ cup cooked cereal or pasta

*A serving of cheese can be used for either the milk or meat group, but not both.

Can the basic four groups be used as a means to secure a balanced diet?

A balanced diet is the primary purpose of the Basic Four Food Group concept. Table 1.4 represents the recommended minimum number of servings from each food group that should provide a balanced intake of essential nutrients for various members of the populations. The number of servings should be adjusted as determined by caloric needs. This point will be discussed further in Chapter 12.

What is an example of a balanced daily menu based on the basic four food groups?

You have a wide variety of foods to select from in order to meet nutrient needs via the four food group approach. Although eggs, pancakes, or cereal are traditionally a part of the breakfast menu in many American homes, there is nothing inherently wrong with having a taco or piece of pizza for breakfast. The nutritional value of the food is the key point. Table 1.5 represents only one example of a daily menu balanced across the Basic Four Food Groups.

How can I tell if my diet is balanced?

Keep track of your food intake over a one-week period. A pocket notebook would be helpful. Record everything you eat, including the amounts. Be sure to note the ingredients of combination foods such as a tuna casserole, which might contain tuna fish, noodles, a vegetable, and a creamed soup (foods representing all four groups). At the end of the week simply consult Table 1.3, tabulate the number of items you consumed in each food group, and see if you have consumed the appropriate number of foods from each group for the week. You should have at least the following amounts, which simply represent seven days times the recommended daily intake for adults.

Meat Group = 14
Milk Group = 14
Bread-Cereal Group = 28
Fruit-Vegetable Group = 28

These figures would be modified for children, teenagers, and pregnant or lactating women. See Table 1.4 for recommended number of servings.

    Computerized analysis of your nutrient intake may be available locally in many hospitals, universities, or commercial organizations. Software packages are also available for those with home computers.

Table 1.5 Example of a daily menu based on the four food groups

Breakfast

Meat	Eggs
Milk	Milk
Bread-Cereal	Toast
Fruit-Vegetable	Orange juice

Lunch

Meat	Ham
Milk	Cheese
Bread-Cereal	Whole wheat bread
Fruit-Vegetable	Apple

Dinner

Meat	Tuna fish
Milk	Yogurt
Bread-Cereal	Noodles, dinner rolls
Fruit-Vegetabale	Lettuce and tomato salad

Snacks

Fruit-Vegetable	Banana

Others

	Margarine
	Salad dressing

Totals

Meat	Two or more
Milk	Two or more
Bread-Cereal	Four or more
Fruit-Vegetable	Four or more

Note: This table presents some common examples of foods within each of the four food groups. As discussed in the text, however, you must select food wisely among and within each group. For example, to avoid excessive amounts of Calories, cholesterol, and saturated fats, you could select egg substitutes, skim milk, lean meats such as turkey and chicken, water-packed tuna fish, low-fat yogurt, and corn oil margarine.

Are there any problems with the basic four food groups or balanced diet concept?

The Basic Four Food Group or balanced diet concept provides a sound basis for assuring nutritional adequacy. However, there may be some problems if the concept is not completely understood. Some of the problems are as follows:

1. It is possible to choose the least nutritious foods from among the four groups, leading to some nutrient deficiency. For example, foods from three groups could be selected containing no vitamin C, and if low vitamin C fruits and vegetables are eaten, a deficiency could be created.

2. With many of the processed foods today, it is difficult to categorize them into one of the four groups. To which group does a pepperoni pizza belong? It has some meat, cheese, bread, and a vegetable. Would this constitute a serving from each of the four groups?

3. It may be possible to overload on one type of nutrient. High fat foods may be selected easily from three of the food groups and contribute an excessive amount of fat calories to the overall diet.

4. Individuals have different metabolic rates and physical activity levels. What might be an adequate intake of calories and nutrients for one person might be too little or too excessive for another. Obesity may be one unfortunate consequence of excessive caloric consumption.

5. The balanced diet may not provide enough iron for women. A recent survey indicated 93 percent of females from ages 10–24 had iron intake below the recommended standard.

6. Those individuals who are on low calorie diets need to exercise special care to insure a balanced intake of nutrients.

7. The terminology used may be inappropriate for the vegetarian who may desire to avoid the meat and milk group altogether. However, knowledge that dried beans may be an alternate food in the meat group helps to alleviate this problem.

Again, with proper understanding of the Basic Four Food Group concept, these problems may be avoided by selection of a wide variety of foods.

Table 1.6 Current dietary intake and proposed dietary goals for Americans expressed in percent of dietary intake

	Current dietary intake	Proposed dietary goals
Fat	42%	30%
Saturated	16%	10%
Monounsaturated	13%	10%
Polyunsaturated	13%	10%
Carbohydrate	46%	58%
Simple	24%	10%
Complex	22%	48%
Protein	12%	12%
Cholesterol	500–1,000 mg	< 300 mg*
Salt	6–18 g	< 3 g*

*Daily cholesterol and salt intake should be restricted to 300 mg and 3 g or less, respectively.

What are the recommended dietary goals for Americans?

Dietary goals for Americans

Although the basic four would appear to be a sound approach to nutrition education, there are some who contend that the general eating habits of Americans represent as critical a public health concern as any now before us. The trend toward increased consumption of fats, simple sugars, and alcohol led to an investigation by a Select Subcommittee on Human Nutrition and Needs of the United States Senate with resultant **recommended dietary goals** for the American public. Table 1.6 presents the current dietary intake and the proposed goals. The values in the table represent the percentage of Calories that come from the three major nutrients.

The major recommended changes include a shift away from fats, particularly saturated fats, toward the complex carbohydrates. Protein intake remains essentially unchanged. Cholesterol and salt consumption should also be restricted. Relative to the four food groups, these goals reflect a need to decrease the use of meat, high fat foods, high cholesterol foods such as eggs, and high simple sugar foods, while at the same time increasing the intake of poultry, fish, fruits, vegetables, and whole grain products. These recommendations are very similar to a recent report to the British public by the Committee on Nutrition of the British Medical Association.

These recommended dietary goals have not been without critics. One of the reasons used to justify a change in American dietary habits is the increasing evidence of degenerative diseases such as coronary heart disease (CHD) and the assumption that such diseases are caused by poor nutrition.

Yet the assumption that dietary changes will help prevent CHD is still being investigated and remains a hypothesis, not a fact. The report has also been criticized due to certain omissions. Although mentioning obesity, it did not discuss the importance of exercise in relation to weight control. And even though the national nutrition survey reported that iron deficiency exists at high incidence levels, the subcommittee report failed to include iron intake as a main goal. Moreover, the recommendation for reduced meat intake may reduce iron consumption since it is one of the best sources of iron in the diet.

Nevertheless, those who criticize the subcommittee report for its shortcomings suggest that it may be a change toward a more healthful diet. Although research has not proven that dietary modification will help to prevent certain diseases such as CHD and hypertension, there is some evidence available to suggest that dietary manipulation may be one of several factors that may serve as a disease-prevention role.

Are there any guidelines that will help you meet the recommended dietary goals?

To make these recommendations more practical for the average American, the following guidelines have been developed to provide a sound means to achieve them.

1. Maintain a normal body weight.

    In order to avoid becoming overweight, you should consume only as many Calories as you expend daily. Methods of maintaining or losing weight are presented in Chapters 12 and 13. Programs to gain weight are presented in Chapter 11.

2. Eat a wide variety of natural foods from among the Basic Four food groups.

    This is the best means to obtain an adequate supply of all the essential nutrients. Of special importance, especially for females and growing children, are foods high in calcium and iron. Milk and other dairy products are excellent sources of calcium, while iron is found in good supply in the Meat and Bread Groups.

3. Eat a sufficient amount of protein.

    The recommended dietary goal for protein is about 12 percent of the daily Calories. This averages out to about fifty to sixty grams of protein per day; the current American intake is about one hundred grams, so we appear to be meeting this dietary goal. However, most of the protein we eat is of animal origin. Although animal products are an excellent source of complete protein, they may also contain substantial quantities of saturated fat and cholesterol.

4. Decrease your consumption of foods that are high in total fat, saturated fats, and cholesterol.

There is no specific requirement for fat in the diet. However, a need exists for an essential fatty acid and vitamins that are components of fat. Since almost all foods contain some fat, sufficient amounts of the essential fatty acid and vitamins are found in the average diet. Even on a vegetarian diet of fruits, vegetables and grain products, about 5–10 percent of your Calories are derived from fat, thus supplying enough of these essential nutrients. Fat, however, currently comprises over 40 percent of our Calories; the recommended dietary goal is less than 30 percent. In addition, the amount of saturated fat in the diet should be 10 percent or less, and cholesterol intake should be limited to 300 milligrams or less per day.

The basis for the reduction in dietary saturated fats and cholesterol is the assumption that they are associated with high blood levels of triglycerides and cholesterol, which is a risk factor associated with atherosclerosis and CHD. There appears to be enough medical evidence to justify a modification of the diet to lower high blood levels of triglycerides and cholesterol, or to prevent their rise in individuals with low to normal levels. The following practical suggestions will help you meet the recommended dietary goal.

    a. Eat less meat that has a high fat content. Avoid hot dogs, luncheon meats, sausage, bacon. Trim off excess fat before cooking. Eat only lean red meat and more white meat, such as turkey, chicken, and fish, which have less fat.
    b. Eat only two to three eggs per week. One egg yolk contains about 250 milligrams of cholesterol, which is close to the limit of 300 milligrams per day. Egg whites have no cholesterol and are an excellent source of high quality protein. You may also use commercially prepared egg substitutes.
    c. Eat fewer dairy products that are high in fat. Switch from whole milk and hard cheeses to skim milk and soft cheeses. Eat other dairy products, such as yogurt and cottage cheese, made from low fat milk.
    d. Eat less butter by substituting margarine made from liquid oils that are polyunsaturated. Try to avoid margarine made from hydrogenated oils.
    e. Eat less commercially prepared baked goods that have been made with eggs and saturated fats. Check the labels for main ingredients.
    f. Broil and bake your foods, rather than fry them. If you must fry other foods, use polyunsaturated liquid oils, rather than hard fats.
    g. Consume less refined sugar and alcohol to help reduce blood triglycerides.

These suggestions should be modified somewhat for young children who may need the excellent nutritional protein of eggs and the Calories of whole milk to help support growth.

5. Reduce your consumption of refined sugar.

   The recommended dietary goal is to reduce consumption of refined sugar from the current level of 24 percent of the daily Calories to 10 percent or less. Excessive consumption of refined sugar has been associated with high blood triglyceride levels. Sticky-type sugars are a major contributing factor to dental cavities. Sugars also significantly increase the caloric content of foods without an increase in nutritional value, so they may contribute to body weight problems.

   In order to meet this goal you should reduce your intake of common table sugar and products that are high in refined sugar. Sugar is one of the major additives to processed foods so check the labels. If sugar is listed first then it is the main ingredient. Look also for terms such as corn syrup, dextrose, fructose, and malt sugar, which are also primarily refined sugars.

6. Increase your consumption of the complex carbohydrates and natural sugars found in vegetables, fruits, and whole grain products.

   The dietary goals recommend that approximately 60 percent of your dietary Calories be derived from carbohydrate, with about 50 percent from the complex carbohydrates. The complex carbohydrates in vegetables and whole grain products are accompanied by significant quantities of vitamins and minerals, with small amounts of protein and little fat. Fruits are a good source of natural sugars, vitamins, and minerals. Increased intake of complex carbohydrates also naturally increases the amount of fiber (regarded as important for a healthy intestinal tract) in the diet.

7. Consume less sodium and high salt foods.

   The recommended dietary goal is to reduce the current sodium intake to less than three grams, which is 3000 milligrams. This lower amount will provide sufficient sodium for normal physiological functioning. Increased sodium intake has been associated with high blood pressure (hypertension), but the National Research Council has indicated there is little or no direct evidence to suggest that high blood pressure can be produced in an individual with normal blood pressure and normal dietary intake of salt. On the other hand, hypertensive individuals may be able to reduce their blood pressure by decreasing the amount of salt in the diet.

   Sodium is found naturally in a wide variety of foods that we eat so it is not difficult to get an adequate supply. Several key suggestions may help you reduce the sodium content in your diet.
   a. Use your salt shaker less often. One teaspoon of salt is 2000 mg of sodium; the average well-salted meal contains about 3000–4000 mg. Put less salt on your food both in your cooking pot and on your table.
   b. Reduce the consumption of obviously high-salt foods, such as pretzels, potato chips, pickles, and other such snacks.

    c. Check food labels for sodium content. If salt is one of the ingredients listed first you have a high sodium food. Salt is a major additive in many processed foods.
    d. Eat more fresh fruits and vegetables, which are very low in sodium. Fruits, both fresh and canned, have less than 8 mg sodium per serving. Fresh vegetables may have 35 mg or less, but if canned may contain up to 460 mg.

8. Use moderation in the consumption of alcohol.

Although this was not a specific recommendation of the Senate report, it is important to include at this point because there are some health implications of alcohol consumption. Alcohol is discussed in Chapter 15.

Carbohydrates—the main energy food

2

Since the early part of this century, scientists have known that carbohydrate is one of the prime sources of energy during exercise. The early research with carbohydrate and physical performance was misinterpreted by the athletic world, and the myth arose that simple sugars such as dextrose and those found in honey would be an immediate source of energy for muscular work. Continued research over the past two decades, both in this country and abroad, has revealed some useful information relative to the beneficial application of carbohydrate nutrition to certain athletic endeavors. In this chapter, we shall explore the nature of carbohydrates, their metabolic fates and interactions in the human body, and their potential application to physical performance.

What are carbohydrates?

Carbohydrates are the basic foodstuffs formed when the energy from the sun is harnessed in plants. They are organic compounds that contain carbon, hydrogen, and oxygen in various combinations.

Carbohydrates are one of the least expensive forms of Calories and hence represent one of the major food supplies for the vast majority of the world.

Types and sources

What are simple and complex carbohydrates?

In general terms carbohydrates may be categorized as either simple or complex. **Simple carbohydrates,** which are usually known as sugars, can be subdivided into two categories, disaccharides and monosaccharides. **Saccharide** means sugar or sweet. Think of saccharin, a noncaloric sweetener. The disaccharides include maltose (malt sugar), lactose (milk sugar), and **sucrose** (cane sugar or table sugar). Upon digestion these disaccharides yield the monosaccharides: **glucose, fructose,** and galactose as follows:

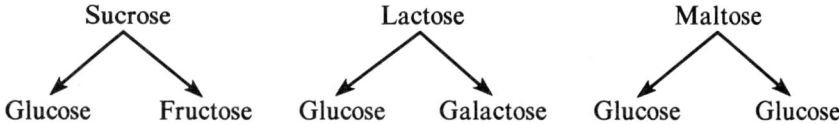

Glucose and fructose also occur widely in nature, primarily in fruits, as free monosaccharides. Glucose is often called dextrose or grape sugar, while fructose is known as fruit sugar.

Table 2.1 Foods high in carbohydrate content

Bread-Cereal group	Fruit-Vegetable group		Milk group
Biscuits	Apples	Oranges	Skim milk
Bread	Applesauce	Peaches	Yogurt
Cereal	Apricots	Pears	Ice milk
Cornbread	Banana	Peas, green	
Crackers	Beans, kidney	Peas, split	
Grits	Beans, lima	Pineapple	**Meat group**
Macaroni	Blackberries	Plums	Dried beans
Muffins	Blueberries	Potatoes	Dried peas
Noodles	Cantaloupe	Raspberries	
Pancakes	Cherries	Squash, winter	
Rice	Corn	Sweet potato	
Spaghetti	Dried fruits	Tangerines	
Waffles	Figs		

The **complex carbohydrates** are the polysaccharides commonly known as starches. The vast majority of carbohydrates that exist in the plant world are in this form. Starches consist of many molecules of glucose bonded together. Of prime interest to us are the plant starches, through which we obtain a good proportion of our daily Calories along with a wide variety of nutrients, and the animal starch, glycogen, about which we shall hear more later.

What are some common foods high in carbohydrate content?

Of the four food groups, the Bread-Cereal and Fruit-Vegetable are the two primary contributors of carbohydrate to the diet. Some foods in the Meat and Milk Groups contain moderate to high amounts of carbohydrate, such as dry beans, dry peas, milk and ice cream. Table 2.1 shows some foods in the Four Food Groups that have high carbohydrate content. Complex carbohydrate foods are accentuated as they are highly recommended under the new American dietary goals.

Foods other than those listed in the table may have appreciable amounts of carbohydrates. Seeds and nuts have moderate amounts in general, dried chestnuts having a high content. Miscellaneous foods such as pies, puddings, candy, cookies, cake with icing, maple syrup, honey, and sugar are rather high in carbohydrates, but primarily the simple type.

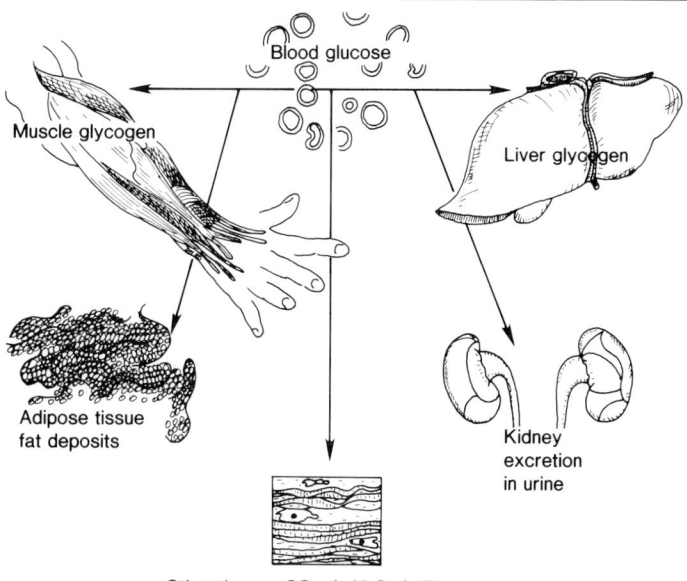

Figure 2.1.
Fates of blood glucose. After assimilation into the blood, glucose may be stored in the liver or muscles as glycogen or be utilized as a source of energy by these and other tissues, particularly the nervous system. Excess glucose may be partially excreted by the kidneys, but major excesses are converted to fat and stored in the adipose tissues.

What happens to dietary carbohydrate in the human body?

Metabolism and function

Carbohydrates are usually ingested in the forms of polysaccharides (starches) and disaccharides (sugars) although some monosaccharides (glucose and fructose) are also found in the diet. It is not necessary to explain all the intricate steps of the digestive process here, but essentially what happens is a breakdown of the polysaccharides and disaccharides to the monosaccharides. The primary site of digestion is the small intestine, and the monosaccharides are then absorbed into the blood.

Of the two monosaccharides, glucose is of most importance to human physiology. It is the blood sugar. The fructose that is absorbed into the blood is eventually transported to the liver where it is converted to blood glucose. The fate of the blood glucose is dependent upon a multitude of factors, with exercise being one of the most important. In essence, however, the following items represent the major fates of blood glucose. Figure 2.1 schematically represents these fates.

1. Blood glucose may be converted to either liver or muscle glycogen. It is important to note that glucose may be converted to liver glycogen, which may later be reconverted to blood glucose. However, this cannot occur to any appreciable extent with muscle glycogen. In essence, glucose is locked in the muscle once it enters, due to the lack of a specific enzyme needed to change its form so it can cross the cell membrane.

    Glycogen is formed in the body when a number of different glucose units are combined. It is not found in plants as such and is found in animal tissues only to a limited extent. Hence, it is not a major source of carbohydrate in our diet, but it does play an important role in human carbohydrate metabolism, especially during exercise. Its role as an energy source will be explored later in this chapter.

2. Blood glucose may be converted to and stored as fat in the adipose tissue. This situation occurs when the dietary carbohydrate, in combination with caloric intake of other nutrients, exceeds the energy demands of the body and the storage capacity of the liver and muscles for glycogen.

3. Blood glucose may be used for energy, particularly by the brain and other parts of the nervous system that rely primarily on glucose for their metabolism.

4. Blood glucose also may be excreted in the urine if an excess amount occurs in the blood due to rapid ingestion of simple sugars.

How much total energy do we store as carbohydrate?

There are three energy sources of carbohydrate in the body—blood glucose, liver glycogen, and muscle glycogen. Since each gram of carbohydrate equals approximately four Calories, an estimate of the energy content of each of these sources may be obtained.

Initial stores of blood glucose are rather limited, totaling only about 5 grams (g) of glucose, or the equivalent of 20 Calories (C). However, blood glucose stores may be replenished from either liver glycogen or absorption of the monosaccharides from the intestine. The liver has the greatest concentration of glycogen in the body. However, since its size is limited, the liver normally contains only about 75 g of glycogen, or 300 C. It is important to note that the glycogen content may be decreased by starvation or increased by a carbohydrate-rich diet. Certain dietary patterns may nearly double the glycogen content of the liver, a condition that may be useful in certain tasks of physical performance.

The greatest amount of carbohydrate stored in the body is in the form of muscle glycogen. This is because the muscles comprise such a large proportion of the body mass as contrasted to the liver. One would expect large differences in total muscle glycogen content between different individuals because of differences in body size. However, for an average-sized man with about 30 kg of his body weight consisting of muscle tissue, one could expect a total muscle glycogen content of approximately 300 g, or 1,200 C. As with liver glycogen, the muscle glycogen stores may also be decreased or increased, with considerable effects on physical performance.

Hence, the total body storage of carbohydrate in this example is only 1,520 C, not an appreciable amount. One full day of starvation could reduce it considerably.

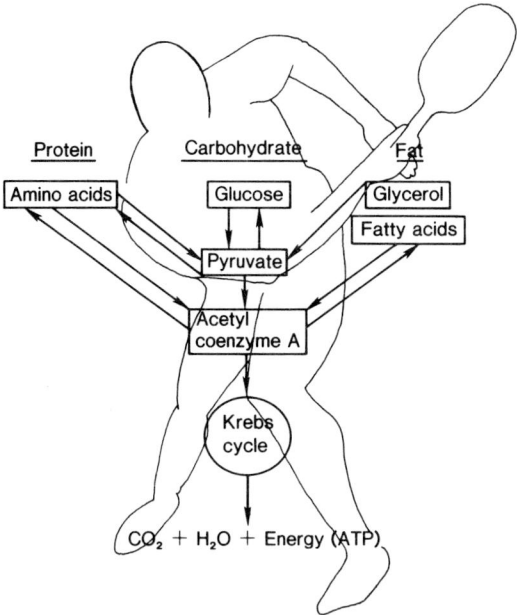

Figure 2.2.
Interrelationships between carbohydrate, fat, and protein metabolism in humans. All three nutrients may be utilized for energy, although the major energy sources are carbohydrate and fat. Excess carbohydrate may be converted to fat; the carbohydrate structure may also be used to form protein, but nitrogen must be added. Fat can not be used to generate carbohydrate to any large extent since acetyl CoA cannot be converted to pyruvate. The glycerol component fat possibly may form very small amounts of carbohydrate. Fats may serve as a basis for the formation of protein, but again nitrogen must be added. Excess protein cannot be stored in the body, but can be converted to either carbohydrate or fat.

Can the human body make carbohydrates from protein and fat?

Since the carbohydrate stores in the body are rather limited, and since glucose is normally essential for optimal functioning of the nervous system, it is important to be able to produce carbohydrate internally if the stores are depleted due to starvation or a zero carbohydrate diet. The body can adapt to a carbohydrate-free diet over a period of several weeks as the nervous system shifts its energy source away from glucose.

Protein may be a significant source of blood glucose. Protein breaks down to amino acids in the body, and certain of these amino acids, notably alanine, may be converted to glucose in the liver. The process is called **gluconeogenesis,** meaning the new formation of glucose.

Fats in the body break down into fatty acids and glycerol. Although there is no mechanism in human cells to convert the fatty acids to glucose, the glycerol may be converted to glucose through the process of gluconeogenesis in the liver. Thus, blood glucose can be derived from protein and fat by liver action on certain of their components.

Figure 2.2 graphically depicts the interactions between the three energy foodstuffs. Further discussion is presented in Chapters 3 and 4.

What are the major functions of carbohydrate in human nutrition?

The major function of carbohydrate in human metabolism is to supply energy. Through a series of biochemical reactions in the body cells, glucose is hydrolyzed, eventually producing water, carbon dioxide, and energy. Details of these energy producing mechanisms are presented in Chapter 8.

The primary carbohydrate source of energy for physical performance is the muscle glycogen, specifically the glycogen in the muscles that are active. As the muscle glycogen is used during exercise, blood glucose may enter the muscles to help maintain muscle glycogen stores. In turn, the liver will release some of its glucose in order to help maintain blood glucose levels.

Monosaccharides in the body can be used also to form other smaller carbohydrate molecules such as trioses and pentoses. These substances may combine with other nutrients and form body chemicals essential to life. Hence, carbohydrate may also serve as a source of material for indispensible components contributing both to structure and function of the human body.

Another function of carbohydrate is to provide fiber, or bulk, to the diet.

What is dietary fiber and what is its importance in the diet?

Carbohydrates and your health

Dietary fiber is the plant carbohydrate resistent to digestive enzymes and hence leaves some residue in the digestive tract. It is found in fruits, vegetables, legumes, and cereals, most notably the bran cereals. Over the past 100 years, the amount of fiber in our diet has decreased considerably, although there are some attempts now being made to increase our dietary fiber content.

The major component of dietary fiber is **cellulose.** Cellulose is found in all plant cells, in marked contrast to animal cells. In general, cellulose is an inert substance that does not break down in the presence of human digestive enzymes. Hence, cellulose adds bulk to our diet as the dietary fiber recommended for prevention of constipation and possible problems in the large intestine. Other forms of dietary fiber include pectin, lignin, gums and mucilages

Based primarily upon a number of epidemiological studies, a decrease in dietary fiber has been associated with a broad spectrum of diseases involving the digestive tract, notably the large intestine and colon. Some have suggested dietary fiber may help prevent atherosclerosis. The suggested underlying mechanisms include the role of fiber in speeding the transit of various materials through the intestines or in helping to decrease the absorption of dietary cholesterol. These claims have not been substantiated totally by experimental research, but the epidemiological data suggests it would be prudent to increase the fiber content of the diet. This increase would be a natural consequence of the high, complex carbohydrate diet recommended as a United States dietary goal in Chapter 1. One precaution should be noted, however. Increased dietary fiber may also be a factor in the decreased uptake of important minerals, notably iron. This could pose a problem to those who have a tendency toward iron deficiency anemia. See Chapter 6 for possible consequences related to physical performance.

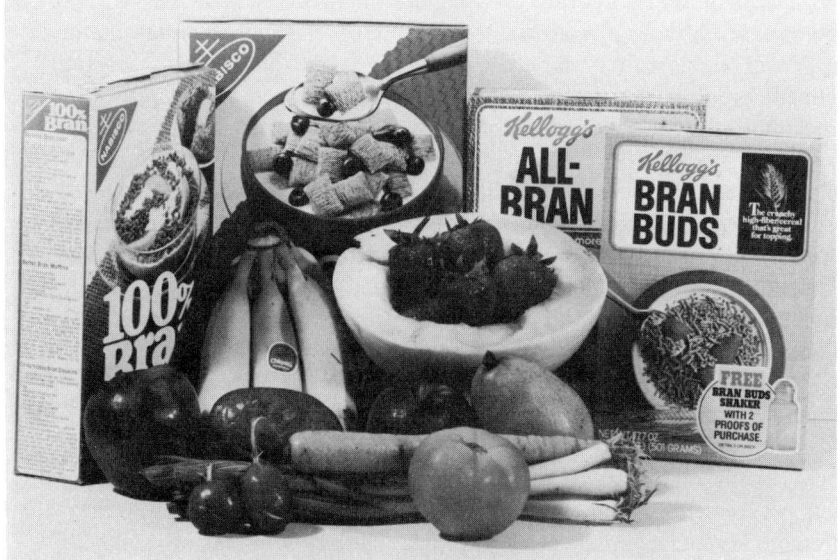

Foods high in dietary fiber.
(David Corona)

What percentage of the diet should be composed of carbohydrates?

The recent dietary goals proposed by the Select Subcommittee on Nutrition and Human Needs of the United States Senate recommend that the carbohydrate content of the diet be raised to 55–60 percent of the total caloric intake. Simple sugars should be limited to 10 percent, while the complex carbohydrates of starches should comprise about 48 percent. However, other diet plans, notably the Pritikin program, recommend that 80 percent of the dietary calories be supplied by carbohydrates, mostly complex and unrefined. A large percentage of the world's population subsists on such a diet high in carbohydrate content. This type of diet will not deter physical performance capacity, as documented by studies of the Tarahumara Indians and their outstanding feats of endurance.

The general recommendation, therefore, is to increase the complex carbohydrate content of the diet. As will be noted later, this may be especially important in certain types of physical performance.

Are there any health benefits or hazards to a high or low carbohydrate diet?

As indicated previously, dietary goals recommend increased consumption of carbohydrate in the diet of most Americans and people of industrialized nations. However, this recommendation is for the complex, not the simple or refined, carbohydrates. Hence, when discussing the health implications of either a high or low carbohydrate diet, one should differentiate between the complex and simple carbohydrates. In general, the diet should be high in complex carbohydrates and low in simple carbohydrates.

The major carbohydrate that has been labeled a villain is sucrose, or table sugar. Although total sugar consumption of Americans has changed little over the past fifty years, the percentage contribution of sugars and refined carbohydrates to the diet has increased as total carbohydrate consumption has decreased. Hence, sugar has been alleged to be a cause of a wide array of health problems ranging from cardiovascular disease to mental illness. However, a number of research studies have investigated the role of sugar as a causative factor in such disease processes, and after an extensive review of such studies, the respected Federation of American Societies for Experimental Biology concluded that there is no evidence that sugar poses a hazard to the public when used at current levels and in the manner now practiced, except for dental caries.

One particular condition of interest to the general population as well as to active individuals is **hypoglycemia,** or low blood sugar, a condition alleged to be caused by high carbohydrate intake. The normal blood glucose level is between 70–100 mg per 100 ml (milliliters) of blood. As this level gets progressively lower, mild to moderate or severe hypoglycemia may develop. Hypoglycemia is often accompanied by symptoms of weakness, trembling, anxiety, headache, and other such signs. In most healthy individuals these symptoms are usually temporary, resulting from the ingestion of a meal high in simple carbohydrates. In essence, the sugars are absorbed rapidly into the bloodstream and cause hyperglycemia, a condition just the opposite of hypoglycemia. This high level of blood sugar triggers the release of excessive amounts of insulin from the pancreas. Insulin is responsible for transporting the glucose from the blood into the tissues, notably the liver and skeletal muscles. As an overreaction occurs, the blood sugar level may fall temporarily and create hypoglycemia. Normally this creates hunger sensations, and upon eating the blood sugar level will return to normal.

Although hypoglycemia has been suggested to be a cause of mental depression, alcoholism, nervous breakdowns, chronic fatigue, and a host of other clinical conditions, a joint committee of several prominent health associations, including the American Medical Association, noted that there is no good evidence that hypoglycemia is a causative factor in such conditions.

It should be noted that hypoglycemia caused by prolonged exercise may be a contributing factor to fatigue, although recent research has suggested that exercise-induced hypoglycemia may not cause fatigue in some individuals. Implications for the active person will be discussed later.

Given the available evidence, it would appear prudent to increase the complex carbohydrate content of the diet and decrease sugar consumption. Dental caries (cavities) are a major consequence of sugar ingestion, particularly sticky-type sugars. Some evidence has shown sugar will increase blood triglyceride levels, possibly a contributing factor to coronary heart disease. Complex carbohydrates and a balanced diet can help avoid symptoms of hypoglycemia. These may be important considerations for reducing sugar intake, but the key point is to replace low nutrient foods, such as sugar, with high nutrient foods.

In what types of activities does the body rely heavily on carbohydrate as an energy source?

Carbohydrate supplies approximately 35–40 percent of the body's energy needs during rest. As one engages in mild to moderate exercise, carbohydrate use increases to 50 percent or more. When exercise becomes more intense, such as when a person is working at 70–80 percent of his capacity, carbohydrate is the preferred fuel. At maximal or supramaximal exercise efforts, it is used almost exclusively. A more detailed discussion is presented in Chapter 8.

Carbohydrate use then is associated with the intensity level of the exercise. The more intense, the greater the percentage contribution of carbohydrate. Of course, the more intense the exercise, the sooner exhaustion occurs. However, dependent upon several factors including the physical fitness level and diet of the individual, carbohydrate may be the prime energy source for events lasting from such time frames as one minute to over an hour. It should be noted that the exhaustion that occurs in high intensity exercise of short duration is not attributed to carbohydrate depletion, but rather to other metabolic processes in the muscle such as an increased acidity level.

Carbohydrates for exercise

Is carbohydrate a form of quick energy for exercise?

Since carbohydrate in the form of sugar is absorbed rather rapidly into the blood, the myth has risen that sugar or similar compounds are quick sources of energy for certain athletic events. In general, however, such is not the case. Although carbohydrate is the prime source of energy for intense activity, the source of this carbohydrate energy is the endogenous glycogen already found in the muscles. The rested individual who has been on a balanced diet will have sufficient muscle glycogen stores for most intense exercises of short duration. Fatigue or exhaustion in such events are due to factors other than muscle glycogen supply. Research has shown that the consumption of glucose, sucrose, or other carbohydrates immediately prior to events of short or moderate duration has a negligible effect upon performance. Adding a gallon of gas to a full tank will not make a car go faster during a short ride. The same is true of sugar to a muscle already filled with glycogen.

However, there may be some beneficial applications of carbohydrate ingestion prior to or during exercise of long duration.

Is it important to consume carbohydrates before or during exercise?

The key point of the answer to this question is the intensity *and* duration of the exercise. This question deals with carbohydrate intake within two hours prior to the exercise; this distinguishes it from carbohydrate loading, to be discussed later.

As expected there is an inverse relationship between intensity and duration of prolonged exercise. If you increase the intensity of your exercise, running speed for example, then the time you are able to continue will decrease. Hence, a well-conditioned person may be able to exercise at 50 percent of capacity for four to five hours, but only one to two hours at 80 percent of capacity. As mentioned previously, more carbohydrate is used when the intensity level is increased. Since the body can store carbohydrate to a limited extent in the muscles and liver, the usefulness of glucose or other carbohydrate intake before or during exercise depends on the adequacy of those supplies already in the muscle and liver to meet energy needs.

In general, muscle glycogen is the major source of carbohydrate energy substrate during the first forty minutes of exercise, but then blood glucose derived from the liver may be used to help sustain the energy demands of the muscle. To what extent can carbohydrate ingested before or during exercise help serve as an energy source?

A number of studies have been conducted on this subject. The interpretation of these studies in order to provide a general answer is difficult since the designs of the studies varied considerably. The amount of glucose ingested, the time prior to the exercise that it was taken, the intensity and duration of the exercise, and the method used to evaluate glucose utilization are some of the important differences between studies. Nevertheless, based upon an overall review of these studies with the given limitations, the following recommendations are made:

1. If the individual is on a balanced diet, glucose feedings are unnecessary for continuous exercise work bouts lasting sixty to ninety minutes or less. The muscle and liver glycogen stores should be adequate to meet carbohydrate energy needs. The critical point is to consume substantial amounts of carbohydrates the day or two prior to the event, not the day of the event, in order to assure ample endogenous glycogen supplies.

2. Simple sugars ingested within one to two hours of an event may speed up muscle glycogen utilization. This may be a disadvantage to the marathoner, for the glycogen levels may be depleted too early in the race.

3. In events of longer duration at a slower speed, glucose feedings may be advisable. The ingested glucose may contribute a significant percentage of the carbohydrate energy source, helping to spare the endogenous liver and muscle glycogen supply and prolonging the exercise bout. The

ingested glucose may also help prevent hypoglycemia and the resultant feeling of weakness often associated with long duration exercise. Although marathoners may benefit from glucose feedings, they are of prime importance to the ultramarathoner, those rare individuals who perform in 50–100 mile races. Recent research has supported the use of **glucose polymer** solutions such as maltodextrin, a complex carbohydrate, prior to prolonged moderate-intensity exercise. Glucose polymers are chains of glucose molecules shorter than starch. Gatorlode® is an example. As noted below, fluid replacement may be a more important concern than glucose replacement.

When and in what form should carbohydrates be consumed?

One aspect of concentrated carbohydrate solutions that may adversely affect physical performance is the effect they may have on concentrating fluids in the stomach. This may be discomforting when attempting to perform at high intensity. Another possible detrimental effect is the hypoglycemic response mentioned previously, the high sugar content creating a condition of hyperglycemia and then a reactive hypoglycemia. In very prolonged bouts of exercise at mild to moderate levels of intensity (4 to 5 hours at 30–50 percent of capacity) carbohydrate feedings in the form of glucose before the exercise bout have been shown to be a significant source of energy, to help maintain normal blood glucose levels, and to prolong the exercise. The glucose was given in a concentrated form, approximately a 20–25 percent solution. In some studies a 60 percent solution was used. The solution was taken within one hour of the exercise. Apparently at these lower intensity levels stomach distress from excess fluids was not a problem. The glucose was ingested in approximately 500 milliliters, or roughly a pint, of fluid. In exercises of this nature, it might be better to ingest such a solution within twenty to thirty minutes of the exercise bout in order to help avoid a hypoglycemic response. Exercise itself will help suppress insulin secretion and thus help to keep blood glucose levels normal or elevated during exercise. However, the type of exercise bout described here is not a very common athletic endeavor.

The most common athletic events or physical performance activities that may benefit from glucose feedings are those associated with long duration at moderate to high intensity levels. Marathon running, cross-country skiing, and soccer matches are some prime examples. The individual participating in these activities, particularly under hot environmental conditions, also has a need to replenish fluid losses incurred through sweating. Electrolytes are lost in sweat. A number of different glucose-electrolyte solutions (GES) have been designed to replenish these losses, and the water-electrolyte aspects will be discussed later. But what of the nature of glucose in these solutions?

A number of studies have been conducted relative to the glucose concentration in certain solutions. In general, the results indicate that if water replenishment is the most critical factor to maintain performance levels, and in most athletic endeavors it usually is, then the glucose concentration should be as low as possible, or about a 1–3 percent solution. Gatorade® is a 5 percent glucose solution, but can be diluted to an acceptable percentage by mixing equal amounts of water. These levels of glucose will not retard the absorption of water, but will provide only limited amounts of glucose. A liter, or a little more than a quart, of a 2 percent glucose solution would provide about 20 g of glucose, or 80 C.

If the critical factor is the replenishment of glucose, then slightly greater glucose concentrations may be utilized. Research has shown that more concentrated solutions may provide slightly more blood glucose during exercise than less concentrated ones, but the difference is low. This may be due to a limited capacity to absorb glucose, as only about 50 g may be absorbed from the stomach in an hour.

More recent research has shown that a glucose polymer solution, a combination of glucose molecules, will result in good glucose uptake without markedly reducing water uptake. Glucose polymer solutions appear to provide the best means to facilitate glucose absorption without hindering fluid absorption.

In summary, glucose solutions may be beneficial during prolonged exercise as they may help prevent hypoglycemia and supply a part of the carbohydrate energy supply to prolong duration of the exercise. The following practical suggestions are offered:

1. Use only a 1–3 percent glucose solution if water replenishment is the major concern. A glucose polymer solution of 5 percent may also be recommended.

2. Use a 5–10 percent solution if glucose replenishment is most important. However, you should experiment with such solutions in practice before using in competition. Defizzed colas are about 10 percent glucose solution. In very long distance bouts, experiment with higher solutions, 50–60 percent. There high concentrations would be useful only to ultramarathoners, but should not be utilized when fluid replacement is of greater concern as in moderate to warm temperatures.

3. Homemade solutions may be used, although care should be taken not to create a solution too concentrated. One rounded tablespoon of sugar per quart will make a 1–2 percent solution and provide approximately 15 g of carbohydrate. Three rounded tablespoons will make a 5 percent solution. Adjust the sugar according to your desired percentage.

Is fructose a better source of carbohydrate energy than glucose?

Fructose is the sweetest of sugars, but it has not been shown to be a better source of energy than glucose. They both contain the same caloric value per gram. Glucose is absorbed more readily than fructose, and even then fructose is converted to glucose by the liver. However, the slower absorption of fructose produces a less abrupt change in blood sugar levels and therefore does not produce the hypoglycemic effect attributed to glucose. Manufacturers have increased the production of fructose, and its use has increased rapidly among the general population. Even though fructose has been suggested to be an advantage for athletes, research has not shown it to be a more effective energy source than glucose. The average individual receives an ample supply of fructose in the diet as it is contained in most fruits and is 50 percent of sucrose, or common table sugar.

What is carbohydrate, or glycogen, loading?

Since carbohydrate becomes increasingly important as a fuel for muscular exercise as the intensity of the exercise increases, and since the amount of carbohydrate stored in the body is limited, then muscle and liver glycogen depletion, as well as low blood sugar, could be factors that may limit performance capacity in distance events characterized by high levels of energy expenditure for an hour or more. A number of research studies have documented the facts that the levels of glycogen stored in the muscle and liver are important determinants of the ability to exercise for prolonged periods of time. Hypoglycemia has also been associated with states of exhaustion, such as in marathon runners, and may be prevented if initial body carbohydrate stores are high. An increase in muscle and liver glycogen stores may be associated with increased endurance performance. Carbohydrate loading might not make you run any faster, but the theory is that you may be able to go further at your optimal speed.

Carbohydrate loading

Carbohydrate loading, then, is simply an attempt to increase significantly the amount of glycogen that is stored in the body.

What type of athlete would benefit from carbohydrate loading?

In general, carbohydrate loading is primarily suited for those individuals who will sustain high levels of continuous energy expenditure for prolonged periods of time. This includes long distance runners, swimmers, and bicyclists, cross-country skiers and similar type athletes. In addition, athletes who are involved in prolonged stop and go activities, such as soccer, lacrosse, and tournament play sports like tennis and handball, may benefit.

It is a well-documented fact that humans have different types of skeletal muscle fibers. In simple terms, they may be called slow twitch and fast twitch. The **slow twitch fibers** are used primarily during long, continuous type activities and are aerobic in nature, whereas the **fast twitch fibers** are used for short, fast type activities and are anaerobic in nature. Consider the differences between a distance runner and a soccer player. The former may run at a steady pace for an hour, whereas the latter will constantly be changing speeds, with many bouts of full speed interspersed with recovery periods of slower running. Research has shown that glycogen depletion patterns of the two different muscle fiber types is related to the type of exercise. Long, continuous exercise primarily depletes glycogen in the slow twitch fibers while fast intermittant bouts of exercise with periods of rest, actually a form of interval training, primarily depletes glycogen in the fast twitch fibers. However, it should be noted that glycogen depletion may occur in both types of fibers in either long continuous or intermittant exercise and may be quite appreciable depending upon intensity and duration of the exercise bouts. If carbohydrate loading works for the specific muscle fiber involved, then both types of athletes may benefit. Both should have greater glycogen stores in the latter stages of their respective athletic contests.

How do you carbohydrate load?

As you might suspect, the key to carbohydrate loading is to switch from the normal balanced diet to one very high in carbohydrate content. In trained runners, recent research has shown that simply changing to a very high carbohydrate diet, combined with one or two days of rest or reduced activity levels, will effectively increase muscle and liver glycogen. This technique will increase muscle glycogen stores as high as the traditional carbohydrate-loading techniques.

The traditional carbohydrate-loading technique involves a glycogen depletion stage by prolonged exercise. For example, a runner might go for an eighteen to twenty mile run to use as much stored glycogen as possible. Another part of the depletion state may be a two to three day period when very little carbohydrate is ingested. Exercises may be continued during this two to three day period in order to keep glycogen stores low. Following the depletion stage, the loading stage begins. During this phase, carbohydrate may contribute 80 or more percent of the caloric input. The intensity and duration of exercise during this phase is reduced considerably. The usual case is to rest fully for two to three days. Thus, the classical carbohydrate-loading pattern involved three stages: depletion, carbohydrate deprivation (high fat-protein diet), and carbohydrate loading.

Table 2.2 represents several methods that have been used to carbohydrate load. Some early research supports method *c,* but more recent evidence suggests that if the total carbohydrate content in each of the diets is the same, then the muscle glycogen content will be similar. Method *c* may be particularly difficult to tolerate, especially if one tries to exercise at high levels during the depletion phase. The lack of carbohydrate in the diet

Table 2.2　Different methods for carbohydrate loading

Method A

1st day	Depletion exercise
2nd day	High carbohydrate diet; little or no exercise
3rd day	High carbohydrate diet; little or no exercise
4th day	High carbohydrate diet; little or no exercise
5th day	Competition

Method B

1st day	Depletion exercise
2nd day	High carbohydrate diet; regular exercise
3rd day	High carbohydrate diet; regular exercise
4th day	High carbohydrate diet; regular exercise
5th day	High carbohydrate diet; little or no exercise
6th day	High carbohydrate diet; little or no exercise
7th day	High carbohydrate diet; little or no exercise
8th day	Competition

Method C

1st day	Depletion exercise
2nd day	High protein-fat diet; low carbohydrate; regular exercise
3rd day	High protein-fat diet; low carbohydrate; regular exercise
4th day	High protein-fat diet; low carbohydrate; regular exercise
5th day	High carbohydrate diet; little or no exercise
6th day	High carbohydrate diet; little or no exercise
7th day	High carbohydrate diet; little or no exercise
8th day	Competition

High carbohydrate diet: 500–600 g per day; about 70–80 percent of diet Calories should be carbohydrate.

Regular exercise: Begin tapering by reducing speed and distance.

combined with the exercise bouts may elicit symptoms of hypoglycemia (weakness, lethargy, irritability). The exercise bouts also may seem extremely difficult, particularly if one tries to maintain the same intensity as prior to depletion. Although some suggest this method be avoided, it may provide a certain degree of mental toughness as the full depletion stage is completed, but it is not necessary from a physiological standpoint.

What is an example of a carbohydrate-loading diet?

Table 2.3 represents a general dietary plan that could be used for either method *a, b,* or *c* described in Table 2.2. The depletion stage diet relates only to method *c.* However, this diet has been modified somewhat from the

Table 2.3 Daily food plan for carbohydrate loading

Sources of fats, proteins and carbohydrates	Depletion stage days 7–4 before event	Loading stage days 3–1 before event
Meat, fish, poultry, eggs, cheese Select low fat items	20–25 oz KCAL: 1500–1875	6–8 oz KCAL: 450–600
Breads and cereals	4 servings KCAL: 280	8–16 servings KCAL: 560–1120
Vegetables	2 servings low calorie vegetables KCAL: 50	4 servings high calorie vegetables KCAL: 360
Fruits and juices	2 servings KCAL: 80	4 servings KCAL: 160
Fats and oils	1–2 tbsp. KCAL: 135–270	1–2 tbsp. KCAL: 135–270
Milk	2 servings KCAL: 160 (skim milk)	2 servings KCAL: 160 (skim milk)
Desserts	1 or 2 servings, unsweetened KCAL: 400	2 servings, sweetened KCAL: 800
Beverages	Nonsweetened, unlimited KCAL: 0	Sweetened, to KCAL level KCAL: 0–360
Water	8 or more servings KCAL: 0	8 or more servings KCAL: 0
TOTAL KCAL	2525–3035	2625–3830

Adapted from Forgac, M. T. "Carbohydrate Loading. A Review." *Journal of the American Dietetic Association* 75 (1979): 42–5.

original, high, fat-high protein diet. It includes about 100 g or 400 C in carbohydrates for the depletion phase. This may help alleviate the symptoms of hypoglycemia previously mentioned. In addition it avoids the high fat content during this stage; fats and oils have been deleted and replaced by low fat foods in the meat group; skim milk is substituted for whole milk.

The total caloric value should be adjusted to individual needs. It is dependent upon the size of the individual and daily energy expenditure in exercise.

Consult Table 2.1 for foods high in carbohydrates, and Table 4.2 for foods high in protein.

Does it matter what type or amount of carbohydrate is eaten to help increase glycogen storage?

Recent research by Dr. David Costill and his associates at Ball State University has revealed that both simple and complex carbohydrates will replace muscle glycogen at about the same rate over a twenty-four-hour

Figure 2.3.
Different possibilities of increasing the muscle glycogen content. Three methods are depicted. First, simply eating a high carbohydrate diet will increase muscle glycogen content. Second, a depletion exercise task followed by a high carbohydrate diet will provide a greater increase. Third, a depletion exercise followed by three days on a high protein-fat diet and then three days of a high carbohydrate diet will provide the greatest increase in muscle glycogen content. (Modified from Saltin, B., and Hermansen, L. 1967. Glycogen stores and prolonged severe exercise. In *Nutrition and physical activity*, ed. G. Blix. Courtesy of Almquist and Weksells, Uppsala, Sweden.

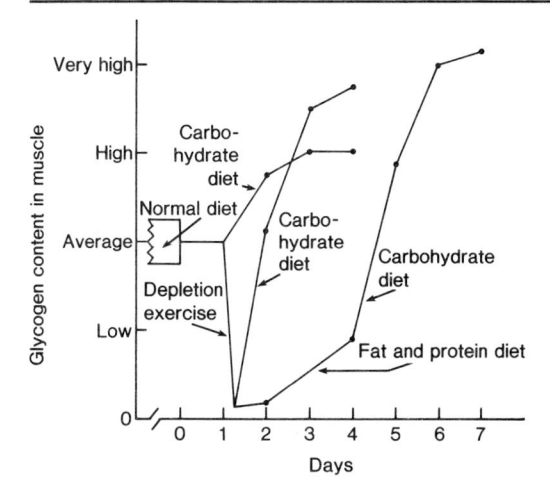

period. However, through forty-eight hours, complex carbohydrates produce a greater muscle glycogen storage than do the simple carbohydrates. Since glycogen loading for long distance events occurs over a two to three day period, it would be wise to stress complex carbohydrates in the diet, but include some simple carbohydrates as well. Moreover, the diet should also include the daily requirements for protein and fat.

Costill's research also revealed, in general, the more carbohydrate eaten, the greater the amount of glycogen storage. Moreover, if the carbohydrate was eaten in two large meals, instead of small ones, glycogen storage would be facilitated.

In a practical sense then, the two to three day glycogen regimen should include large amounts of carbohydrate, primarily the complex type, consumed in two large meals per day. The total carbohydrate intake should be about 500–600 g per day. The last meal should be about fifteen hours prior to race time, possibly topped off with a simple carbohydrate snack before retiring for the night. A light carbohydrate breakfast such as orange juice, toast, and jelly may be eaten three to four hours prior to competition. This overall dietary regimen should help to maximize muscle and liver glycogen stores.

How long does it take muscle and liver glycogen to return to normal levels following depletion?

Following a normal daily exercise bout, muscle and liver glycogen levels usually return to normal within twenty-four hours, even on a balanced diet containing about 50–60 percent carbohydrate. However, following glycogen depletion, two to three days on a high carbohydrate diet with little or no exercise may be necessary.

Does carbohydrate loading work?

As a method of increasing the glycogen stores in the muscles and liver, the answer is yes. See figure 2.3 for the effects of the different methods. Body glycogen stores will return toward normal on a regular balanced diet during a twenty-four-hour recovery period, and even if no food is ingested some slight increase in muscle glycogen stores has been noted. However, in order to get the maximal supercompensation effect during recovery, you must consume a high carbohydrate diet. Glycogen content in the muscle has been reported to increase two to three times beyond normal and liver glycogen content nearly doubled.

As a means of increasing endurance performance, the answer is a qualified yes. Some laboratory studies have noted that work time to exhaustion is closely associated with the amount of energy the subject derives from carbohydrate. When performance is compared after subjects have been on either a high fat-protein diet, a mixed balanced diet, or a high carbohydrate diet, performance on the high fat-protein diet is worse than on the other two, but there is little difference in performance on the latter two diets. However, the performance tests in these studies often were not possibly long enough for the individual to derive the full benefit from carbohydrate loading. We still await sound laboratory experimentation to document whether or not the carbohydrate-loading technique will benefit an individual in running faster in a distance—for example, a 26.2-mile marathon. On the other hand, several laboratory and field studies with runners and cross-country skiers have shown increased performances. In general, carbohydrate loading, in contrast to a mixed diet, did not enable these athletes to go faster during the early stages of their events, but the high glycogen levels enabled them to perform longer at a given speed.

How do you know if your muscles have increased their glycogen stores?

The most accurate way would be to have a muscle biopsy taken (a needle is inserted into the muscle and a small portion is extracted and analyzed), but this is not very practical. However, keeping an accurate record of your body weight, which should be recorded every morning as you arise and after you urinate, may help you determine the answer to this question. For each gram of glycogen that is stored, approximately 3 g of water are bound to it. Hence, your body weight should increase 2–3 pounds above your normal training weight during the loading phase. This is indicative that the carbohydrate loading has been effective.

Are there any possible detrimental effects relative to carbohydrate loading?

From a health standpoint there may be some potential hazards to individuals with certain conditions. Although diabetics have been known to carbohydrate load, they should consult their physician prior to using the technique. Individuals with high blood lipid or cholesterol levels should avoid the high fat-protein diet phase of the depletion stage. Blood serum lipids and cholesterol have been reported to rise significantly during this phase. In addition, these individuals should eat mostly complex carbohydrates during the loading phase since an increased intake of simple carbohydrates may raise blood lipid levels. In addition, hypoglycemia may occur during the high fat-protein phase.

There have been one or two reports of individuals suffering a heart attack or having blood in the urine after carbohydrate loading. However, no cause and effect relationship has been established. In general, the carbohydrate-loading technique, which at the most is only a seven-day dietary regimen, poses no significant health hazards to the normally healthy individual. Dr. Steven Blair has reported that the classic carbohydrate-loading method had no adverse effects on blood lipids or ECGs in marathoners.

From a performance standpoint, the extra body weight associated with the increased water content may serve to be a disadvantage. In activities where lifting the body weight is important, extra energy will be required to move the extra 2–3 pounds of body water. However, in most performance events for which carbohydrate loading is advocated, the benefits from the energy aspects of the increased glycogen should more than offset the additional water weight. Moreover, if the individual is performing in a hot environment, the extra water will be available as a source of sweat and may be helpful in controlling body temperature during exercise in the heat.

Fat—an additional energy source during exercise

Although fat is one of the most criticized nutrients, it does play a rather significant role in human nutrition and in human physiological functioning. In this chapter, we will look at the nature of fat and the associated compound cholesterol, the role of fat during exercise, the health implications of diets high in fat and cholesterol, and the effects of diet and physical training programs upon fats in the body.

What are fats?

Fats, also known as lipids, represent a general term for a number of different compounds found in the body in the forms of both solid fat and liquid oils. The three major classes are triglycerides, sterols, and phospholipids. The fats of major interest are the triglycerides, or neutral fats, for this is the primary form in which fats are eaten and stored in the human body. **Triglycerides** are composed of two different compounds—fatty acids and glycerol (there are three fatty acids attached to each glycerol molecule). Figure 3.1 represents a diagram of a triglyceride.

Types and sources

What is the meaning of such terms as saturated, monounsaturated, polyunsaturated, and hydrogenated?

Fatty acids, one of the components of fat, are chains of carbon, oxygen and hydrogen atoms that vary in the degree of saturation with hydrogen. A **saturated fatty acid** contains a full quota of hydrogenated ions while **unsaturated fatty acids** may absorb more hydrogen; these latter fatty acids may be classified as monounsaturated, capable of absorbing two more hydrogen ions, and **polyunsaturated,** capable of absorbing four or more hydrogen ions. Saturated fats are usually solid while unsaturated fats are usually liquid. Figure 3.2 represents the structural difference between a saturated and unsaturated fatty acid.

Hydrogenated fats or oils have been treated by a process that adds hydrogen to some of the unfilled bonds, thus hardening the fat or oil. In essence, the fat becomes more saturated. The health implications of these different types of fats will be discussed later.

What are some common foods high in fat content?

The fat content in foods can vary from 100 percent, as found in most cooking oils, to minor trace amounts, less than 1 percent, as found in most fruits and vegetables. The fat content of some foods is obvious, such as

Figure 3.1.
Structure of a triglyceride. Three fatty acids combine with glycerol to form a triglyceride.

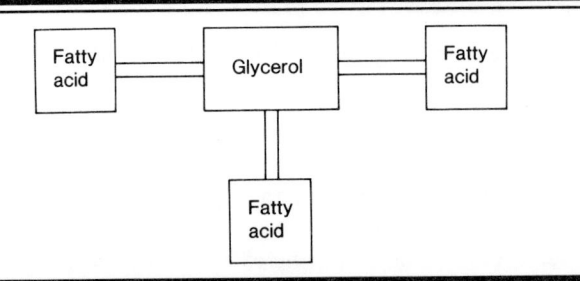

Figure 3.2.
Structural differences between saturated and unsaturated fatty acids. Note the double bonds between carbon atoms in the unsaturated fatty acid, indicating that more hydrogen atoms may be added. The R represents the radical or the presence of many more C–H bonds.

Saturated fatty acid

Unsaturated fatty acid

butter, oils, shortening, mayonnaise, and margarine. However, in other foods the content may be high but not as obvious. For example, meat, milk, cheese, nuts, desserts, and some vegetables and cereals may contain considerable amounts of fat.

Both animal and vegetable fats are triglycerides; however, the nature of the fatty acids in each is different. Animal fats are composed mainly of saturated fats, while vegetable fats are primarily unsaturated.

Table 3.1 represents the percent of food energy that is derived from fat in some common foods; the percentages are indicated for both total fat and saturated fats.

Is fat necessary in the diet?

There is no specific requirement for fat in the diet; no RDA have been established for fat. However, a need exists for certain essential fatty acids that are components of fat. Most fatty acids may be synthesized in the body, but according to the National Research Council, linoleic fatty acid must be supplied in the diet. Since almost all foods have some fat, sufficient amounts of this essential fatty acids are found in the average diet. Even on a vegetarian diet of fruits, vegetables, and grain products, about 5–10 percent of your total calories would be derived from fat.

Table 3.1 Percentage of total fat Calories and saturated fat Calories in some common foods

Food	% Calories total fat	% Calories saturated fat
Meat group		
Bacon	80	30
Beef, lean and fat	59	29
Beef, lean only	32	13
Ham	70	23
Hamburger, regular	62	29
Chicken, breast	23	8
Lamb, lean and fat	74	40
Lamb, lean only	38	19
Liver	41	—*
Pork, lean and fat	43	28
Sausage, pork	79	29
Veal cutlet	39	24
Fish		
Haddock	32	6
Salmon	37	7
Eggs, whole	67	22
Milk group		
Milk, whole	45	28
Milk, skim	trace	trace
Cheese, cheddar	62	39
Cheese, cottage		
Creamed	35	20
Uncreamed	3	3
Cream, whipping	81	46
Ice cream	49	28
Ice milk	31	18
Yogurt, partially skimmed milk	29	14
Dried beans and peas; nuts		
Beans, dry, navy	4	—
Beans, dry, lima	4	—
Peanuts	77	17
Peanut butter	76	19
Peas, split, dry	3	—

*Dashes indicate no value was found although it is believed an appreciable value is present.

Table 3.1 *Continued*

Food	% Calories total fat	% Calories saturated fat
Vegetables		
Asparagus	trace	trace
Beans, green	trace	trace
Broccoli	20	—
Carrots	trace	trace
Peas, green	10	—
Potatoes	trace	trace
Squash	trace	trace
Fruits		
Apples	trace	trace
Bananas	trace	trace
Oranges	trace	trace
Pineapples	trace	trace
Breads-Cereals		
Bread { White	12	—
Bread { Whole wheat	12	—
Cake, plain sheet	31	8
Grits	trace	trace
Crackers	18	—
Doughnuts	43	7
Macaroni	5	—
Macaroni and cheese	46	20
Oatmeal	13	—
Pancakes, wheat	30	—
Pie, apple	39	10
Rice	trace	trace
Rolls, dinner	22	7
Spaghetti	5	—
Wheat, shredded	10	—
Fats and oils		
Butter	99	54
Lard	99	38
Margarine	99	19
Oil, corn	100	10
Salad dressings { French	68	14
Salad dressings { French, special dietary low fat	trace	trace

Table 3.2 Calculation of the percentage of Calories in foods that are derived from the total fat and saturated fat

Data from food energy, fat, and saturated fat.

Bacon, 2 slices
   Food energy = 90 C
            Fat = 8 g
   Saturated fat = 3 g

1. To calculate percentage of food Calories that consists of fat, use caloric value for fat of 1 g = 9 C
   fat = 8 g   8 g × 9 = 72 C
   72 ÷ 90 = .80
   .80 × 100 = 80% of the Calories in bacon are supplied by fat

2. To calculate percentage of food that consists of saturated fat
   saturated fat = 3 g   3 g × 9 C = 27 C
   27 ÷ 90 = .30
   .30 × 100 = 30% of the Calories in bacon are supplied by saturated fat

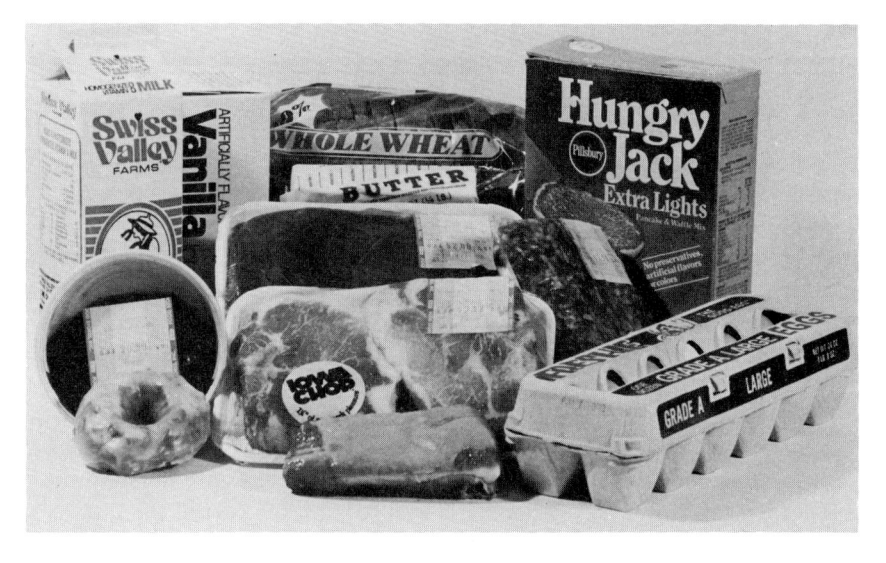

Foods high in cholesterol.
(David Corona)

What is cholesterol?

Cholesterol is not a fat, but it is a fatlike pearly substance found in animal tissues. It is a sterol. Cholesterol is found only in animal products and is not found in fruits, vegetables, nuts, grains or other nonanimal foods. However, cholesterol can be manufactured in the body not only from fatty acids, but also from the breakdown products of carbohydrate and protein—glucose and amino acids. Cholesterol is used in the formation of several hormones in the body and is a component of certain tissues, such as the covering for nerve fibers.

Cholesterol

Fat—an additional energy source during exercise

Cholesterol is vital to human physiology, but since it may be manufactured in the body from either fats, carbohydrate, or protein, there is apparently little need for us to obtain it in the foods we eat. Since a positive relationship has been established between blood cholesterol levels and coronary heart disease, reduction of dietary cholesterol has been advocated by a number of health related associations. This topic will be discussed later in this chapter.

What foods are high in cholesterol content?

Cholesterol is found only in animal foods, not in plant products. Table 3.2 represents some foods from the Meat and Milk Groups with the cholesterol content in milligrams. Several foods from the Bread-Cereal Group are also included, indicating that the preparation of some bread-cereal products may add cholesterol by including some animal product with cholesterol, mainly eggs.

What happens to dietary fat in the human body?

Metabolism and function

The major dietary source of fat is the triglycerides, being about 95 percent. The other 5 percent of dietary fat is sterols and phospholipids. The ingested fat is digested primarily in the small intestine by the action of enzymes (lipases) with the assistance of bile. They are broken down into free fatty acids (FFA), glycerol, cholesterol, and phospholipids, which are then absorbed into the cells of the intestinal wall. Here they are recombined into a fat droplet called a **chylomicron,** which contains a large amount of triglyceride and smaller amounts of cholesterol, phospholipids, and protein. The chylomicron is then absorbed into the lymph and eventually flows into the bloodstream.

The subsequent fate of this chylomicron depends on the nutritional state of the individual. The enzymes that can convert the triglyceride back to fatty acids and glycerol for absorption into body tissues are found in the arteries. In general, if the individual is well fed, a large part of the fatty acids and glycerol are deposited into the fat (adipose) cells of the body and converted back to triglyceride. This adipose tissue is the major storage depot of energy in the human body, averaging about 100,000 C. If the individual is in a fasted state, the fatty acids and glycerol enter the muscle cells where they can either be stored for future energy use or be used immediately as a source of energy. Hence, after a meal with a high fat

Table 3.3 Cholesterol content, in milligrams for some common foods

	Amount	Cholesterol
Meat group		
Beef	1 oz	25
Pork, ham	1 oz	25
Poultry	1 oz	23
Fish	1 oz	21
Shrimp	1 oz	45
Lobster	1 oz	25
Sausage	2 links	45
Tuna, salmon	1 oz	0
Frankfurter	1	50
Bacon	1 strip	5
Eggs	1	253
Liver	1 oz	120
Milk group		
Milk, whole	1 cup	27
Milk, 2%	1 cup	15
Milk, skim	1 cup	7
Butter	1 tsp	12
Margarine	1 tsp	0
Cream cheese	1 tbsp	18
Ice milk	1 cup	10
Ice cream	1 cup	85
Bread-Cereal group		
Bread	1 slice	0
Biscuit	1	17
Pancake	1	40
Sweet roll	1	25
French toast	1	130
Doughnut	1	28
Cereal, cooked	1 cup	0

Fruits, vegetables, grains, and nuts have no cholesterol.

Figure 3.3.
Diagrammatic representation of the chemical composition of the major plasma lipoprotein classes. The large VLDL contain triglyceride as the major constituent with small proportions of cholesterol. LDL are intermediate in size and contain high proportions of cholesterol and phospholipids. The small HDL carry major proportions of cholesterol, phospholipids, and protein. *TG*, triglycerides; *C*, cholesterol; *PL*, phospholipids; *P*, protein. (From Wood, P. et al. 1977. Plasma lipoprotein distributions in male and female runners. *Annals of The New York Academy of Sciences* 301:758. Reprinted with permission of The New York Academy of Sciences.)

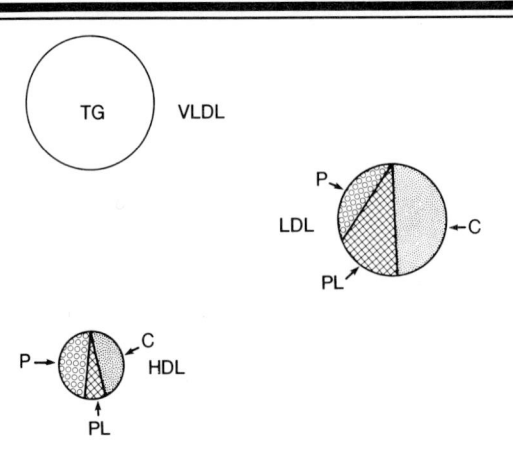

content is ingested, the fat level of the blood, known as the blood **serum lipid level,** will rise. However, the serum lipid level will return to normal as the chylomicrons deposit their triglycerides and cholesterol in the adipose tissue, muscles, and liver.

The liver plays a central role in fat regulation. It is primarily responsible for regulating the major lipids in the blood plasma. The level of lipids in the plasma is determined not only by those absorbed from the intestine, but also by those lipids released from the liver into the plasma.

The liver is a clearinghouse in human metabolism. As the blood passes through, its cells take the basic nutrients and convert them into other forms. As mentioned in Chapter 2, it converts fructose to glucose. It also clears most drugs from the body. Pertinent to our discussion here is its role in lipid metabolism. In essence, the liver can take fatty acids directly from the blood or form new fatty acids from other compounds such as glucose, amino acids, or alcohol. These fatty acids are then combined with glycerol, cholesterol, phospholipids, and a protein complex and returned to the blood plasma as a complex triglyceride. Hence the major lipids in the blood—triglycerides, cholesterol, and phospholipids—do not circulate as free compounds, but are bound to a protein complex. This complex is known as a **lipoprotein.**

These lipoproteins, as represented in Figure 3.3, may be grouped into a number of classes. The three major classes are:

VLDL—Very low density lipoproteins. Consists primarily of triglycerides, which are transported to the tissues to provide fatty acids and glycerol.

LDL—Low density lipoproteins. Contain a high proportion of cholesterol and phospholipids. LDL may be taken up by the muscle cells in the artery walls and have been implicated in the development of atherosclerosis. In general, LDL transport cholesterol from the liver to the other body cells. They are often referred to as "bad" cholesterol.

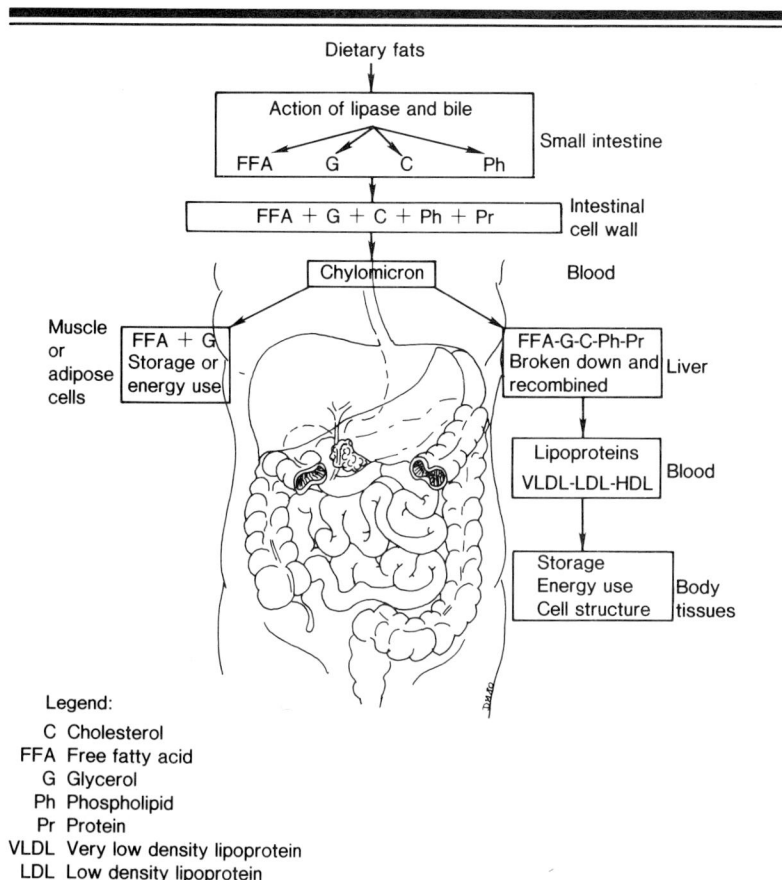

Figure 3.4.
Simplified diagram of fat metabolism. After digestion, fats are carried in the blood as chylomicrons. Through the metabolic processes in the body fat may be utilized as a major source of energy, used to help develop cell structure, or stored as a future energy source.

Legend:
- C   Cholesterol
- FFA Free fatty acid
- G   Glycerol
- Ph Phospholipid
- Pr Protein
- VLDL Very low density lipoprotein
- LDL Low density lipoprotein
- HDL High density lipoprotein

HDL—High density lipoproteins. HDL also consists of high proportions of cholesterol. However, the HDL transport cholesterol in the reverse direction of the LDL; HDL remove cholesterol from peripheral cells and return it to the liver for possible degradation. HDL have been associated with lower incidence levels of coronary heart disease and are often referred to as the "good" cholesterol.

A simplified schematic of fat metabolism is presented in Figure 3.4. It should be mentioned that a small amount of FFA is transported in the plasma attached to a protein. These FFA, as shall be seen, are important sources of energy during mild to moderate exercise.

Can the body make fat from protein and carbohydrate?

As noted in Figure 2.2, the amino acids of protein may be converted to acetyl CoA, which can then be converted into fat. Carbohydrates may also be converted to fat via acetyl CoA. It is important to understand that the body will take excess amounts of both these nutrients and convert them to body fat when caloric expenditure is less than caloric intake. Thus, it is not necessarily what you eat, but rather how much, that determines whether or not you gain body fat.

What are the major functions of fats in human nutrition?

Dietary fats help to provide energy supplies, the essential fatty acid, and the fat soluble vitamins A, D, E, and K for the regulation of human metabolism. Fat may also be synthesized in the body. In the body, fat depots in the adipose tissues are used as insulators and shock absorbers to protect various organs. Fats are integral components of many body structures. In general, however, body fat is primarily a very concentrated form of energy. Each gram of fat contains approximately 9 C, or more than twice the amount of carbohydrate or protein. Most of this energy, the amount depending on body fat stores, is contained in the adipose tissue.

The present view of adipose tissue is one of a highly metabolically active tissue regarding the uptake and release of fat. The adipose tissue is constantly synthesizing and degrading triglycerides. As mentioned previously, energy balance of the individual determines whether or not fat stores increase or decrease.

During rest, triglycerides break down into fatty acids and glycerol as they enter the body tissues. These products are then used by the cell to produce energy. During rest, nearly 60 percent of the energy supply is provided by metabolism of fats.

What percentage of the diet should be composed of fats?

Fats, exercise, and your health

For reasons associated with health, as mentioned in Chapter 1, the percentage of fat in the diet should be reduced to less than 30 percent of the total caloric intake. Saturated fats should not be more than 10 percent. Cholesterol should be less than 300 mg daily. Others have suggested that the total fat content be reduced to 10 percent or less of the total daily caloric intake. Even with this low percentage, the essential fatty acids and fat soluble vitamins would still be received.

Are fats used as an energy source during exercise?

Fats may be an important source of energy during mild to moderate levels of exercise. The muscle cells possess the necessary enzymes to convert the energy of free fatty acids (FFA) to a form that may be used by the muscle.

Fatty acids for energy production may come from a variety of sources. They may be delivered to the muscle from the plasma by any of the three major lipid transport mechanisms, namely the chylomicrons, lipoproteins, and the FFA. Or they may be derived from local storage pools, primarily those stores within the muscle themselves. However, the plasma FFA and the triglyceride stores in the muscles appear to be the main sources of fat energy during prolonged mild to moderate exercise. They supply about 50 percent of the total energy, the remaining 50 percent being derived from carbohydrate. The FFA are mobilized primarily from the adipose tissue, where the triglycerides in the adipose cell are hydrolized to FFA and glycerol and released into the blood. The FFA are then delivered to the muscle cell for oxidation and release of energy. The muscle triglycerides go through a similar metabolic fate in the muscle cell itself.

As long as the exercise is not too intense, the FFA can continue to serve as a major energy source. However, once the exercise intensity reaches a certain level, about 60–65 percent of VO_2 max in the untrained subject, FFA release from the adipose tissue decreases, and the muscle cell begins to rely more and more on carbohydrate as the major energy source, mainly muscle glycogen.

As noted previously, the amount of energy that may be obtained from muscle and liver glycogen is rather limited. Hence, within about an hour or so of high intensity exercise, glycogen stores approach very low levels. As this happens, the body shifts to an increasing usage of fats leading to a decrease in the intensity of the exercise.

Should the active individual supplement the diet with fat?

An interesting physiological change occurs in humans following a physical fitness training program based on cardiovascular endurance exercise. At levels of exercise that are of mild to moderate intensity, the percentage of energy derived from fat increases. If you ran an 8-minute mile both before and after a two-month training program you would use the same amount of caloric energy each time. However, after training, more of that energy would be derived from fat. Hence, training helps you to become a fat burner, so to speak, which may help to spare some of the glycogen in your muscles.

Some other interesting studies have shown the importance of FFA as an energy source during exercise. In one study, when the vitamin niacin was administered to block the release of FFA from adipose tissues, the time a person could perform prolonged work was shortened. In another study, a chemical was given to subjects to increase the FFA in the blood. The greater the concentration of FFA in the blood, the more the muscle cells would take in and use for energy. Less muscle glycogen was used. This has been labeled the glycogen sparing effect of FFA. In yet another study, caffeine was administered to subjects in order to increase plasma FFA. There was an increase in performance that was attributed to the glycogen sparing effect. This role of caffeine will be explored later in Chapter 15.

So what does all of this mean to the physically active person? Should you increase your fat intake? Of course the answer is no. As you have probably found out by now, the body has a substantial supply of fat calories stored in the adipose tissue as triglycerides. The body can also manufacture triglycerides from protein and carbohydrate. During exercise, these triglycerides may be hydrolyzed to FFA, which will be sufficient to meet your energy needs. In addition, the relationship between high intakes of saturated fats and cholesterol with atherosclerosis suggests it would be prudent to reduce fat intake, not increase it.

Although some studies have shown a glycogen sparing effect of high levels of plasma FFA, more research with humans needs to be done before any definite conclusions may be drawn relative to increased endurance performance. The only practical method available to elevate plasma FFA would be the ingestion of caffeine. Other techniques such as the ingestion of a high-fat meal followed by injection of a chemical into the veins that facilitates the breakdown of triglycerides to FFA naturally have limitations.

In summary, current evidence suggests that the complex carbohydrates are the preferential fuel for the active individual, not excess dietary fats. During exercise, carbohydrate is the most efficient fuel for it produces more energy per unit of oxygen than fat or protein.

Are there any health benefits or hazards to a high or low fat and cholesterol diet?

The most significant cause of death in the United States involves disorders to the cardiovascular system, primarily atherosclerosis of the blood vessels in the heart, the coronary arteries. **Atherosclerosis** is a condition wherein the inner layers of the arterial wall develop a buildup of yellow plaque consisting of cholesterol and other lipid material. The internal channel narrows and the blood flow is reduced considerably. When this condition occurs in the coronary vessels it is characterized as coronary heart disease (CHD) and may cause symptoms ranging from mild discomfort upon exertion to death.

Since CHD is so prominent in industrialized society, it has received considerable attention and resultant research. A variety of research approaches have been used, including epidemiological studies of large populations, genetic studies of families predisposed to CHD, experimental studies with animals, and therapeutic studies using both animals and man. The results of this research have revealed a number of risk factors associated with CHD. Among these factors are such items as diet, serum lipids, serum cholesterol, physical inactivity, obesity, high blood pressure, smoking, age, heredity, sex, stress, and several others.

Of interest to our discussion are the risk factors of high serum cholesterol levels and high serum triglyceride levels. Both may be caused by high dietary intake of fat and cholesterol. CHD and these two associated risk factors are part of the rationale underlying the general recommendation to reduce fat and cholesterol content in the diet. Thus, there appears to be no significant benefits to a diet high in fat and cholesterol, but possibly some healthful consequences may result from a reduction.

Dr. William B. Kannel has reported that an increased ratio of total cholesterol to HDL cholesterol will increase the probability of CHD. The risks associated with these ratios are as follows:

Risk	*Men*	*Women*
1/2 Average	3.43	3.27
Average	4.97	4.44
2 × Average	9.55	7.05
3 × Average	23.39	11.04

Thus a man with a total cholesterol of 240 and an HDL level of 70 would have a ratio of 3.42 (240 ÷ 70). He would have a risk of getting CHD one-half the average rate.

It must be noted, however, that a risk factor simply indicates a statistical relationship between two items such as high serum cholesterol and CHD; it does not mean that a cause and effect relationship exists. Nevertheless, it would appear prudent at this time to modify lifestyle in order to decrease or eliminate those risk factors that may contribute to CHD. You have control over several of them. You may stop smoking, lose excess body weight, and reduce your blood pressure. Of what importance are diet and exercise?

Can diet effectively reduce blood lipids and cholesterol?

In a review paper on nutrition and atherosclerosis, S. Dayton noted a clear relationship between high serum lipid concentrates, such as cholesterol and triglycerides, and the development of coronary atherosclerosis. He also noted there exists high suspicion, but something less than certainty, that this is a causal relationship. There appears to be enough evidence to justify the prophylactic measure of reducing both high blood cholesterol (**hypercholesteremia**) and high blood triglyceride (**hypertriglyceridemia**) levels. For individuals with normal blood lipid levels, dietary modifications may be helpful in maintaining normal or low levels. A generally recommended goal is to reduce both serum cholesterol and serum triglycerides to levels of 180 mg/100 ml blood or less.

Although authorities are still debating the effectiveness of lower serum triglyceride levels in preventing coronary heart disease, a recent study by the National Heart, Lung and Blood Institute revealed that lowering serum cholesterol levels will help to prevent coronary heart disease. The following dietary modifications have been shown to effectively lower serum cholesterol or serum triglycerides.

1. Adjust the caloric intake to achieve and maintain ideal body weight. One of the most common causes of high triglyceride levels is overweight. In many cases, simply losing body weight or reducing caloric intake will reduce these levels.

2. Reduce simple sugars and alcohol in the diet. Dietary sucrose (table sugar) provokes higher triglyceride concentrations than do the complex carbohydrates. Again, the value of complex carbohydrates in the diet is stressed. Moderate alcohol intake would be two drinks per day.

3. Decrease the amount of dietary cholesterol. Even though only about 35–40 percent of dietary cholesterol is absorbed, blood serum levels go up with increasing amounts in the diet. The average American intake is approximately 600–800 mg/day. It is recommended this amount be reduced to 300 mg/day or less.

4. Reduce the total amount of fats in the diet, particularly saturated fats. This dietary modification would help reduce both serum cholesterol and serum triglycerides. The ratio of polyunsaturated fats to saturated fats is important in controlling cholesterol levels. Saturated fats raise serum cholesterol levels; polyunsaturated fats help lower them.

In practical terms, what does this mean? In essence, eat less butter, fatty meats, organ foods such as liver and kidney, eggs, whole milk, cheeses, ice cream, shrimp, gravies, creamed foods, or desserts with animal fats. Eat more fish, poultry, fruits and vegetables, breads and cereal products, lean meats, and vegetable oils, which are high in polyunsaturates. Avoid simple carbohydrates and excessive alcohol intake. The hints and guidelines presented in Chapter 12 are relevant. In addition, an example of a polyunsaturated fat, low cholesterol diet plan is presented in Appendix H.

Dr. William B. Kannel has noted that a 100 mg reduction in dietary cholesterol per day will equal a 5 mg reduction in blood serum cholesterol. He suggests seven steps to a diet low in saturated fats and cholesterol.

1. Eggs—Only two per week.

2. Meats—six to seven ounces per day, primarily poultry, veal, and fish. Eat lean red meat and trim off excess fat. Avoid hot dogs, lunch meats, bacon, and sausage.

3. Dairy products—Watch out for whole milk and hard cheese. Switch to skim milk and soft cheeses. Use hard cheese only as a substitute for meat.

4. Margarine—Use polyunsaturated margarine instead of butter.

5. Baked goods—Avoid commercially prepared goods made with eggs and saturated fats.

6. Vegetables—Eat more fruits, vegetables, and whole grain products.

7. Cooking oil—Use oils instead of hard fats.

Can exercise effectively reduce blood lipids and cholesterol?

Physical inactivity, or lack of exercise, has been identified as one of the risk factors associated with incidence of CHD. Hence, exercise programs stressing aerobic endurance-type activities have been advocated as a means to reduce CHD incidence levels. However, the precise mechanism whereby exercise may help reduce the morbidity and mortality of CHD has not been identified. Therefore, many authorities believe that the beneficial effect may not be due to exercise itself, but rather the effect it may have on other possible risk factors such as smoking behavior, body weight, high blood pressure, and serum levels of triglycerides and cholesterol.

A large number of older, as well as contemporary, studies have revealed that exercise programs with proper intensity and duration may effectively lower serum triglycerides. However, the lowering effect of exercise on total serum cholesterol had not been established. Thus, exercise training was believed to effectively reduce one possible lipid risk factor, but not the main culprit, serum cholesterol.

In recent years, cholesterol has been shown to exist in several different forms in the blood. As mentioned previously, cholesterol may be carried primarily in either the low density lipoproteins (LDL) or high density lipoproteins (HDL). Research findings from the Framingham heart disease research program have revealed that high levels of LDL may contribute to CHD whereas high levels of HDL may serve a prevention role.

In a recent review of worldwide research on this subject, Peter Wood and William Haskell of the Stanford heart project have noted a consistent pattern between exercise and blood lipids. In general, increased levels of exercise are associated with lower plasma levels of triglycerides and LDL and higher levels of HDL. These findings have also been supported in major reviews by Dufaux and Tran. Although the precise biochemical mechanisms have not been identified, researchers have found that physically trained males and females possess increased activity levels for an enzyme that may produce the higher HDL levels.

What type of exercise program is necessary? Generally speaking, aerobic endurance activities such as running, swimming, or bicycling are advisable. The amount of exercise may be an important variable. The exercise equivalent of about 10–15 miles of running per week has been recommended to be sufficient to produce desirable changes. However, other research findings support a more beneficial effect of greater distances such as 40–45 miles per week.

In summary, interpretation of the available evidence suggests it would be wise to modify current diet and exercise habits in many Americans, including our children, to help reduce serum lipid levels and aid in the prevention of coronary heart disease. Additional guidelines will be presented in Chapters 12 and 13.

Protein—the tissue builder

4

Since most feats of human physical performance involve strenuous muscular activity in one form or another and since muscle tissue is comprised of protein, it is no wonder that protein has persisted throughout the years as the food of the athlete. The protein-muscle-strength relationship has been exploited by numerous commercial firms extolling the virtues of their particular product, including such names as "Protein-Energizers," "Protein-Powerizers," and "Protein-Weight Gainers." The implications are that extra protein is needed in the diet of the active person for energy, to gain strength and power, and to increase body weight.

Indeed, protein is one of our most essential nutrients. It has a wide variety of physiological functions that are essential to optimal physical performance. But, does the active individual need more protein in the diet for any of the reasons advanced above? Hopefully the information presented in this chapter may provide some basic answers relative to protein and its metabolism in the human body, and in the process hopefully eradicate some of the myths associated with protein and physical performance.

What is protein?

Protein is a complex chemical structure containing carbon, hydrogen and oxygen—just as carbohydrates and fat do. Protein has one other essential element—nitrogen. These four elements are combined into a number of different structures called **amino acids,** each one possessing an amino group (NH_2), an acid group (COOH), and the remainder being different combinations of carbon, hydrogen, oxygen and, in some cases, sulfur. There are twenty amino acids (peptides), all of which can be combined together in a variety of ways to form the proteins necessary for the structure and functions of the human body. Figure 4.1 depicts the formula of **alanine,** an amino acid discussed later.

Proteins are formed when two amino acids link together and form a peptide bond; hence, a dipeptide is formed. As more amino acids are added, a polypeptide is formed. Most proteins are polypeptides, the number of combined amino acids ranging up to 300.

Protein is contained in both animal and plant foods. Humans obtain their supply of amino acids from these two general sources.

Types and sources

Figure 4.1.
The chemical structure of alanine, an amino acid. The amino group (NH$_2$) contains nitrogen, while the acid group is represented by COOH.

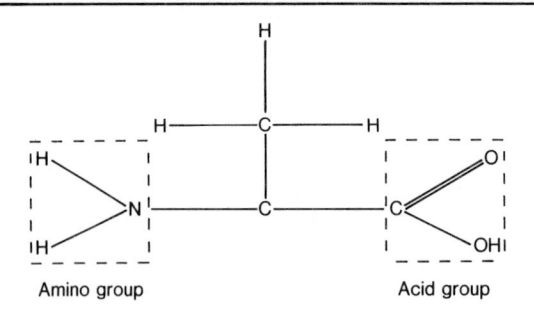

Amino group   Acid group

What are essential and nonessential amino acids?

Humans can synthesize some amino acids in their bodies, but cannot synthesize others. Amino acids that cannot be manufactured in the body are called **essential amino acids** and must be supplied in the diet. It should be noted that all twenty amino acids are necessary and must be present simultaneously for optimal maintenance of body growth and function. The utilization of the term essential in relation to amino acids is to distinguish those that must be obtained in the diet. For those interested, the essential amino acids may be found in Table 1.1. The **nonessential amino acids,** which may be formed in the body, are as follows:

alanine	glycine
aspartic acid	glutamine
arginine	proline
aspartamine	serine
cystine	tyrosine
glutamic acid	

What are the basic differences between animal and plant protein?

In general, the proteins ingested as animal products are superior to those found in plants. This is not to say that an amino acid found in a plant is inferior to the same amino acid found in an animal. They are the same. However, when we look at the distribution of all the amino acids in the two food sources, we can then see why animal protein is called a high quality protein whereas plant protein is of lower quality.

    The reasons for the superiority of animal protein are twofold. First, it is a complete protein since it contains all the essential amino acids. Secondly, it also contains the essential amino acids in the proper proportion. As noted above, all amino acids must be present simultaneously in order for the body to synthesize them into necessary body proteins. If one essential amino acid is in short supply, protein construction may be blocked. Having the proper amount of animal protein in the diet is a good way to ensure receiving a balanced supply of amino acids. Excellent sources include milk, cheese, meat, and eggs.

Vegetable proteins usually exist in smaller concentrations in plant materials and may be lower in three of the essential amino acids—lysine, methionine, and tryptophan. Most individual vegetables are usually unable to meet human nutrition needs. However, if vegetables are eaten in proper combinations, then the individual may receive a balanced supply of amino acids. Some populations receive most of their protein from plant sources. A good combination that represents a complete protein is rice and beans. This balanced intake is of extreme importance to strict vegetarians.

How much protein do you need?

The amount of protein necessary in the diet varies in different stages of the life cycle. During the early years of life, the child is manufacturing protein tissue during rapid growth stages, the rate of growth varying from infancy through late adolescence. In young adulthood, the protein requirement stabilizes. However, throughout the life cycle, the protein requirement established in the RDA is based upon the body weight of the individual. As a person goes through the life cycle, the amount of protein per unit body weight decreases.

Table 4.1 presents the amount of protein needed per kilogram of body weight for different age groups. To calculate your requirement, simply determine your body weight in kilograms, find the proper ratio in the table, and multiply. One kilogram equals 2.2 pounds. As an example, compute the protein requirement for a 165 pound, twenty-three-year-old male:

165 ÷ 2.2 = 75 kg
.8 g protein/kg × 75 kg = 60 g protein day

To be in protein balance, this individual should average about 60 g of protein intake daily. Table 4.2 illustrates how easy it is to meet this requirement if proper foods are chosen.

Table 4.1 Grams of protein needed per kilogram body weight during the life cycle

Age	Grams/kg body weight
0.0–0.5	2.2
0.5–1.0	2.0
1–3	1.8
4–6	1.5
7–10	1.2
11–14	1.0
15–18	0.9
19–22	0.8
23–up	0.8

The minimum necessary intake of protein is much less than the RDA. If all proteins were the same quality as egg protein, then the RDA would be approximately 0.34 g protein/kg body weight per day. Allowances are made for the fact that there exists individual variability in the need for protein, that the biologic quality of all dietary protein is not as good as egg protein, and that the efficiency of utilization decreases at higher dietary protein intake levels. Hence, the RDA is adjusted upward to account for these factors.

What are some common foods that are high quality protein?

Foods in the Milk and Meat Groups generally have high protein content. Mature dry beans and peas, nuts, and related products also have a high protein content. Fruits, vegetables, and grain products all have some protein, but the content varies; generally speaking, the protein content is low. Table 4.2 presents some common foods in each of these groups with the number of grams of protein in each. Notice the effect combination type foods have on protein content, for example, macaroni and cheese versus plain macaroni.

Table 4.2 Common foods in each of the food groups with grams of protein in each

	Amount	Grams of protein
Milk group		
Milk, whole	1 cup	9
Milk, skim	1 cup	9
Cheese, cheddar	1 ounce	7
Cheese, cottage	1 ounce	5
Custard, baked	1 cup	14
Ice cream	1 cup	6
Yogurt	1 cup	8
Meat group		
Beef, lean	1 ounce	8
Hamburger, lean	1 ounce	8
Chicken, breast	1 ounce	8
Ham, lean and fat	1 ounce	6
Luncheon meat	1 ounce	5
Fish	1 ounce	7
Tuna fish	1 ounce	8
Eggs	1	6

Table 4.2 *Continued*

	Amount	Grams of protein
Dry beans group		
Navy beans, cooked	1/2 cup	7
Lima beans, cooked	1/2 cup	8
Peanuts, roasted	1/2 cup	18
Peanut butter	1 tablespoon	4
Peas, split	1/2 cup	10
Vegetable group		
Beans, green	1/2 cup	1
Broccoli	1/2 cup	2
Carrots	1	1
Corn	1 ear	3
Peas, green	1/2 cup	4
Potato, baked	1	3
Fruit group		
Apple	1	trace
Banana	1	1
Grapefruit	1/2	1
Orange	1	1
Orange juice	1 cup	2
Pear	1	1
Breads-Cereals		
Bread, wheat	1 slice	3
Bread, white	1 slice	2
Bran flakes	1 cup	4
Cupcake	1	1
Grits	1 cup	3
Doughnuts	1	1
Macaroni	1 cup	6
Macaroni and cheese	1 cup	17
Noodles	1 cup	7
Spaghetti	1 cup	5
Spaghetti with meat balls	1 cup	19

Foods high in protein include meats, milk, and plants such as legumes.
(David Corona)

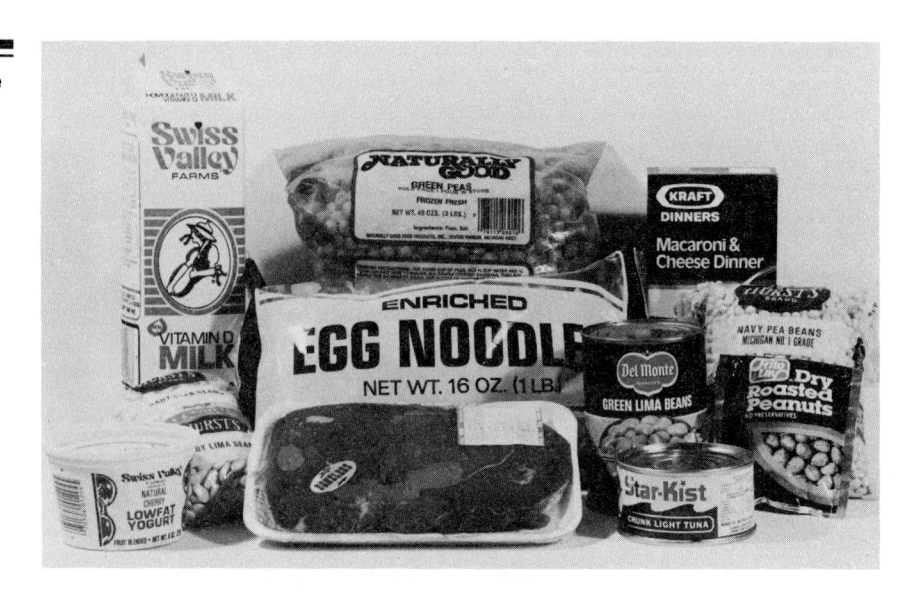

What happens to protein in the human body?

Metabolism and function

The amino acids in the diet of humans are present as proteins and must be released through the digestive process. Enzymes in the stomach and small intestine break the complex protein down into polypeptides and then into individual amino acids. The amino acids are absorbed through the small intestine wall, pass into the blood, and then to the liver. The liver is a critical center in amino acid metabolism. It is constantly synthesizing a balanced amino acid mixture for the formation of the diverse protein requirements of the body. The main metabolic fate of protein is this conversion into bodily tissues and functional compounds.

When the body is in protein balance, excess protein may be channeled into the metabolic pathways of carbohydrate and fat. The liver is the main organ where this conversion occurs. A schematic representation is presented in Figure 2.2. In essence, some of the amino acids are said to be glucogenic, that is, glucose forming. At various stages of the energy transformations within the liver, the **glucogenic amino acids** may be converted to glucose. The process is gluconeogenesis. Other amino acids are known as **ketogenic** and can also enter certain biochemical pathways in the liver and be converted to fat. The glucose and fat thus produced may be transported to other parts of the body to be used. Thus, although excess protein cannot be stored as amino acids in the body, the energy content is not wasted for it is converted to either carbohydrate or fat.

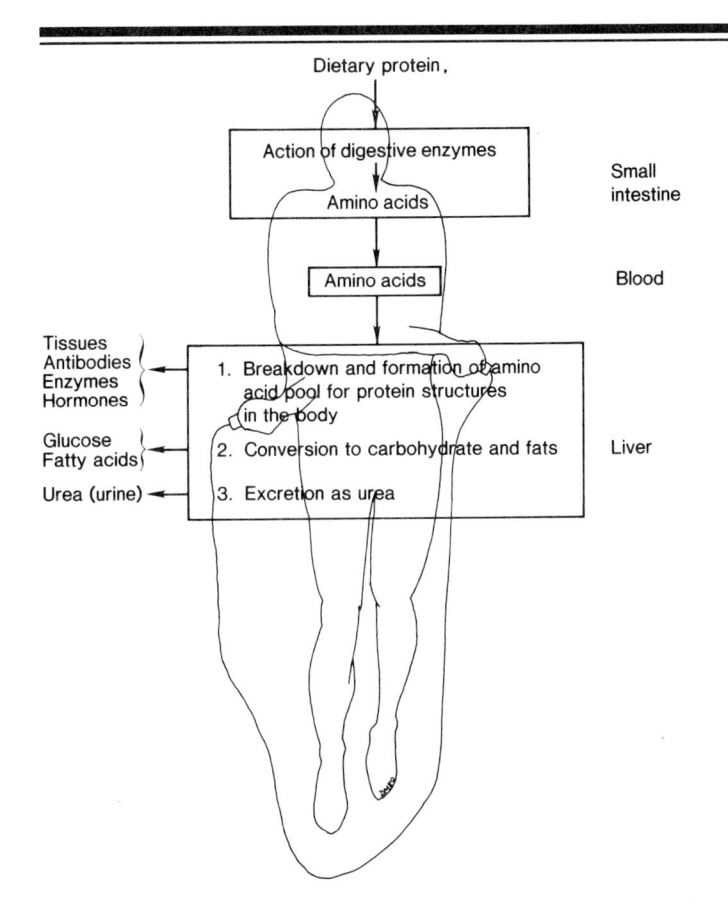

Figure 4.2.
Simplified diagram of protein metabolism. After digestion, amino acids are metabolized in the liver, either forming amino acids needed for new protein synthesis, being converted to glucose or fatty acids, or converted to urea. These by-products are then transported by the blood for body use or in the case of urea, excretion.

Dietary protein

Action of digestive enzymes → Amino acids — Small intestine

Amino acids — Blood

Liver:
1. Breakdown and formation of amino acid pool for protein structures in the body → Tissues, Antibodies, Enzymes, Hormones
2. Conversion to carbohydrate and fats → Glucose, Fatty acids
3. Excretion as urea → Urea (urine)

During the process of converting excess protein to carbohydrate and fat, the nitrogen component of protein must be eliminated, for carbohydrate and fat do not contain nitrogen. In essence, the liver forms ammonia from the excess nitrogen; the ammonia is converted into urea, which passes into the blood and is eventually eliminated by the kidney into the urine.

Figure 4.2 presents a summary of the fates of protein in human metabolism.

Can protein be formed from carbohydrates and fats?

Yes, but with some limitations. Protein has one essential element, nitrogen, which is not possessed by either carbohydrate or fat. However, if the body has an excess of one particular amino acid, the liver may be able to save the nitrogen from this excess amino acid and combine it with some of the carbon, hydrogen, and oxygen elements found in carbohydrates and fats.

The net result is the formation in the body of one of the nonessential amino acids using carbohydrates and fats as part of the building materials. Figure 2.2 illustrates that pyruvate and acetyl Co-A, products that are the result of fat and/or carbohydrate metabolism, may be used to help form amino acids. Keep in mind that nitrogen must be present for this to occur, and its source is through dietary protein.

What are the major functions of protein in human nutrition?

As has been alluded to in previous questions, the main function of protein is to provide the building materials for most body structures and to provide functional biochemical compounds. In one way or another protein is involved in almost all body functions. Its individual roles are beyond the scope of this text, except where they are of dietary importance to the active individual. The following represent just some of its major functions:

1. Forms most body tissues.
2. Forms the structural basis for all enzymes controlling body functions.
3. Forms antibodies.
4. Forms hormones.
5. Helps to maintain water balance.
6. Helps to maintain acid-base balance.
7. Helps control the blood clotting process.
8. Carries nutrients in blood as lipoprotein.
9. Carries nutrients into cells.
10. Carries iron and oxygen in the blood.

Although protein is not a major energy source for humans, it can serve such a function under several conditions. As noted above, excess protein may be converted to carbohydrate or fat and then enter metabolic pathways. During periods of starvation or semistarvation when adequate amounts of carbohydrates and fats are not available, protein is utilized for energy purposes since energy takes precedence over tissue building in metabolism. Hence, if the active individual desires to maintain lean body mass, it is essential to have sufficient carbohydrate and fat calories in the diet in order to provide a **protein sparing effect.** In other words, carbohydrate and fat calories will be utilized for energy production, thus sparing utilization of protein as an energy source and allowing it to be used for its more important metabolic functions.

What percentage of the diet should be composed of protein?

There is an RDA for protein that as noted above, is based upon body weight of the individual at different ages. If you would take the recommended energy intake in Calories for each age group, say 2,700 C for an adult male, and calculate the percentage of this value that the RDA for protein supplies, the values are less than 10 percent for each age group. This value is less than the recent 12 percent recommendation of the Senate Select Subcommittee on Nutrition and Health Needs. A proportion of 10–12 percent protein Calories in the diet should meet most individual needs.

One point to consider, however, is the fact that protein in many foods is often accompanied by substantial quantities of fat. You should be selective in the types of protein foods eaten. For example, a glass of whole milk and a glass of skim milk both have 9 g of protein, but the whole milk also has 9 g of fat compared to none in the skim milk. Nutritionally, skim milk is 40 percent protein Calories while the whole milk is 22.5 percent. Further examples are provided in Appendix B. Check for nonfat and low fat milk products and low fat meats.

Are there any health benefits or hazards to a high or low protein diet?

Since protein is the source of essential amino acids, a deficiency could be expected to cause serious health problems. Such is the case in certain parts of the world where protein intake is inadequate due to political, economic, or other reasons. Protein-Calorie insufficiency is one of the major nutritional problems in the world today. Protein deficiency may also occur in individuals who abuse sound nutritional practices, such as drug addicts, chronic alcoholics, and extreme food faddist groups.

Protein intake in the United States appears to be more than adequate to meet the nutritional requirements of the average American. On the other hand, individuals who are on a low protein diet plan or young men who are on modified starvation diets to lose weight for such sports as wrestling, may experience periods of protein insufficiency. During this time, the individual may be in negative nitrogen balance, that is, more nitrogen is being excreted from the body than is being ingested. Hence, body tissues such as muscles and hemoglobin may be lost with possible decreases in strength and endurance capacity. Adequate protein intake is essential for proper physiological functioning, both in the inactive and active individual.

The RDA for protein in the average adult is approximately 50–60 g per day. High protein diets may contain up to 200 g per day, or about four times the RDA. In general, a high protein diet will not be harmful to the average healthy individual. As mentioned before, excess protein may be converted to carbohydrate and fat either to be stored or used as an energy source. However, saturated fats and cholesterol, which normally accompany animal protein, should be restricted by wise selection of protein foods. High protein diets may also be potentially dangerous to individuals who have a history of kidney or liver disease. Gout, an aggravation of joint inflammation, may be aggravated by high protein diets. Large quantities of fluid should be consumed by anyone on a high protein diet in order to help the kidney excrete the waste products of protein metabolism. Very high protein diets may lead to dehydration if fluid intake is not adequate.

Although they appear to no longer be in vogue, be aware of the potential dangers associated with commercially advertised **liquid protein diets.** Liquid protein products often consist of predigested (in the laboratory) protein with vitamin and mineral supplements. They were advertised to contain all the essential nutrients with low caloric intake and hence be very effective in weight loss programs. However, some of these products contained low-quality protein. Unfortunately, prolonged intake of these products resulted in some electrolyte imbalances and other medical problems in certain individuals and resulted in some fatalities. Anyone using similar products for weight control should be under the careful supervision of a physician.

In one carbohydrate-loading regimen there is a three-day depletion phase that consists of a high protein diet combined with very little carbohydrate intake. This phase may often be associated with periods of weakness and lethargy, which may be attributed more to the low carbohydrate intake than the high protein consumption.

Are proteins used for energy during exercise?

Proteins and exercise

Although protein may serve as a source of energy during rest under certain conditions such as starvation, its utilization as a major source during exercise is rather limited. Carbohydrates and fats are the primary energy sources, protein contributing only approximately 1–2 percent during normal exercise.

A recent report has revealed that alanine, an amino acid, is released by the active muscles during exercise and that the output increases in proportion to the severity of the exercise performed. Even in prolonged exercise of two to four hours, alanine output continues. This amino acid is one of the prime contributors to gluconeogenesis, the formation of new glucose. Hence, during exercise alanine may be transported to the liver and be converted to glucose. The glucose is released into the blood and eventually find its way to the contracting muscle to be used as an energy source. Although this may be one means whereby protein may be used for energy during exercise, it does not appear to be a highly significant factor. However, it may become an important source of blood glucose during prolonged exercise. Research has shown that protein may contribute about 4 percent of the energy demand during prolonged exercise when a person has normal glycogen stores. The percentage contribution may be as high as

10 percent if the person is depleted of glycogen, for example, during the last part of a marathon. Thus, carbohydrate loading may have a protein sparing effect for distance runners. This increased protein utilization could easily be replenished by the extra protein Calories the individual would consume during recovery the following day.

Does strenuous exercise tear down body protein?

Several authorities have reported there is no conclusive evidence at the present time that indicates that muscular activity increases destruction of cellular protein in individuals who are on a balanced diet. On the other hand, others have suggested that exercise may increase protein breakdown. They noted that the mechanisms underlying the protein loss, measured primarily by nitrogen losses in the urine, are not fully understood, but may be due to the breakdown of amino acids that have leaked from the muscles during exercise. Small amounts of amino acids are also found in sweat from exercise.

As noted in response to the previous question, exercise does cause the loss of protein from the exercising muscle, primarily as the amino acid alanine. At the same time the exercising muscles are also absorbing other amino acids from the blood, which may have been formed in the liver. Whether or not there is a net loss of cellular protein, such as muscle tissue, during exercise has not been established. The small amount of muscle tissue that might be lost during exercise would be replaced during the next day of recovery, as research has shown an increased muscle protein synthesis during recovery from exercise.

An important finding was revealed in this research with protein and exercise. The consumption of glucose during exercise reduced the rate of amino acid uptake by the liver. Since the glucose intake could be used itself in the energy processes, the demand for production of new glucose by protein breakdown was not as great. Hence, carbohydrate intake during exercise may be helpful to spare protein loss, even though the loss may be very small and insignificant.

Do individuals in strenuous physical training, including the developing adolescent athlete, need more protein in the diet?

Those who recommend increased protein intake during physical training have suggested it is necessary for three reasons. The first reason is to prevent a condition known as sports anemia; the second is to increase muscle mass; and the third is to replace possible protein losses incurred during moderate exercise for prolonged periods of time.

Some Japanese studies have revealed that during the early stages of training, the hemoglobin levels dropped in many individuals. The condition has been labelled **sports anemia.** Indeed, when an individual undergoes the transition from a sedentary life-style to a more physically active one, there are some bodily adaptations that require the incorporation of protein.

Muscle tissue may increase in size, while enzymes and other protein compounds in the cell may increase in size and number to meet the new metabolic demands of exercise. As the theory goes, the use of protein for these adaptations takes precedence over its use for hemoglobin production. Hence, hemoglobin levels fall and sports anemia occurs, which may handicap physical performance. In order to counteract these effects, a protein intake of 2 g/kg body weight has been recommended during the early stages of training.

Athletes or others who are training for strength usually utilize a program with weights in order to help increase body weight and muscle mass. Since the solid constituent of muscle is protein, the general recommendation for weight trainers in this country as well as abroad ranges from 2.0–2.5 g protein/kg body weight. Theoretically, this increased protein content in the diet will facilitate an increase in body weight and development of muscle mass. In this regard, many weight lifters and body builders are notorious for the amount of protein supplements they ingest.

In prolonged exercise, such as the long distance running and bicycling, protein has been shown to make a contribution, albeit minor, to the energy demands during training. In addition, nitrogen losses in the sweat may require additional protein in the diet, but only about a total of 7–8 g. Some authorities recommend that the endurance athlete obtain about 2.5–3.0 g protein/kg body weight in order to replace these losses.

What are the general conclusions of the research conducted relative to these three problems? First, sports anemia has not been shown to occur in all subjects initiating a strenuous training program, particularly if on a balanced diet. Some have reported that there may be a drop in hemoglobin concentration, but this may be explained by an increase in the plasma of the blood with no loss of total hemoglobin. However, a recent report did note the development of sports anemia in those individuals with low protein intake (0.5 g/kg) as contrasted to others undergoing training with normal or high protein intakes.

Second, recent research has indicated that individuals undertaking hard physical training and consuming the amount of protein normally found in the American diet (100 g) retained more of this protein as muscle than did a group who had an intake of only 40–50 g. They did not retain all the additional protein, but enough to make a difference in body weight and muscle mass. It should be noted however, that no differences in physical performance were found between these two groups on different protein intakes. In a review of the research conducted relative to protein requirements and physical activity, J. V. G. A. Durnin noted that the evidence causes skepticism about any requirement of protein of much more than 1 g/kg body weight per day.

Third, there is little data available relative to the effect of high protein diets upon endurance capacity. One recent report did note that low protein intake, only 4 g per day, did not lower maximal endurance capacity over a

Table 4.3 Calculation of grams protein/kilogram body weight

Body weight: 70 kilograms
One gram protein = 4 Calories

Daily caloric intake:	3,500–4,000	3,500–4,000
Percent protein	15	20
Calories in protein	525–600	700–800
Grams of protein	131–150	175–200
Grams protein/kilogram	1.9–2.1	2.5–2.9

ten-day period. Other research has suggested that normal dietary protein intake should be sufficient to replace small amounts lost during training to maintain endurance capacity.

The general conclusion from this brief overview is that prolonged low protein intake may have adverse effects upon physical performance, but intakes above those normally found in the American diet will not increase performance capacity. It should be noted that of those individuals who recommend protein intakes on the order of 2.0–2.5 g/kg, many are noted authorities in the fields of exercise and nutrition. Is there a conflict between their recommendations and the available research? Let us look at the protein RDA and the actual intake of most active individuals.

Most strenuous physical training occurs during adolescence and early adulthood, although the increasing popularity of exercise in the United States finds people participating at all age levels. For most people the RDA ranges from 0.8–1.0 g protein/kg body weight. Based on moderate activity levels, the average 70 kg male would be in protein balance with 56 g daily. However, according to the suggested recommendations of 2.0–2.5 g/kg, he would need 140–175 g daily if involved in a strenuous training program. The same would be true of an adolescent going through a physical training program.

The average caloric intake for a moderately active male averages 2,700–3,000 C. This caloric intake may be increased through physical training as more Calories are expended. Thus, caloric intake would be increased to approximately 3,500–4,000 C. If the protein content of the dietary Calories averaged 15 percent, which represents the approximate intake in the United States, then the intake of protein would approximate 1.9–2.1 g/kg. Increasing the protein content to 20 percent would provide a value of 2.5–2.9 g/kg. The mathematics are presented in Table 4.3 These values approach those recommended for individuals in training.

In summary, expensive protein supplements are not necessary for individuals undertaking strenuous exercise programs. Wise selection of quality protein foods will provide adequate amounts through balanced diets to meet bodily needs during the early and continued stages of training. Additional points on this subject are covered in Chapter 11 under the topic of gaining weight.

5

Vitamins—the organic regulators

Vitamins continue to be one of the most used and abused nutrient supplements in the United States today, not only by physically active individuals such as athletes, but also the general public as well. The vitamin industry is a multimillion dollar business. M. Tatkon, in his excellent book entitled *The Great Vitamin Hoax,* indicated that vitamin pill manufacturers and advertisers have perpetuated the myth that the average American diet contains insufficient amounts of vitamins, a potential cause of many common diseases. Vitamin supplements are on the market shelves that have been designed, or so the manufacturers say, to help us combat the stress of everyday life, to help prevent the common cold, and to provide optimal energy for athletic performance. To be sure, vitamins are necessary nutrients. However, exaggerated claims by those with economic interests in vitamin supplements, especially those aimed at the active individual, need to be challenged by factual data. Moreover some misinformed individuals are publishing articles in leading sports magazines extolling the virtue of a particular vitamin. In a recent issue of *Runners World,* one such individual raved about the benefits of vitamin E to the athlete. He used a rather outdated report as the basis for comments, even though this report had been repudiated by the original author. Thus, the purpose of this chapter is to present an overview relative to the requirements of vitamins, particularly for active individuals.

A slightly different approach is used in this chapter and the next one. Several general overall questions relative to vitamins will be answered, and then each individual vitamin will be discussed in terms of RDA, food sources that provide ample amounts, metabolic functions in the body with particular reference to the active individual, the need for supplements, and potential hazards of high dosages.

What are vitamins and how do they work?

Vitamins represent a number of extremely complex organic compounds that are found in small amounts in most foods. They are essential for the optimal functioning of a great number of diverse physiological processes in the human body. The activity levels of many of these physiological processes are increased greatly during exercise, and an adequate bodily supply of vitamins must be present for these processes to function in an optimal manner.

Basic facts

In order for the fundamental physiological processes of the body to proceed in an orderly controlled fashion, a number of complex chemicals known as enzymes are necessary for the regulation of these diverse reactions. Several hundred **enzymes** have been identified in the human body. Enzymes are necessary to digest our foods, to make our muscles contract, to release the energy stores in our body, to help us transport body gases such as carbon dioxide, to help us grow, to help clot our blood, and so on. Enzymes serve as catalysts; that is, they are capable of inducing changes in other substances without changing themselves. For example, the digestive enzymes will speed up the breakdown of fats, carbohydrates, and protein into simpler compounds. Once these simpler compounds are produced, the enzymes are left unchanged and are able to work on new materials.

Enzymes are chemicals that generally consist of two parts. One part is a protein molecule and to it is attached the second part, a **coenzyme.** In order for the enzyme to function properly, both parts must be present. The coenzyme often is a vitamin or some related compound. It is now known that most vitamins are essential in human nutrition because of their role in the formation of many body enzymes.

The enzyme is not used up in the chemical process that it initiates or participates, but enzymes may deteriorate with time. The coenzymes also may be degraded through body metabolism. A fresh supply of vitamins, particularly the water soluble vitamins, is constantly needed.

Although vitamins are indispensible for regulating many body functions and for the maintenance of optimal health, it should be noted that they are not a source of energy. They do not have any caloric value. Moreover, they make no significant contribution to the structure of the body, as do protein and some minerals.

The existence of the vitamins was discovered by their physiological actions before their chemical structures had been identified. In assigning names to vitamins, the alphabet was used in relation to their time of discovery. In some cases, a large time gap existed between the discovery of the vitamin and the determination of its chemical structure. In others, the chemical nature was discovered rapidly, and the chemical name came into early use. There may be two different terms for some vitamins, and only one for others.

Table 5.1 lists those vitamins and interchangeable synonyms often used. There are two general classes of vitamins, those that are soluble in fat and those that are soluble in water. The former are stored to a greater degree in the human body than are the water soluble vitamins.

Table 5.1 Essential vitamins with synonymous terms

Vitamin name	Other terms
Fat soluble vitamins	
Vitamin A	Retinol; carotenoids
Vitamin D	Calciferols
Vitamin E	Tocopherols
Vitamin K	Phylloquinone
Water soluble vitamins	
Vitamin B$_1$	Thiamin
Vitamin B$_2$	Riboflavin
Niacin	Nicotinamide; nicotinic acid
Vitamin B$_6$	Pyridoxine
Pantothenic acid	
Folacin	Folic acid
Vitamin B$_{12}$	Cyanocobalamin; corrinoids
Biotin	
Vitamin C	Ascorbic acid

Can some vitamins be formed in the body?

In general most vitamins must be obtained in the food we eat. However, certain vitamins may be formed in the body. Vitamin A may be synthesized from carotene (provitamin A); however, the carotene must be obtained in the diet. Vitamin D may be formed through a complex series of body reactions that are triggered by the action of the ultraviolet rays in sunlight upon the skin. The actions of intestinal bacteria are responsible for formation of vitamin K, and one of the B vitamins, niacin, can be formed from tryptophan, an essential amino acid that must be obtained in the diet.

Is there any difference between a natural and a synthetic vitamin?

The major difference between a natural and a synthetic vitamin is how they are made. Natural vitamins are often called organic vitamins, and this is the way they exist in nature in the foods we eat. Natural vitamins also may be extracted from plants. We may get natural vitamins through our daily diet or by purchasing special preparations in health stores. A synthetic vitamin, simply put, is a manmade vitamin; it is a manufactured product.

If the chemical structures of these two types of vitamins are compared, no difference would be noted. They have the same chemical composition and structure. One of the known facts of human nutrition and functioning is that the body cells do not recognize foods per se, they recognize only simple chemical compounds. Since the two types of vitamins are of the same chemical structure, the body cells cannot differentiate between them and will be able to use one just as effectively as the other. To emphasize this point, the Food and Drug Administration noted that there is no nutritional difference between a vitamin provided by a natural source and the same vitamin provided by a synthetic, or manufactured, source.

Although there is no difference between a natural and a synthetic vitamin, it is probably better to get your vitamins in their natural state as they exist in plants and animals. In this way, other nutrients, particularly minerals, will be obtained at the same time as they also are natural constituents of the food we eat. Vitamins often work in conjunction with minerals, such as vitamin D and calcium, vitamin B_6 and magnesium, and vitamin E and selenium. By obtaining vitamins through selection of a balanced diet, we may be assured of receiving sufficient amounts of other nutrients necessary for optimal physiological functioning.

On the other hand, there may be certain situations when a synthetic vitamin may possess some advantages. For example, alcoholics may have a deficiency of vitamin B_6 and folacin, and research has shown that these vitamins in pure synthetic form were absorbed more readily than the same vitamins in foods.

Supplements and megadoses

Are vitamin supplements recommended?

The vitamin industry, through its advertising media, has attempted to convince the American public that we are not receiving an ample supply of vitamins in the foods we normally eat and thus experience certain diseases because of vitamin deficiency. Moreover, some have used subtle advertisements to suggest that vitamin supplements are essential to increased physical performance. In general, however, there is no solid evidence to indicate that the average healthy American on a balanced diet is suffering from vitamin deficiency and related diseases. Nor is there any substantial evidence to support the use of vitamin supplements with well-nourished athletes or other highly active individuals. A well-balanced diet contains all the necessary vitamins for the average individual. However, there may be certain situations where vitamin supplements are recommended.

Some recent national surveys have noted slight deficiencies in several nutrients, particularly iron and the water soluble vitamins, in the diets of some Americans. Surveys with some athletic groups have revealed similar

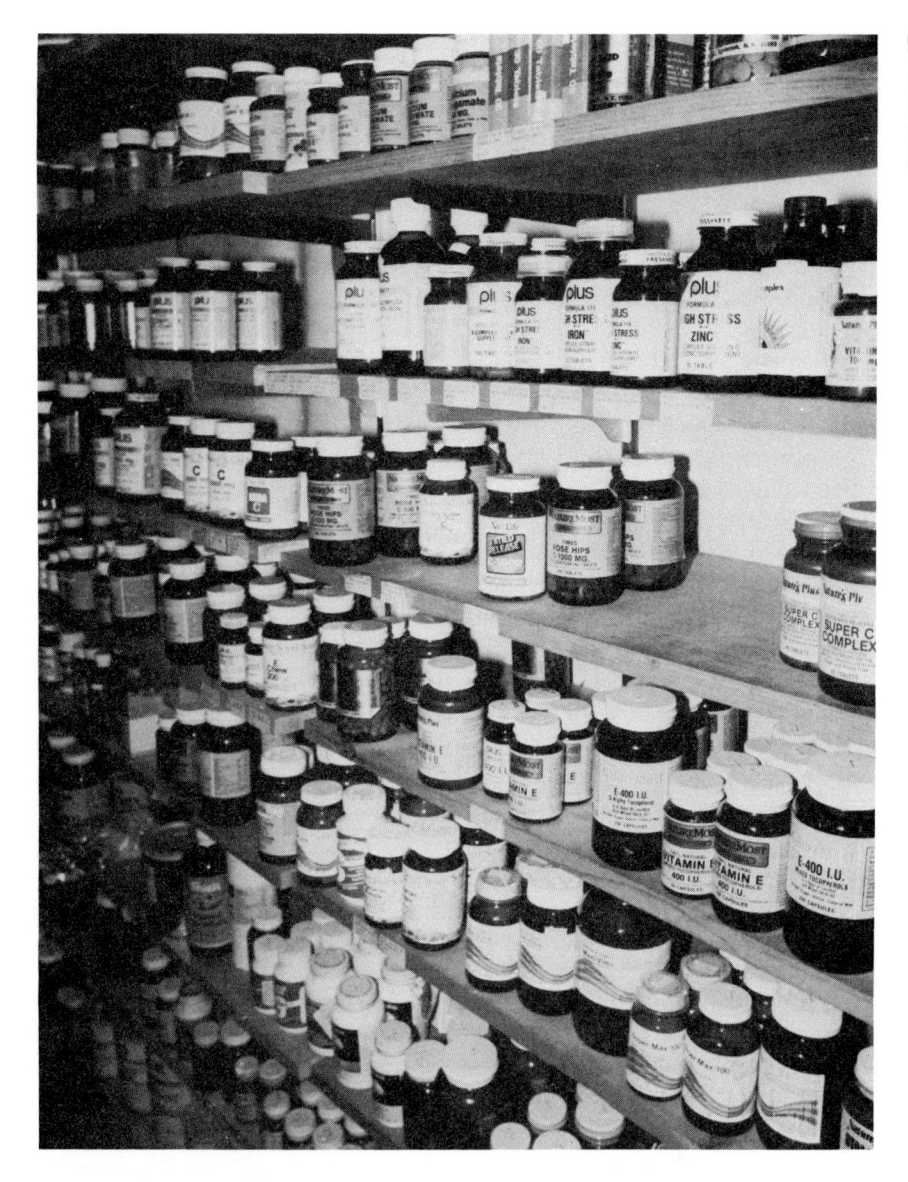

Active individuals generally do not need vitamin supplements.
(Michael DiSpezio)

findings. However, these surveys only indicated a deficiency in reference to the RDA, and did not report any disease symptoms or lower physical performance capacity. If an individual feels he is not receiving a balanced diet for some reason, a simple balanced vitamin supplement will not do any harm. There are a number of preparations on the market that contain the daily RDA of most vitamins. The only damage of consuming such products is to the individual's pocketbook, for a balanced diet will provide all the necessary vitamins.

In certain types of sports, such as wrestling and boxing, participants may go through prolonged periods of time on semistarvation or starvation diets. This is not a recommended procedure, but some athletes may do it in order to lose substantial amounts of body weight. In such cases, when the caloric intake may be well below 1,200 C per day, the athlete may not be receiving adequate vitamin intake. Recent research has suggested that vitamin depletion, mainly the water soluble vitamins, can occur rapidly in humans on low-Calorie diets and should be replaced daily. A vitamin supplement may be helpful to prevent a vitamin deficiency in such individuals.

Some individuals may have increased needs for a specific vitamin as a consequence of a particular drug they may be taking or some other factor in their life. For example, alcohol may retard the absorption of vitamins B_6, B_{12}, and folacin; oral contraceptives may increase the need for the same three vitamins and vitamin C; smoking and aspirin may increase vitamin C needs. Other such drug-vitamin interactions exist. In such cases, physicians may recommend specific vitamin supplements.

One particular vitamin, B_{12}, is not found in plant foods. A strict vegetarian will need a B_{12} supplement, but his foods will provide the other essential vitamins.

In summary, the average individual, physically active or not, should receive an adequate amount of vitamins if the diet is well balanced. The typical one-a-day vitamin supplement will certainly do no harm and may be recommended in those special cases noted above. But what about the use of large amounts of vitamins as often recommended by the health food industries?

What value, if any, do vitamin megadoses have?

For those individuals who feel they are not receiving a balanced intake of vitamins, taking a daily capsule with the RDA of each will do no harm. However, many individuals, particularly so in athletics, believe that if a little is good, then a lot is better. Hence, we have some athletes consuming 10,000 mg of vitamin C daily when the RDA is only 60 mg. Are there any benefits or hazards to such practices?

Vitamin deficiencies are rare in the United States. If and when they do occur, megavitamin dosages may be appropriate therapy to correct the deficiency state.

On the other hand, if the vitamin content of the body is adequate, then excess vitamin intake does not serve any useful purpose and may even be harmful in certain situations. As noted previously, vitamins have a primary function as coenzymes. When a vitamin enters the body, it will travel through the bloodstream to a particular body cell and then form part of the enzyme complex within that cell. Now the cell has a limited capacity to produce these enzymes, and when that capacity is reached, the vitamin cannot be used for its rightful purpose. It may now have other fates. It may be excreted from the body if it is in excess, particularly if it is a water soluble vitamin; it may be stored in some body tissues; or it may assume a chemical, rather than a vitamin, function.

Victor Herbert, Director of the Hematology and Nutrition Laboratory at the Bronx Veterans Administration Hospital, noted that megadoses of vitamins may have undesirable side effects due to the fact that the enzyme systems in which they participate are saturated, and therefore, the megadose excess may begin to act as a chemical. Dr. Herbert cites a number of instances where vitamin megadoses may be harmful. Where relevant, these megadose effects will be noted for each vitamin in the remainder of this chapter.

The individual vitamins

Vitamin A **Vitamin A** is a fat soluble, unsaturated alcohol, which exists mainly in mammals and saltwater fish as preformed vitamin A, or retinol. It also may be formed in the body from its precursor, carotene, which is found in many fruits and dark green and yellow vegetables.

The RDA for vitamin A is 1,000 retinol equivalents (1 mg) for adult males and 800 retinol equivalents (.8 mg) for adult females. Slightly lesser amounts are needed by children. The RDA for specific ages may be found in Appendix A. One milligram of vitamin A equals 1,000 Retinol units (R.E.) or 5,000 I.U. Hence, to convert from I.U. to R.E., simply divide the I.U. value by 5.

Vitamin A, as retinol, is found in substantial amounts in whole milk, butter, cheese, egg yolks, cod liver oil, and fortified milk. Provitamin A, as carotene, is found in green leafy and yellow vegetables as well as in some fruits as oranges, limes, pineapples, prunes, and cantaloupes. Vitamin A is not destroyed by ordinary cooking temperatures.

Vitamin A is essential for maintenance of the epithelial cells, those cells covering the outside of the body and lining the body cavities. It is also essential for normal growth and development and the prevention of night blindness. Mild deficiencies may retard growth, increase susceptibility to infection, cause skin lesions and night blindness. A severe deficiency may lead to blindness due to destruction of the cornea.

Excessive amounts of vitamin A, normally caused by self-medication with megadoses, can cause a condition known as hypervitaminosis A. Symptoms may include headache, loss of appetite, vomiting, disorders of bone tissue, and peeling of skin.

Vitamin A supplementation to the diet of the active individual has no sound theoretical basis. Moreover, the research conducted with vitamin A and physical performance has shown no beneficial effect. Hence, there appears to be no advantage for the active individual to supplement the diet with vitamin A, particularly not so with megadoses that may have undesirable effects.

Vitamin B₁ (Thiamine) Vitamin B₁ is a water soluble vitamin. It is a component of the vitamin B complex.

The RDA for vitamin B₁ varies during various stages of the life cycle; the adult male needs approximately 1.5 mg/day while the adult female needs about 1.1 mg/day. See Appendix A for other age groups.

Vitamin B₁ is widely distributed in both plant and animal tissues. Good sources include whole grain cereals, eggs, milk, cheese, peas, beans, nuts, and many fruits and vegetables. It is not readily destroyed by ordinary cooking temperatures.

Vitamin B₁ has a central role in the metabolism of carbohydrates and is essential for the normal functioning of the nervous system. Deficiencies could prove to be detrimental to the active individual who might rely on high levels of carbohydrate metabolism for energy. In addition, nervous system functions could be disturbed resulting in impaired performance.

Megadoses of thiamin appear to have no detrimental effect. The excess will be excreted from the body in the urine.

Physical activity, particularly high level endurance-type activity, will increase the need for thiamin in the diet as well as increase the need for caloric intake. With proper selection of foods, the increased thiamin need and caloric need may be met by the content in the additional foods eaten.

Since the role of vitamin B₁ in energy metabolism and nervous system functioning has been known for over thirty years, a number of studies have been conducted to evaluate the effect of thiamin supplementation on physical performance. Following a careful review of these studies, many with problems in establishing a proper experimental design, there appears to be no conclusive evidence to support the contention that vitamin B₁ intake above and beyond the normal RDA will enhance performance.

Vitamin B₂ (Riboflavin) Vitamin B₂, riboflavin, is a water soluble vitamin. It is a component of the vitamin B complex.

The RDA for riboflavin is similar to that of thiamin, only slightly higher. It averages about 1.7 mg for the adult male and 1.3 mg for the adult female. Appendix A contains the RDA for other age groups.

Riboflavin is distributed widely in foods. Good sources include liver, eggs, green vegetables, wheat germ, milk, cheese, yeast, and enriched foods. It is not destroyed in ordinary cooking processes.

Riboflavin is important for the formation of a number of enzymes involved in the energy transformations occurring in the body cells. It is also necessary for normal growth. Deficiencies are rare and have been associated with impaired growth and feelings of weakness. Cracks at the corner of the mouth also may be evident.

No adverse effects of riboflavin megadoses have been reported. Excess riboflavin is apparently excreted from the body.

The National Research Council has noted there is no evidence that riboflavin requirements are increased with exercise, although some recent research suggested an increased dietary intake in women who start a jogging program. However, no reputable research has been uncovered that has studied the effects of riboflavin supplementation upon physical performance. Based on theoretical considerations, the available research data, and the absence of riboflavin deficiency in most individuals, one must conclude that riboflavin supplementation to the diet will not enhance physical performance.

Niacin   Niacin is also known as nicotinic acid, nicotinamide, or the antipellagra vitamin. It is one of the B complex vitamins.

The RDA for niacin is about 16–19 mg of niacin equivalent (N.E.) for adult males and about 13–14 mg N.E. for adult females. The requirement varies for other age groups and specific values may be obtained from Appendix A. Since niacin may be synthesized in the body from tryptophan, an essential amino acid, humans do not have a requirement for niacin per se, but rather for an N.E. One N.E. equals 1 mg of niacin or 60 mg tryptophan, since 1 mg niacin can be produced from that amount of tryptophan.

Niacin is distributed widely in plant and animal sources. It is most abundant in poultry, lean meats, fish, organ meats, whole grain cereal products, legumes, peanuts, peanut butter, and enriched foods. Milk and eggs are almost completely empty of niacin, although both are good sources of tryptophan from which niacin can be made in the body. Niacin is not destroyed in ordinary cooking.

The major function of niacin is to serve as a component of two coenzymes concerned with energy processes within the cell. One of these enzymes is important in the process of glycolysis, which is a means to produce energy rapidly without the presence of oxygen. Hence, a lack of niacin may be theorized to block this process and impair physical performance. Niacin is also involved in cellular respiration and the synthesis of fat. A deficiency of niacin may cause pellagra, gastrointestinal disturbances, and mental disturbances.

Large doses of niacin may cause symptoms of flushing with burning and tingling sensations around the face, neck, and hands. Taken over long periods of time, niacin may contribute to liver problems and peptic ulcers. Large doses also have been shown to decrease the plasma level of free fatty acids (FFA). Since FFA are a source of energy during prolonged submaximal work, this effect may have some implications for physical performance.

During the past forty years, a number of experiments have been conducted relative to niacin supplementation and physical performance capacity. A theoretical base existed. Niacin could possibly facilitate glycolysis and provide more energy by this route, or it could block FFA and thus force the muscle to use carbohydrate as a fuel, which might be more efficient. However, research failed to substantiate any beneficial effect of niacin on physical performance. As a matter of fact, its use is not suggested as a supplement, particularly in long endurance type exercise such as marathon running. Niacin may block the FFA and thus the muscle glycogen may be used at a faster rate, resulting in a more rapid depletion of this important energy source.

Vitamin B_6 (pyridoxine)   Vitamin B_6 is a collective term for three naturally occurring substances that are all metabolically and functionally related. They are pyridoxine, pyridoxal, and pyridoxamine. Pyridoxine is most often used as a synonym. Vitamin B_6 belongs to the B complex.

The adult RDA for vitamin B_6 is 2 mg/day. Slightly different amounts are needed at different age levels. Consult Appendix A for specific RDA. Requirements may increase for those women who are taking oral contraceptives.

Vitamin B_6 is widely distributed in foods. The best sources are meats, poultry, fish, potatoes, wheat germ, whole grain products, yeast, blackstrap molasses, eggs, and seeds. The heat of cooking may be destructive to this vitamin.

Vitamin B_6 plays a central role in the metabolism of certain amino acids, helping cells convert nutrient amino acids into particular amino acids necessary for their own activities. It has been reported to be important in the formation of protein compounds essential to oxygen processes in the body. Theoretically then, B_6 deficiency could adversely affect endurance activities dependent upon oxygen. Also, the requirement for B_6 increases with protein intake, which may have some implications for those on high protein diets. However, since it is found in protein products, it should be easily obtainable in a high protein diet.

Megadoses of B_6 have been regarded as harmless; however, a recent report suggested they may contribute to loss of peripheral sensory input and an impaired gait.

There have been several recent studies relative to B_6 and physical performance, but the data available conclude that supplementation to a balanced diet will not increase performance.

Pantothenic acid   **Pantothenic acid** is a water soluble vitamin. It is a factor in the B complex. The Food and Nutrition Board does not list the RDA of pantothenic acid in the main table, but they do recommend 4–7 mg daily as a safe and adequate intake.

Pantothenic acid is distributed widely in foods. It is found in all animal products, eggs, yeast, and whole grains.

Pantothenic acid is an essential component of a compound called acetyl CoA, which plays a central role in energy and tissue metabolism within the cell. Deficiencies have been reported to cause a variety of symptoms, including fatigue, muscle cramping, and impairment of motor coordination. Theoretically, then, pantothenic acid appears crucial to the active individual. However, recent research has found that large dosages of pantothenic acid, over 100 times the RDA, exerted no effect upon endurance capacity. At the present time we must conclude that supplementation is not necessary for the individual who is on a balanced diet.

Folacin (folic acid) **Folacin,** or **folic acid,** is a water soluble vitamin. It is part of the B complex.

The RDA for folacin is 0.4 mg/day, or 400 micrograms (μg), for adults. A microgram is a millionth of a gram. Slightly different amounts are set for children and for women during pregnancy and lactation. See Appendix A.

Folacin derives its name from foliage because it is found in green leafy vegetables like spinach. It is also found in organ meats such as liver and kidney, dry beans, and whole grain products.

Folacin serves as a coenzyme that plays a critical role in the formation of DNA, the genetic material that regulates tissue processes. It also is essential for maintenance of normal red blood cell production. One of the outcomes of folacin deficiency is anemia, which could create a severe impairment in the performance ability of endurance-type athletes. Folacin deficiency may also produce diarrhea. Individuals who consume large quantities of alcohol and women who take oral contraceptives may experience deficiencies in folacin, as these drugs may impair absorption of the vitamin.

Megadoses are usually considered harmless. However, they may counteract the effect of certain drugs taken for conditions such as epilepsy and may mask a deficiency of vitamin B_{12}.

No evidence is available to support the theory that supplementation with folacin will benefit physical performance. To be sure, anemia resulting from a folacin deficiency could have serious consequences for endurance performance, but a balanced diet should prevent this condition from developing.

Vitamin B_{12} (cyanocobalamin) **Vitamin B_{12}, cyanocobalamin,** is a water soluble vitamin. It is part of the B complex.

The adult RDA for B_{12} is 3 μg per day. The average diet contains about 5–15 μg. Slightly different allowances are made for other age groups. See Appendix A.

Vitamin B_{12} is not found in plant foods, that is fruits, vegetables, beans and grains. Only meat and other animal products such as cheese, eggs, and milk may serve as good sources. Hence, a strict vegetarian may need supplementation.

Vitamin B_{12} is present in all body cells and is essential in the metabolism of DNA. Like folacin, it has an important role in the development of red blood cells. Deficiencies may cause several types of disorders, but anemia has major implications for the active person. As mentioned for folacin, endurance-type activity could be impaired. The use of certain drugs such as alcohol, oral contraceptives, and other steroids may increase the needs for this vitamin.

Megadoses of vitamin B_{12} are considered to be relatively harmless.

Vitamin B_{12} is one of the most abused vitamins in the athletic world, with some reports of athletes receiving large amounts by injection just prior to competition. The belief probably exists that if a little vitamin B_{12} can prevent anemia, then a lot of it will do something magical to increase performance capacity. However, several well-controlled studies have been conducted with B_{12} supplementation with the general conclusion that it will not help to increase performance. It may be an effective medical treatment for a particular type of anemia, but it will not benefit the active individual on a balanced diet.

Biotin Biotin is found mainly in peas, beans, meats, and vegetables. It is a coenzyme necessary for the synthesis of fat and glycogen. It is also involved in amino acid metabolism. It could have important implications for carbohydrate-loading programs. The recommended safe and adequate daily dietary intake is 100–200 μg. There is no evidence that biotin supplementation will increase physical performance capacity.

Other B-complex factors Several other water soluble compounds are found in the B complex, although they are not considered to be vitamins. They are choline, inositol, and para-aminobenzoic acid (PABA).

Choline is found in foods containing phospholipids, such as egg yolk, liver, grain products, and dried beans. No RDA has been established. It is involved in the formation of several body chemicals. No evidence is available to support supplementation of this vitamin to athletes.

Inositol and PABA are not recognized by the Food and Nutrition Board as essential to human health although experimentation with these compounds has been done in animals. There is little theoretical or experimental evidence to support their uses as supplements to the diet of the athlete.

Vitamin C (ascorbic acid) Vitamin C, or ascorbic acid, is a water soluble vitamin. It is one of the most controversial vitamins today.

The adult RDA for vitamin C is 60 mg/day. Slightly lower amounts are recommended for children. See Appendix A. Smoking, aspirin, oral contraceptives, and stress may increase the need for this vitamin. The body can accumulate a pool of vitamin C that may total 2–3 g.

The best sources of vitamin C are citrus fruits and vegetables such as green peppers, potatoes, broccoli, tomatoes, and salad greens. One orange contains the RDA. However, vitamin C may be lost in the cooking process, especially if the water in which the food was cooked is discarded.

Vitamin C has a number of different functions in the body, some of which have important implications for the active individual. Vitamin C is an important antioxidant, preventing the oxidation of certain compounds in the body. It is essential to the maintenance of such body tissues as cartilage, tendon, and bone—the connective tissues of the body. It may be important in the healing of wounds through the development of scar tissue. It helps absorb iron from the intestinal tract. Vitamin C is also involved in the formation of certain hormones, such as epinephrine, that are secreted during stressful situations such as exercise. The major deficiency sign is scurvy, which is primarily a disintegration of the connective tissue in the gums, skin, tendons, and cartilage. Another sign would be impaired healing. Accompanying vitamin C deficiency are such symptoms as weakness and anemia, which may be caused by inadequate iron absorption.

Megadoses of vitamin C have been reported to be relatively harmless. The body may be able to handle relatively large doses since excess amounts may be excreted. However, excessive amounts of vitamin C, such as 5–10 g daily, have been reported to produce some undesirable side effects such as diarrhea, predisposition to gout creating pain in the joints, formation of kidney stones, destruction of vitamin B_{12} in the diet, and excess excretion of vitamin B_6.

The effect of vitamin C on physical performance has received considerable attention over the past forty years, mainly because it is one of the vitamins that athletes consume in rather substantial quantities. A number of different theories have been advanced relative to its beneficial effect, most of them suggesting that it may be useful in endurance-type performance by facilitating the transport and utilization of oxygen in the body.

A careful review of both the older and more contemporary research with vitamin C has revealed conflicting results. In general, it may be concluded that vitamin C supplementation does not increase physical performance capacity. No solid experimental evidence supports the use of megadoses of 5–10 g that some athletes take. However, since exercise is a stressor, the active individual may need slightly more vitamin C than the RDA. Some respected investigators in the area of vitamin C and physical performance have recommended values of 200–300 mg/day. This amount could easily be obtained by wise selection of foods high in vitamin C content.

Vitamin D (cholecalciferol) **Vitamin D** is a fat soluble vitamin. It represents a number of different compounds in the body related to bone formation. Cholecalciferol is the naturally occurring compound in the skin formed by exposure to sunlight. The liver and kidney help to transform cholecalciferol into the final form of vitamin D, which is classified by some as a hormone.

The adult RDA for vitamin D, given as cholecalciferol, is about 10 μg for males and 5–7.5 μg for females; 10μ is equal to 400 I.U. Children need 10 μg, but the recommended amounts are lower for older adults. See Appendix A for particulars.

Good sources of vitamin D include eggs, dairy products, fortified milk and margarine, fish liver oils, tuna, salmon, and liver. It is also formed in the skin by the action of sunlight.

Vitamin D has a central role in the growth and mineralization of bones through the deposit of calcium and phosphorus. It helps absorption of calcium and phosphorus from the intestinal tract. Deficiencies may lead to inadequate calcium metabolism and bone deformities, especially in children. Some view vitamin D as a hormone rather than a vitamin.

Since vitamin D is fat soluble, megadoses may lead to increased storage in the body, and pathological results have been reported. Hypervitaminosis D may lead to vomiting, diarrhea, loss of weight, loss of muscle tone, and possible kidney damage. As with vitamin A, there appears to be sound medical reasons not to utilize vitamin D supplementation with healthy individuals.

Only a few studies have been conducted with vitamin D supplementation and physical performance, and they revealed no beneficial effect, either through single megadoses or supplementation over a two-year period of time.

Vitamin E (alpha-tocopherol) **Vitamin E** is a fat soluble vitamin. Its activity is derived from a series of tocopherols of plant origin, alpha-tocopherol being the most active.

The adult RDA for vitamin E, given in alpha-tocopherol units, is 10 mg for males and 8 mg for females. The amount is slightly less for children. See Appendix A for specific values. Ten mg is 15 I.U.

Good sources of vitamin E include wheat germ oil, seeds, green leafy vegetables, margarine, dried beans, and nuts. Vitamin E is stable at normal cooking temperatures.

Vitamin E serves primarily as an antioxidant in the body. It helps prevent the oxidation of fatty acids, which protects the structure of cell membranes from damage. Other claims have been made that vitamin E exerts a beneficial effect upon the circulatory system, but these claims are not well documented. Vitamin E deficiency, although absent in humans, has been found to cause anemia in animals. Damage to the membrane of the red blood cell may be the cause. Although there is no evidence of vitamin E deficiency anemia in humans, some have used this as rationale for supplementation to athletes.

The general consensus suggests megadoses of vitamin E are relatively nontoxic. However, since it is a fat soluble vitamin, excess consumption is not recommended.

The diet of the average American appears to contain ample vitamin E, for deficiency states are nonexistent. However, vitamin E ranks with vitamin C as one of the most ingested nutrients among sedentary and active individuals alike. There are many claims for this vitamin, such as a slowing of the aging process, an improvement in sexual potency, and an increase in physical performance. These claims are not substantiated by reputable research.

A careful review of those studies concerned with vitamin E supplementation and athletic performance has been conducted by Dr. Roy Shephard, an eminent researcher in the area of physical performance. His general conclusion is that vitamin E supplementation, even with megadoses, will not increase physical performance of those individuals on a balanced diet who perform at sea level. However, there is some data available which show a beneficial effect on performance at altitudes above 5000 feet.

Vitamin K (phylloquinone) **Vitamin K** is a fat soluble vitamin. The RDA for adults is about 70–140 μg per day. Although it is found in such foods as green leafy vegetables, corn, tomatoes, eggs, whole grain products, and meats, the main supply appears to be formed in the intestines by bacterial action.

Vitamin K is important to the blood clotting process. Deficiency states are rare. Megadoses are considered to be nontoxic but are not recommended.

There is no evidence available that supports vitamin K supplementation to active individuals.

Are vitamin supplements needed by active individuals?

Vitamins for athletes

As is evident from the preceding review regarding vitamins and physical performance, the active individual who is on a balanced diet has no need for vitamin supplementation. Although individual studies with vitamin supplementation have not been cited in this review, the overwhelming majority of sound research shows that physical performance is not improved.

However, it is recommended that the active individual be selective relative to foods chosen for the diet. The stress of exercise can increase the utilization of some water soluble vitamins, but these can be replaced easily if the extra calories expended during exercise are replaced by foods with high nutrient density. Table 5.2 presents a quick overview of the major vitamins and foods containing substantial amounts of these vitamins.

Table 5.2 High vitamin content foods

Vitamin A	Beef liver, fish liver oils, egg yolks
	Milk, butter, cheese, fortified margarine
	Yellow vegetables (carrots, sweet potatoes)
	Green vegetables (spinach, collards)
Vitamin B$_1$	Pork, legumes (dried peas and beans)
(Thiamin)	Milk
	Nuts, peanuts
	Whole grain and enriched cereal products (bread)
	All vegetables
	Fruits
Vitamin B$_2$	Meats, liver, kidneys, eggs
(Riboflavin)	Milk, cheese
	Whole grain and enriched cereal products
	Wheat germ
	Green leafy vegetables
Niacin	Lean meats, organ meats (liver), poultry
	Legumes, peanuts, peanut butter
	Whole grain and enriched cereal products
Vitamin B$_6$	Meat, poultry, fish
(Pyridoxine)	Whole grain cereals, seeds
	Vegetables
Pantothenic acid	Meats, poultry, fish
	Milk, cheese
	Legumes
	Whole grain products
Folacin	Meats, liver, eggs
	Milk
	Legumes
	Whole wheat products
	Green leafy vegetables
Vitamin B$_{12}$	Meats, poultry, fish, eggs
(Cyanocobalamin)	Milk, cheese, butter
	(not found in plant foods)
Biotin	Meats, liver, egg yolk
	Legumes, nuts
	Vegetables
Vitamin C	Citrus fruits, oranges, grapefruit, melons, berries, tomatoes
	Broccoli, brussel sprouts, cabbage, salad greens, green peppers, cauliflower

Minerals—the inorganic regulators

You may recall the periodic table hanging on the wall in your high school or college chemistry class containing all the known **elements** on earth. At latest count there were 103 known elements, 90 of them occurring naturally and the remainder being manmade. A number of the natural elements were incorporated in humans through the process of evolution and became essential to bodily structure and function.

In this chapter we shall discuss briefly the nature of minerals and their function in the human body, particularly those that may be of interest to the active individual. Since sodium (Na), potassium (K), and chloride (Cl) are the primary elements found in sweat, a detailed discussion of these electrolytes will be presented in Chapter 14, "Exercising in the Heat."

This chapter will have a format similar to the preceding one. After several introductory questions, each of the major minerals will be discussed relative to RDA, good dietary sources, metabolic functions in the body with reference to the active individual where relevant, the need for supplements, and potential hazards of high dosages. For those trace elements where little research has been done relative to human physical performance, data will be presented in a table.

What are minerals and what is their importance to humans?

A **mineral** is an inorganic element found in nature, and the term is usually reserved for those elements that are solid. Hence a mineral is an element, but an element is not necessarily a mineral. In nutrition, the term mineral is used to list those elements essential to life processes.

Of the 103 elements in the periodic table, 25 are known currently to be essential in animals. These elements have a wide variety of functions in the body. Seven of the elements (carbon, oxygen, hydrogen, nitrogen, sulfur, calcium, and phosphorus) are used as the building blocks for body tissues such as bones, teeth, muscles, and other organic structures. Other elements are important components of enzymes and hormones, similar to the role of vitamins. Minerals are also important in a number of regulatory functions in the body. Some of the physiological processes regulated or maintained by minerals include muscle contraction, nerve impulse conduction, acid-base balance of the blood, body water supplies, blood clotting, and normal heart rhythm.

Basic facts

What minerals are essential to human nutrition?

As mineral salts are excreted daily from the body by sweat, urine, or feces, they must be replaced. Since they are widely distributed in foods, dietary deficiencies are rare. Table 6.1 lists those nutrients considered to be essential to humans. The RDA or the estimated safe and adequate daily dietary intakes, as suggested by the Food and Nutrition Board of the National Research Council, is also listed. Carbon, oxygen, hydrogen, and nitrogen are not listed as they are the prime elements of our energy foodstuffs—carbohydrate, fat, and protein.

The six **major minerals** are calcium, phosphorus, sodium, potassium, chloride, and magnesium. They are classified as major minerals because the RDA is greater than 100 mg per day. For the purpose of this discussion, iron is construed to be a major mineral in the sense that it is one of the minerals most likely to be deficient in the diet.

The individual minerals

Calcium (Ca) Calcium is a silver-white metalic element. The RDA for calcium is 800 mg/day for young children and adults, but 1,200 mg/day for youngsters aged eleven to eighteen. Calcium content is high in such foods as milk, cheese, dried peas and beans, and dark green vegetables. One cup of milk supplies about one third of the RDA.

Calcium exerts considerable influence over human metabolism. The vast majority, 99 percent, is found in the skeleton, and a large part of dietary calcium is used for bone and tooth formation. The remainder exists in an ionic state. **Ions,** or **electrolytes,** are small particles carrying electric charges. Calcium ions (Ca^{++}) are involved in muscle contraction both in heart and skeletal muscle, nerve impulse transmission, blood clotting, and as part of lipase, an enzyme that digests fats. It should be noted that the skeletal content of calcium is not inert. The body functions, such as nerve cell transmission, take precedence over formation of bone tissue. If the diet is low in calcium for a short period of time, the body can mobilize some from the skeleton.

Although calcium deficiency is rare in the United States, symptoms such as stunted growth in children, **osteoporosis** (a softening of bones) in adults, and muscle cramps may occur on a diet low in calcium. This underscores the need to have dairy products in the diet, as they are one of our most readily available sources of calcium. The body normally gets rid of excess calcium in the diet, but in some individuals excess amounts may accumulate in the blood and may contribute to abnormal heart rhythm. There are a few medical conditions where excess calcium intake may be harmful, but in general there is no evidence to suggest that excess dietary calcium intake will be detrimental to the health of the average individual.

The central role that calcium plays in regard to the muscles and nerves is indicative of its importance to movement. However, no research has been uncovered that has studied the effect of calcium supplements upon physical

Table 6.1 Minerals essential to humans with RDA or safe and adequate daily dietary intakes for adults*

Mineral	Symbol	RDA (mg) Male	RDA (mg) Female	Amount in adult body (g)
Calcium	Ca	800	800	1,500
Phosphorus	P	800	800	850
Sulfur	S	**	**	300
Potassium	K	1,875–5,625		180
Chloride	Cl	1,700–5,100		75
Sodium	Na	1,100–3,300		65
Magnesium	Mg	350	300	25
Iron	Fe	10	18	45
Fluoride	F	1.5–4.0		2.5
Zinc	Zn	15	15	2
Copper	Cu	2–3		0.1
Silicon	Si	not established		0.024
Vanadium	V	not established		0.018
Tin	Sn	not established		0.017
Nickel	Ni	not established		0.010
Selenium	Se	0.05–0.2		0.013
Manganese	Mn	2.5–5.0		0.012
Iodine	I	0.15	0.15	0.011
Molybdenum	Mo	0.15–0.5		0.009
Chromium	Cr	0.05–0.2		0.006
Cobalt	Co	not established		0.0015

A range of values (represented by a dash) is appropriate for both males and females.
*See Appendix A for extended table values.
**Provided by amino acids containing sulfur.

performance. Based upon current knowledge of calcium metabolism in the average individual, there appears to be no rationale for active individuals to take calcium supplements. A balanced diet should supply ample amounts.

On the other hand, calcium supplements may help prevent softening and brittleness of the bones in elderly individuals, particularly women. Recent research has revealed that calcium and vitamin D supplements may help prevent osteoporosis in inactive elderly females. Moreover, it should be noted that exercise, in and by itself, also helped prevent osteoporosis in elderly females. However, although both exercise and the supplement alone were effective, there was no additive effect of combined supplement and exercise treatments. Thus, either of these two treatments may be recommended for women, particularly those entering middle age, as a means to help prevent osteoporosis. Some nutritionists are recommending 1200–1500 mg for adult women.

Phosphorus (P) **Phosphorus** is a nonmetalic element. The adult RDA is 800 mg for both men and women. Higher amounts are needed during adolescence. Specific values for different age groups may be found in Appendix A. Phosphorus is distributed widely in foods, mainly in conjunction with protein. Excellent sources include milk, cheese, meats, eggs, nuts, dried beans and peas, grain products, and a wide variety of vegetables.

Phosphorus is extremely important in human metabolism. Although the vast majority of bodily phosphorus is used in conjunction with calcium for the formation of bones and teeth, about 10–15 percent is found in other forms, primarily as phosphate in combination with various organic substances. These phosphate compounds are involved in a number of metabolic functions, but three are of prime importance to the active individual. First, phosphates are essential to the normal function of several of the B vitamins involved in the energy processes within the cell. Second, they are also part of the high energy compounds found in the muscle cell that are needed for muscle contraction. Third, phosphates are part of a compound abbreviated as 2,3-DPG, which is important in oxygen delivery to the tissues.

Since phosphorus is distributed so widely in foods, deficiency states are rare. Extreme muscular exercise may increase phosphorus excretion in the urine, but has not been reported to cause a deficiency state. Individuals who use antacid compounds for long periods of time may experience deficiency symptoms as the antacid decreases the absorption of phosphorus. Symptoms might include loss of calcium and bone material and weakness. Excesses of phosphorus in the body are excreted by the kidney. Phosphorus excess per se does not appear to pose any problems, but if the ratio of phosphorus to calcium intake gets too large, problems may develop. The normal phosphorus-calcium ratio is 1:1, but if the diet is low in calcium products such as milk and other dairy products and excessively high in phosphorus products such as meat protein and soft drinks, the ratio may be higher. Calcium may then be lost from the bones. This is not a common problem in the average American diet. The body usually adapts to minor deviations in the phosphorus-calcium ratio.

Phosphates, the salts of phosphoric acid, are found in association with several alkaline elements; sodium phosphate and potassium phosphate are two examples. These compounds have been alleged to relieve fatigue in German soldiers during World War I and still appear to be a favorite among European athletes. Extensive advertisement aimed at the athlete continues, stressing their beneficial qualities as components of body energy sources. Most of the older studies that investigated phosphates and physical performance were not well designed, but a recent report suggested phosphate salts may increase the 2,3-DPG level is the red blood cell which facilitated the release of oxygen to the muscle and increased aerobic capacity.

Lecithin is a fatty substance that contains phosphorus; it is found mainly in animal tissues. It has been reported to have therapeutic properties, due to its phosphorus content, and has been recommended for

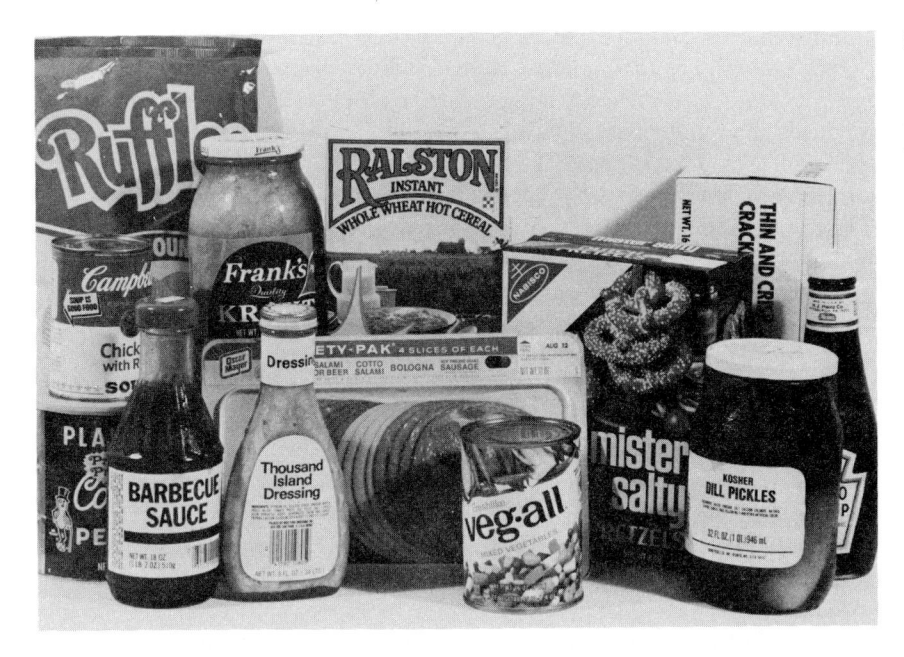

Foods with high salt (sodium) content should be reduced in the diet. Be aware of foods that have large amounts of hidden sodium.
(David Corona)

athletes to help increase their performance. However, a review of the relevant research conducted with lecithin has revealed that its effectiveness has not been documented adequately.

Sodium (Na)   **Sodium** is one of the principal ions, or electrolytes, in the body. The RDA is 1,100–3,300 mg/day, although the amount may be greater in individuals who lose excessive amounts of sweat through exercise or their occupation. Although table salt (sodium chloride) is a major source of sodium in the diet, sodium also is distributed widely in other foods. Humans have a natural appetite for salt, assuring adequate sodium intake.

As the principle **cation** (positive ion), sodium (Na^+) is an important element in several body functions. It is found mainly in fluids outside the body cells. It serves primarily to help maintain normal body fluid volume and is involved in nerve impulse transmission and muscle contraction. It is also a component of several compounds such as sodium bicarbonate, which help maintain normal acid-base balance.

The body has an effective regulatory mechanism allowing for a wide range of dietary sodium intake. One of the hormones from the adrenal gland, aldosterone, helps control sodium balance in the body by regulating its excretion by the kidney. If the blood level of sodium is too high, the kidney excretes the excess; the kidney will conserve more sodium when the blood levels are low. Deficiency states are not common, but may occur due to excessive loss of salt through sweating. An individual who exercises in hot weather for a prolonged period of time and replaces lost body fluids with only water may experience symptoms of salt depletion. These may include nausea, loss of appetite, weakness, and muscle cramps, which can be particularly debilitating to the active individual.

Increased sodium intake has been associated with high blood pressure (hypertension), but the National Research Council has indicated there is little or no direct evidence to suggest that high blood pressure can be produced in an individual with normal blood pressure and normal dietary intake of salt. On the other hand, hypertensive individuals may be able to reduce their blood pressure by decreasing the amount of salt in the diet. The recent recommendations of the Senate Select Subcommittee on Nutrition and Health Needs has recommended a daily intake of about 1–3 g. The average well-salted meal contains about 3–4 g of sodium, and the average daily intake today is 6–12 g. Since sodium is found in a wide variety of foods, and since it is used extensively in the preparation of the foods we eat, it would probably be wise to use the saltshaker less often. The substitution of potassium chloride for sodium chloride has been recommended.

The major concern of the active individual is the replacement of sodium that may be lost through prolonged sweating. As other electrolytes and water may also be lost during exercise in the heat, with possible severe consequences, this subject is covered separately in Chapter 14.

Potassium (K) **Potassium** is one of the principal cations in the body. The RDA is 1,875–5,625 mg/day. This amount may be greater in individuals who lose potassium through excessive sweating. Potassium is found in most foods and is especially abundant in oranges, grapefruit, bananas, fresh vegetables, meat, and fish.

As the major electrolyte inside the body cells, potassium works in close association with sodium and chloride to maintain body fluids and the acid-base balance of the blood. Potassium plays an important role in the conduction of nerve impulses, and a proper balance with calcium and magnesium is essential for normal functioning of muscle tissue. It also plays an important role in the energy processes within the muscle cell, including the formation of muscle glycogen and the production of high energy compounds.

As with sodium, the body possesses efficient control mechanisms to regulate blood levels of potassium. Since the average daily dietary intake is about 2–6 g, potassium deficiency is unlikely under normal circumstances. However, several reports have indicated that potassium deficiency may be common in those with diarrhea, vomiting, or poor dietary practices. Moreover, potassium losses are increased through excessive sweat losses. Resultant low potassium levels in the blood may interfere with muscle cell nutrition and produce muscle weakness and fatigue, which could be detrimental to physical performance capacity. Excess body potassium is not too common, occurring primarily in conjunction with several disease states.

Since potassium depletion may have serious consequences for the active individual, it is important to have an adequate supply in the diet. This is especially true of those individuals who may incur large daily losses of sweat. Further discussion of the potassium needs of the active person is presented in Chapter 14.

Chloride (Cl) **Chloride** is one of the major electrolytes in the body; it is an **anion** (a negative ion). The RDA for chloride is 1,700–5,100 mg/day. The dietary intake of chloride is closely associated with that of sodium, notably in the form of common table salt.

Chloride is allied with sodium in the regulation of normal body water and electrolyte balance. It is also used in the formation of gastric juices.

Under normal circumstances, the loss of chloride from the body parallels the loss of sodium, and the symptoms are similar, including weakness and muscular cramps. Also, as the need and intake for chloride is similar to that of sodium, problems with excessive intakes of chloride parallel those associated with the excess sodium intake.

As with sodium and potassium, chloride losses may be increased during exercise under high environmental temperatures. This aspect of electrolyte balance in active individuals will be covered in Chapter 14.

Magnesium (Mg) **Magnesium** is another principal electrolyte found in the body; it is a positive ion and is related to calcium and phosphorus. The adult RDA for magnesium is 350 mg for men and 300 mg for women. Slightly different amounts, found in Appendix A, are required by children and adolescents. Magnesium is widely distributed in foods, particularly whole grain products, green leafy vegetables, and other fruits and vegetables.

Magnesium is indispensable to humans because it activates a number of enzymes and may be involved in the regulation of protein synthesis, muscle contraction, and body temperature. Substantial quantities of magnesium are stored in the skeletal system, which may serve as a reserve during short periods of dietary deficiency.

The National Research Council has reported that magnesium deficiency is rare because of its availability in a variety of foods. Several investigators have reported a substantial drop in blood magnesium levels following prolonged periods of exercise. However, sweat losses failed to account for this drop, as the loss of magnesium in sweat is relatively low. As others have noted, the magnesium is not lost from the body but enters the muscle tissue where it may be involved in increased cellular activity during exercise. Other health conditions such as chronic diarrhea may contribute to excessive magnesium losses. A deficiency state may lead to weakness and muscular cramps. Excess magnesium in the diet may contribute to diarrhea. The usual cause is the ingestion of magnesium salts, such as found in milk of magnesia.

Although several reports have recommended that individuals undergoing hard physical training should increase their daily intake of magnesium, the current dietary intake in the United States is within range of those recommendations. The extra Calories consumed as a result of increased energy expenditure during exercise should provide the additional magnesium. In addition, no evidence is available to suggest that magnesium supplementation will increase the physical performance capacity of individuals on a balanced diet. There is some evidence that magnesium salts may be effective in the treatment of leg cramps developing from prolonged exercise.

Figure 6.1.
Simplified diagram of iron metabolism in humans. After digestion, iron is used in the formation of hemoglobin, myoglobin, and certain cell enzymes, all of which are essential for transportation of oxygen in the body.

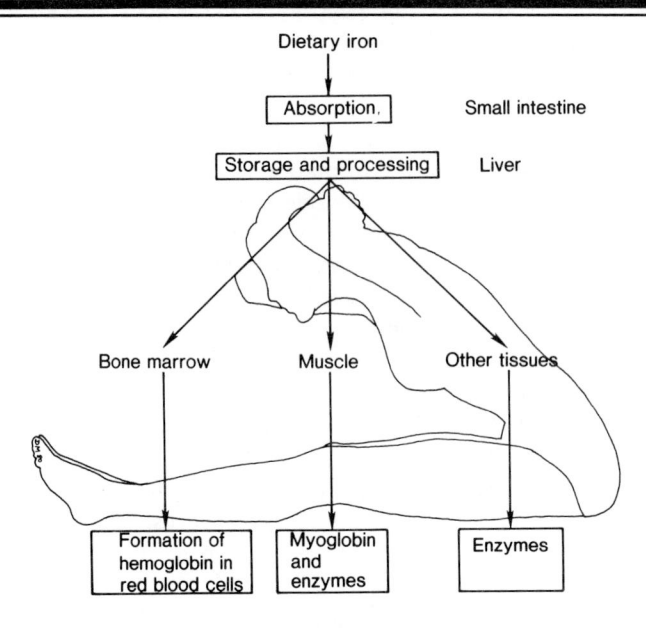

Iron (Fe)   Iron is a metallic element that exists in two general forms, ferrous (Fe^{++}) and ferric (Fe^{+++}). The RDA is 10 mg for men and 18 mg for women and teenagers of both sexes. Slightly different amounts are needed by other age groups and may be found in Appendix A. Excellent sources of dietary iron include liver, heart, lean meats, oysters, dried apricots, and beans. Although iron is widely distributed in foods, the iron found in animal products is more effectively absorbed than that found in plants. Meat is a very reliable source of dietary iron. The iron found in meat products is called heme iron, while that in plants is known as non-heme iron. On a balanced diet about 6 mg iron is provided for in every 1,000 C ingested.

The major function of iron in the body is the formation of compounds essential to the transportation of oxygen. The vast majority is used to form hemoglobin, a protein-iron compound that transports oxygen from the lungs to the body tissues. Other iron compounds include myoglobin and various enzymes located in the cells, primarily muscle tissues, which help use oxygen at the cellular level. The remainder of body iron is stored in the tissues, principally as a compound called ferritin. Since iron is so critical to oxygen use in humans, it is essential that those individuals engaged in endurance type exercises have an adequate dietary intake. Figure 6.1 represents a brief outline of iron metabolism in humans.

It should be noted that copper, manganese, and cobalt are necessary for the proper utilization of iron. A brief summary of these trace elements is found in Table 6.3.

Iron is one of the few nutrients commonly found to be slightly deficient in the diet of humans, particularly in women and teenagers. The body normally loses very little iron through such routes as the skin, hair, and sweat. About 1 mg/day will replace these losses. Females also lose some additional iron in the blood flow during menstruation. They need about 1.8 mg/day to replace their total losses. Adolescent boys also need 1.8 mg/day as they are increasing muscle tissue and blood volume during this rapid period of growth. As noted above, the RDA is ten times this amount; this is so because only about 10 percent of the iron in the diet is absorbed. Some nutrients, like vitamin C, can help absorb more iron, while other substances such as phytates in grain products and oxalates in spinach non-heme have been shown to decrease absorption of non-heme iron.

With 6 mg Fe/1,000 C, the adult male has no problem meeting his requirement of 10 mg/day. With a normal intake of 2,700–2,800 C he will receive 16.2–16.8 mg, of which about 1.6 mg would be absorbed. Teenage boys would be slightly deficient at this level of iron consumption. With 2,000–2,100 C, the average intake for females, only 12.0–12.6 mg iron would be provided. This is far short of the 18 mg needed. Only 1.2 mg would be absorbed at the 10 percent absorption level. Although iron deficient individuals have been reported to have a better level of absorption, a number of survey reports substantiated iron deficiency, particularly in American women.

The problem of concern to the inactive individual, which may be a major problem to the endurance athlete, is the development of iron-deficiency anemia. Symptoms include paleness and lower vitality. A number of studies have shown that anemia will cause a significant reduction in the ability to perform prolonged high-level exercise. The donation of blood causes a drop in hemoglobin, which may also decrease performance capacity. This is, of course, related to the decreased ability to transport and use oxygen in the body.

Some athletes, particularly long distance runners and especially female long distance runners, may be susceptible to iron deficiency. Possible causes may be large sweat losses of iron in those who sweat profusely, hematuria due to the rupturing of red blood cells upon foot contact or ruptured muscle cell membranes, or increased losses through the intestinal tract caused by exercise.

Although remote, there may be some danger associated with excess iron in the body. This may result from prolonged consumption of large amounts of iron or a disturbance in iron metabolism. Iron then tends to accumulate in the liver in a form that may cause cirrhosis and the possible ultimate destruction of that organ.

Several studies have been conducted in order to assess the effect of iron supplements upon physical performance capacity. In general, if the individual suffers from iron-deficiency anemia, then iron therapy could help correct this condition and concomitantly increase performance capacity. Recent research with several distance runners with iron deficiency anemia reported improved performance after iron supplementation corrected the

Table 6.2　Foods rich in some major mineral elements

Mineral	Food source
Calcium	Egg yolk, dried beans, peas Milk, cheese, cream Dark green vegetables, cauliflower
Phosphorus	All protein products Meat, poultry, fish, eggs Milk, cheese Dried beans and peas Whole grain products
Sodium chloride	Common table salt Peanuts, salt pork, salted foods
Potassium	Beef, fish, milk Fruits and vegetables, especially avocado, bananas, cantaloupe, honeydew melons, nectarines, raisins, grapefruit juice, oranges, and baked potatoes
Magnesium	Whole grain products Fruits and vegetables, especially green leafy vegetables
Iron	Liver, meats, eggs Dried beans and peas Whole grain products Green leafy vegetables Dried apricots, dates, figs, raisins

condition. On the other hand, if the individual has normal hemoglobin levels, iron supplementation will not offer any additional benefits. Some recent well-controlled research has shown that iron supplementation to highly active females in physical training did not raise their hemoglobin levels or the percent of hemoglobin saturated with iron if they had normal levels.

Research with iron-deficient, but nonanemic, athletes, although observing no improvement in endurance capacity, has suggested that aerobic metabolism in the muscle cells may be enhanced through iron supplementation.

In summary, it would be wise for the developing adolescent male and the female of all ages to be aware of the iron content in their diet. This concern is especially important to endurance athletes, although it would appear that the extra Calories they eat to meet the additional energy requirements of training would provide the necessary iron. All active males and females should be aware of iron-rich foods and be sure to include them in the daily diet. Moreover, iron supplementation by commercial preparations may be recommended for certain individuals, including females who experience heavy menstrual blood flow, those individuals who are on restricted caloric intake and those who incur heavy sweat losses. The usual vitamin pill with iron contains about 18 mg iron, which is 100 percent of the RDA for females and adolescent boys.

Table 6.3 Brief summary of essential trace minerals for active persons

Mineral	Food source	Major body functions	Deficiency effects	Excess effects	Recommended as diet supplement
Chromium (Cr)	Meat, liver, vegetable oils, fats, spices, stainless steel cookware	Functions in glucose metabolism in cells; related to insulin action	Lessened ability to metabolize glucose	Skin and kidney damage	No
Cobalt (Co)	Meat, liver, milk	Component of vitamin B_{12}; promotes development of red blood cells	Not found in humans	Nausea, vomiting, death	No
Copper (Cu)	Meat, vegetables, drinking water	Function with iron in formation of hemoglobin and iron enzymes	Anemia, weakness, impaired growth	Rare	No
Fluoride (F)	Milk, egg yolk, drinking water, seafood	Helps form bones and teeth	Higher incidence of dental cavities	Discolored teeth	No
Iodine (I)	Iodized salt, seafood, vegetables	Helps in formation of thyroxine, a thyroid hormone	Goiter, an enlarged thyroid gland	Depress thyroid gland activity	No
Manganese (Mn)	Whole grain products, dried peas and beans, leafy vegetables, bananas	Many enzyme functions; bone formation; fat synthesis	Poor growth	Weakness; nervous system problems	No
Molybdenum (Mo)	Liver, organ meats, whole grain products, dried beans and peas	Required in several enzymes	Not found in humans	Rare	No
Nickel (Ni)	Whole grain products, vegetables	Not known, under study	Not found in humans; large amounts in sweat	Industry exposure; pneumonia	No
Selenium (Se)	In protein foods: meat, fish, whole grain products	Functions with vitamin E; involved in liver function	Rare in humans	Not a significant problem in humans	No

Table 6.3 *Continued*

Mineral	Food source	Major body functions	Deficiency effects	Excess effects	Recommended as diet supplement
Silicon (Si)	Whole grain products, vegetables	Involved in formation of connective tissue	Not found in humans	Industrial poisoning; silicosis	No
Sulfur (S)	Essential amino acids in diet, meat, fish, poultry, milk, cheese, whole grain products	Formation of body tissues, enzymes	Protein deficiency	Rare	No
Tin (Sn)	Meats, fish, whole grains, fruits, vegetables	Not known, under study	Not found in humans	Industrial exposure; vomiting	No
Vanadium (V)	Whole grain products, bread, nuts, root vegetables, vegetable oils	Not known, under study	Not found in humans	Industrial exposure; lung irritation	No
Zinc (Zn)	In protein foods: beef, chicken, grain products, vegetables	Component of many enzymes	Slower rate of growth, poor appetite, small sex glands	Relatively nontoxic	No

What dietary recommendations will help insure adequate amounts of mineral nutrients in the diet?

Dietary recommendations

In general, as with all other nutrients, a balanced diet is essential. Table 6.2 presents a brief summary of those foods high in some of the major mineral nutrients. Notice that a diet stressing the four food groups will provide insurance that you will obtain adequate amounts of these elements. Table 6.3 presents some good dietary sources of the **trace elements,** and again a balanced diet is the critical factor. If you select a diet to provide the major minerals, you will receive adequate amounts of the trace elements at the same time.

7

Water—the medium

Water is a clear, tasteless, odorless fluid. It is a rather simple compound being composed of two parts hydrogen and one part oxygen (H_2O). With its simple chemical composition, it is a very stable compound. Water is just about everywhere. Of all the compounds essential in the chemistry and functioning of living forms, it is the most important. Most of the other nutrients essential to life can be used by the human body only because of their reaction to water. It provides the medium within which the other nutrients may function.

Water is an essential nutrient, even though it provides no food energy. Under optimal conditions humans may survive only about ten days without water. Short-term loss of body water through dehydration may also be hazardous to health and could prove to be fatal. For the active individual, water losses can be detrimental to physical performance capacity, particularly in those events characterized by prolonged endurance. Since this situation occurs most often during exercise in hot weather and is associated with both water and electrolyte losses, the effects of exercise-induced dehydration in the heat will be covered more thoroughly in Chapter 14.

This brief chapter will provide an overview of water needs in humans.

How much water do you need per day?

The requirement for body water depends upon the body weight of the individual. The requirement will vary in different stages of the life cycle. Under normal environmental temperatures and activity levels, the average adult needs about 2,000 ml (2 liters) of water per day; this is slightly more than 2 quarts. This amount will help maintain adequate water balance in the body.

Body water balance is maintained when the input of water matches the output of body fluids. Urinary output is the main avenue for water loss, and a small amount is lost in the feces and through the exhaled air in breathing. **Insensible perspiration,** which is not visible, is almost pure water and makes a significant contribution to body water losses. Sweat losses may be increased considerably during exercise and/or hot environmental conditions. Fluid intake by beverages is the main source of water to replenish losses. However, solid foods also contribute as a water source, and in two different ways. First, food contains water in varying amounts; certain foods such as lettuce, celery, melons, and most fruits contain about 90 percent water and

Metabolism and function

Table 7.1 Daily water loss and intake for water balance

Water loss

Urine output	1,100 ml
Water in feces	100 ml
Lungs—exhaled air	200 ml
Skin—insensible perspiration	600 ml
Total	2,000 ml

Water intake

Fluids	1,000 ml
Water in food	700 ml
Metabolic water	300 ml
Total	2,000 ml

many others contain more than 60 percent; even bread, an outwardly appearing dry food, contains 36 percent water. Second, the metabolism of foods for energy also produces water. Fat, carbohydrate, and protein all produce water when broken down in energy. You may recall the reaction when glucose is metabolized to produce energy:

$$C_6H_{12}O_6 + 6O_2 \rightarrow Energy + 6CO_2 + 6H_2O$$

The water is often called **metabolic water.** One additional point: Carbohydrate stored in the body as glycogen also has considerable amounts of water bound to it and may prove to be an advantage as discussed in Chapter 2. Table 7.1 summarizes the daily water loss and intake for the maintenance of water balance. As shall be seen later, however, these amounts may change drastically under certain conditions.

Where is water stored in the body?

Water comprises about 60 percent of the body weight. It is stored in various body compartments although there is a constant movement of water between these compartments. The vast majority of the body water is stored inside the body cells, the **intracellular water.** The remainder is outside the cells and is termed the **extracellular water;** the extracellular water is further subdivided into the **intercellular** (interstitial) **water** between or surrounding the cells, the **vascular water** within the blood vessels, and miscellaneous water compartments such as the cerebrospinal fluid, water in the eye, and similar compartments. Figure 7.1 represents the distribution of water in the body.

Proper water and electrolyte balance within these compartments is of extreme importance to the active individual. Decreases in blood volume and cellular dehydration both could contribute to the onset of fatigue.

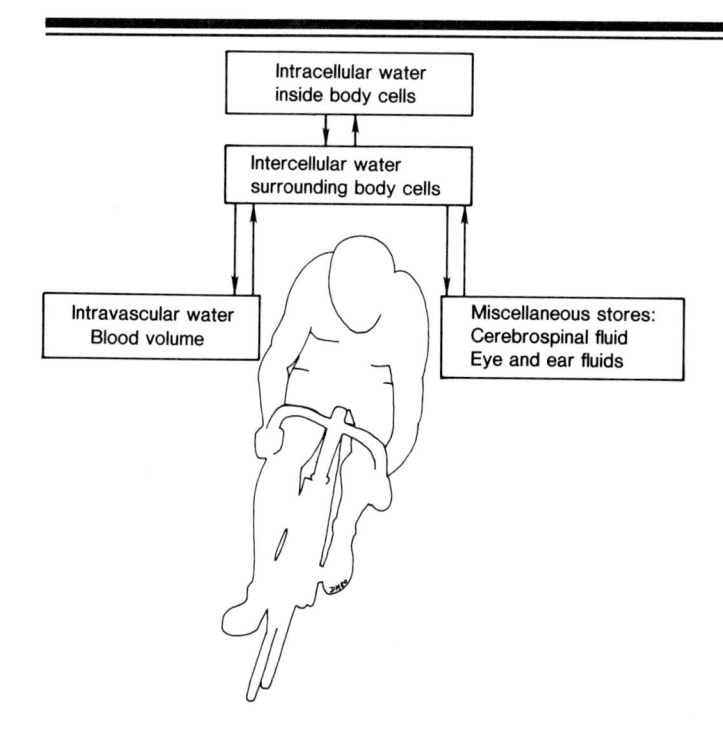

Figure 7.1.
Body water compartments. There is a constant interchange among the different body water compartments. The water inside the body cells, the intracellular water, is important for cell functions. The other three compartments are known collectively as the extracellular water. Decreases in blood volume may adversely affect endurance capacity.

What are the major functions of water in the body?

As mentioned previously, water is essential if the other nutrients are to function properly within the human body; it is the solvent for life. It has a number of diverse functions and they are summarized as follows:

1. It provides the essential building material for cell protoplasm, the essence of all living matter.

2. It is essential in the control of the osmotic pressure in the body, or the maintenance of a proper balance between water and the electrolytes. The major and minor electrolytes are dissolved and ionized in water, and any major changes in their concentration may adversely affect cellular function. A serious departure from normal osmotic pressure cannot be tolerated by the body for long.

3. Water is the main transportation mechanism in the body, conveying oxygen, nutrients, hormones, and other compounds to the cells for their use and waste products of metabolism away from the cells to various organs such as the lungs and kidney for excretion from the body.

4. Water is essential for the proper functioning of our senses. Hearing waves are transmitted by fluid in the inner ear. Fluid in the eye is involved in the reflection of light for proper vision. In order for the taste and smelling senses to function, the foods and odors need to be dissolved in water.

Water—the medium

5. Water, in close association with the major electrolytes, also helps to regulate the acid-base balance in the body.

6. Of primary importance to the active individual is the role that water plays in the regulation of body temperature. Water is the major constituent of sweat and through its evaporation from the surface of the skin can help to dissipate excess body heat. An extended discussion of this role is presented in Chapter 14.

How is body water regulated?

Since water is so essential to life, it is indeed fortunate that the body possesses an efficient mechanism to maintain proper water balance. **Homeostasis** is the term used to describe the maintenance of a normal internal environment so that the body has the proper distribution and use of water, electrolytes, hormones, and other substances essential for life processes. These homeostatic mechanisms are usually rather complex, and a full discussion is beyond the scope of this book. However, in essence, all homeostatic mechanism work by a series of feedback devices. If these feedback devices are functioning properly then the body usually has no problem in maintaining a state of relative constancy of the body fluids relative to their physical and chemical composition. For example, if too much salt is ingested and the sodium content of the blood is elevated, certain hormones will then act on the kidney to help it excrete more sodium, eventually returning the blood level to normal. On the other hand, if salt content is low, the kidney will retain more sodium in order to conserve the body supply.

Body water is maintained at a normal level through kidney function. Normal body water level is called **normohydration.** Loss of body water by dehydration results in a state of **hypohydration. Hyperhydration** results from increased consumption of fluids and the body has an excess of fluids. Normal kidneys function by eliminating excess water during hyperhydration and conserving water during hypohydration through feedback mechanisms.

To briefly illustrate the feedback mechanism for control of body water, let us look at what happens when you become dehydrated due to excessive body water losses or lowered water intake. The body fluids then become more concentrated, or hypertonic. Certain cells in the brain, called osmoreceptors, are sensitive to changes in the composition of the body fluids. These cells react to the more concentrated body fluids by stimulating the release of a hormone from the pituitary gland, the so-called master gland of the body. This hormone is called the **antidiuretic hormone (ADH).** The increased ADH travels by the blood to the kidneys and directs them to reabsorb more water. Hence, urinary output of water is diminished

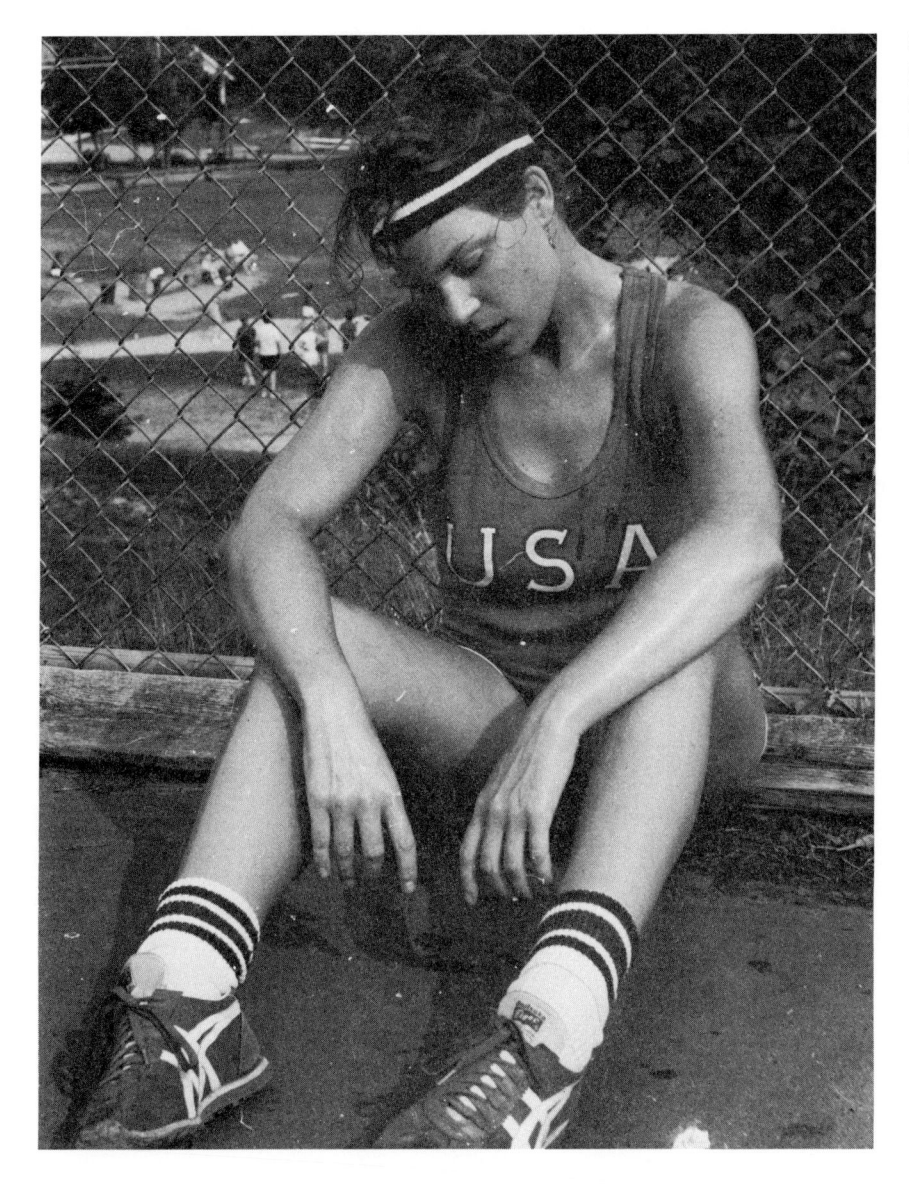

Body water loss can be very rapid during exercise in warm or hot weather.
(Michael DiSpezio)

considerably. The reverse process would occur during hyperhydration, which would produce a hypotonic condition in the body fluids.

The sensation of thirst is usually a good guide relative to body water needs and is effective in restoring body water to normal over a period of time. However, as shall be noted in Chapter 14, thirst may not be an accurate indicator of the need for water replacement during exercise in a hot environment.

Water and exercise

What is the importance of adequate water intake for the active individual?

As is obvious, hot environmental conditions make us thirstier due to the loss of body water through sweating. Physical activity under such conditions can contribute to enormous sweat losses amounting to a gallon or more during prolonged exercise. In hot weather, runners, football players, tennis players, and other active individuals have been known to lose 8–10 pounds over a two-hour period. Less than one pound of this is body fat so the vast majority consists of body fluids. Since a pint of water, or 16 ounces, weighs one pound, then 8–10 pints may be lost. If body fluids are not replaced, these losses could have disastrous effects upon performance and even the health of the individual. Of all the nutrients, water is the most important to the active person and is one of the few that may have beneficial effects on performance when used in supplemental amounts before or during exercise. Hence, the active individual should know what is necessary to help maintain proper fluid balance, a topic covered in Chapter 14.

Human energy sources and human energy systems

8

Energy is essential to all forms of life. Through technological processes, man has harnessed a variety of energy sources such as wind, waterfalls, the sun, wood, and oil in order to operate the machines invented to make life easier. However, humans can not use any of these energy sources for their own metabolism, but must rely on food sources found in nature. The food we eat must be converted into forms the body can use, and the use of these forms may vary considerably when comparing rest with exercise.

The purpose of this chapter is to review briefly the major human energy sources and how they are utilized in the body under different exercise conditions. This chapter will help establish the basis for several chapters that follow.

What is energy?

For our purposes, **energy** represents the capacity to do work. **Work** is one form of energy, often called mechanical energy. When we throw a ball or run a mile, we have done work; we have produced mechanical energy.

Energy exists in a variety of other forms in nature, such as the light energy of the sun, nuclear energy in uranium, electrical energy in lightning storms, heat energy in fires and chemical energy in oil. The six forms of energy—mechanical, chemical, heat, electrical, light, and nuclear—are all interchangeable according to various laws. We take advantage of these laws every day. One such example is the use of chemical energy of gasoline to produce mechanical energy, or the movement of our cars.

In the human body, four of these types of energy are important. Our bodies possess stores of chemical energy that can be used to produce electrical energy for creation of electrical nerve impulses, to produce heat and help keep our body temperature at 98.6° F even on cold days, and to produce mechanical work through muscle shortening so that we may move about.

The human body is constantly using energy, even during resting situations. Your body needs energy to digest food, form hormones and secrete them into the blood, create nerve impulses for thinking, break down and create new tissues, help enzymes function, and a host of other physiological processes occurring automatically.

The optimal intake and output of energy is important to all individuals, but especially so for the active person. In order to perform to capacity, body energy stores must be used in the most efficient manner possible.

Measures of energy

Eight ounces of orange juice will provide enough chemical energy to enable an average man to produce enough mechanical energy to run about one mile.
(David Corona)

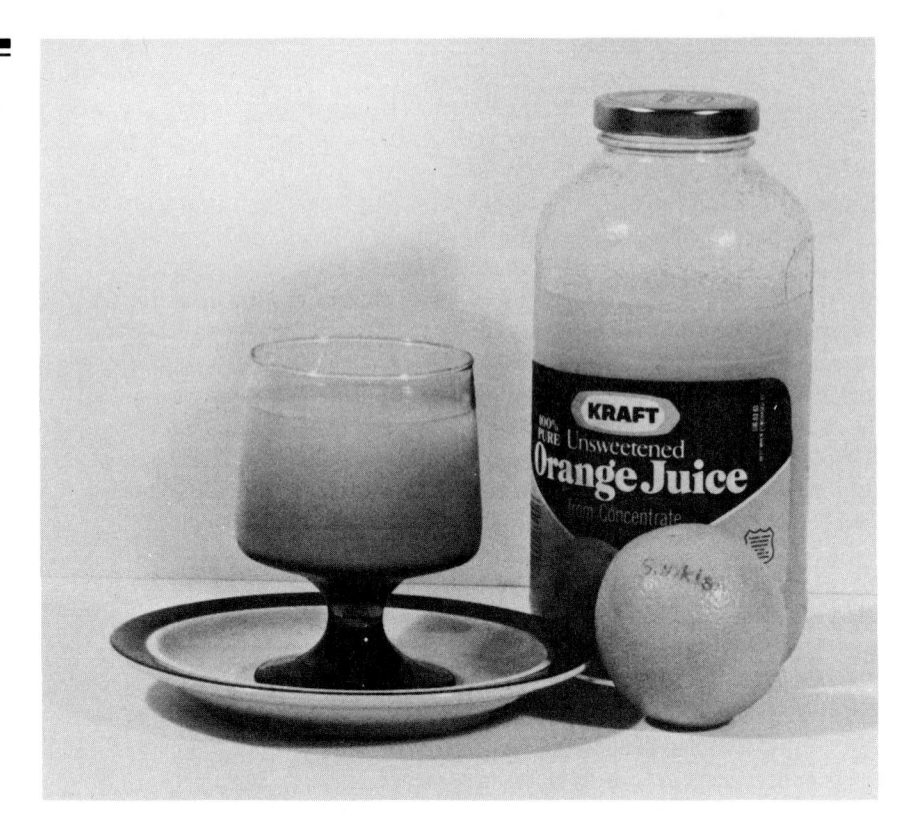

How do we measure energy?

Energy has been defined as the ability to do work. According to the physicist's definition, work is simply the product of force times distance, or in formula format W = F × d. When we speak of how fast work is done, the term *power* is used. **Power** is simply work divided by time, or P = W/t.

Two major measurement systems have been utilized in the past to express energy in terms of either work or power. The metric system has been in use by most of the world while we have used the English system. The following terms have been in use and still continue to be used in a number of books.

	Metric System	*English System*
Mass	kilogram	slug
Distance	meter	foot
Time	second	second
Force	newton	pound
Work	kilogram meter	foot-pound
Power	watt	horsepower

The nutrition for fitness answer book

In an attempt to provide some uniformity in measurement systems around the world, the **International Unit System (SI)** has been developed recently. In this system the unit of work is the **joule** and the unit of power is the **watt.** The basic units and some of their interrelationships are given below:

International Unit System (SI)

Mass—kilogram
Distance—meter
Time—second
Force—newton
Work—joule
Power—watt

1 newton-meter = 1 joule
1,000 joule = 1 kilojoule
1 watt = 1 joule/sec

It will take some time before this system becomes part of our everyday language. As the conversion to the metric system continues, some of the terms may become more prevalent, such as kilogram and meter. For our purposes in this text, when needed, we shall use the terms **foot-pound** and **kilogram-meter (KGM)** to express work. For example, if you weigh 150 pounds and climb a 20-foot flight of stairs, you have done 3,000 foot-pounds or work. One KGM is equal to 7.23 foot-pounds, so you would do about 415 KGM. Relative to power we would have to know the time needed to climb the stairs. Let us say that you ran up the stairs in 4 seconds; your rate of work is then 750 foot-pounds/second (3,000 ÷ 4). Since one horsepower (HP) is equal to 550 foot-pounds/second, then you have worked at the rate of 1.36 horsepower (750 ÷ 550). Some interrelationships among the metric and English system are noted below. Other equivalents between the two systems may be found in Appendix D.

Weight:

1 kilogram = 2.2 pounds
1 kilogram = 1,000 grams
454 grams = 1 pound
1 pound = 16 ounces
1 ounce = 28.4 grams

Distance:

1 meter = 3.28 feet
1 meter = 1.09 yards
1 foot = 0.30 meters
1,000 meters = 1 kilometer (km)
1 kilometer = .6215 mile

In essence then, to measure work we need to know the weight of an object and the distance through which it is moved. This is fine according to the formal definition of work, but are you doing work while holding a weight stationary out in front of your body? According to the formal definition, the answer is no since the distance moved is zero. How about when you come down stairs as compared to going up? It is much easier to

Figure 8.1.
A bomb calorimeter. The food in the calorimeter is combusted via electrical ignition. The heat (calories) given off by the food raises the temperature of the water, thus providing data relative to the caloric content of specific foodstuffs.

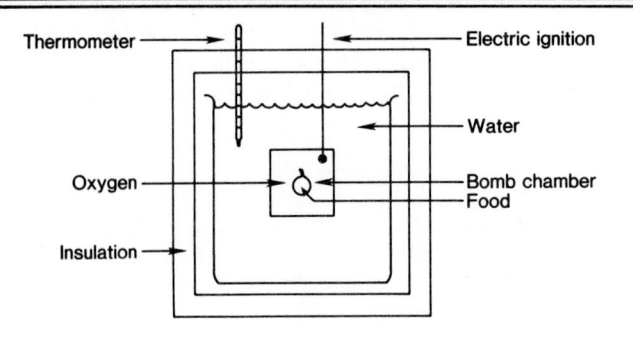

descend the stairs and yet according to the formula you have done the same amount of work. Therefore, we need to have other means to express the energy expenditure of the human body other than simply the amount of work done.

Without going into much detail, look briefly at two different methods for measuring energy production in humans. First, a device known as a **calorimeter** may be used to measure the energy content of a given substance. Figure 8.1 is an example of a bomb calorimeter. For example, a gram of fat may be placed in the calorimeter, oxidized completely, and the heat it gives off is recorded. We then know the heat energy of one gram of fat and can equate it to work units if needed. There are large expensive calorimeters available that can accommodate human beings and measure their heat production under differing conditions of exercise.

A second more commonly used method is to determine the amount of oxygen an individual consumes. In general, humans need oxygen in order to produce energy by helping to metabolize the various nutrients in the body. It is known that when oxygen combines with a gram of carbohydrate, fat, or protein, a certain amount of energy is released. If we can accurately measure the oxygen consumption (and carbon dioxide production) of an individual, we can get a pretty good measure of energy expenditure. The amount of oxygen used can be equated to other forms of energy, such as work done in foot-pounds or KGM and heat produced as in Calories.

What is the Calorie concept?

The Calorie concept of energy

Although there are a number of different ways to express energy, the most common term used in the past and still most prevalent and understood in the United States at the time of this writing is the Calorie. It is used as the energy requirement in the 1980 RDA.

A calorie is a measure of heat. One **small calorie** represents the amount of heat needed to raise the temperature of one gram of water 1° Celsius; it is sometimes called the **gram calorie**. A **large Calorie,** or **kilocalorie,** is equal to 1,000 small calories. It is the amount of heat needed to raise 1 kg of water (1 L) 1° Celsius. In human nutrition, the kilocalorie is the main expression of energy. It is usually abbreviated as *kcal, kc, C,* or capitalized as *Calorie.* Throughout this book, Calorie or C will refer to the kilocalorie.

According to the principles underlying the first law of thermodynamics, energy may be equated from one form to another. Thus, the Calorie, which represents thermal or heat energy, may be equated to other forms. Relative to our discussion concerning physical work such as exercise and its interrelationships with nutrition, it is important to equate the Calorie with mechanical work and the chemical energy stored in the body. As will be explained later, most of stored chemical energy must undergo some form of oxidation in order to release its energy content.

The following represents some equivalent energy values for the Calorie in terms of mechanical work and oxygen utilization. Some examples using several of the interrelationships will be used in later chapters.

1 C = 3,086 foot-pounds of work
1 C = 4.2 kilojoules (kj)
1 C = 200 ml oxygen (approximately)

For our purposes, then, the Calories in food represent a form of potential energy to be used by our bodies to produce heat and work.

What is the caloric equivalent of the various nutrients?

Through the use of a calorimeter, the energy content of the basic nutrients has been determined. Vitamins, minerals, and water, although actively involved in the energy processes within the body, do not contain energy themselves. Although an advertisement for a vitamin-mineral supplement may suggest it will help increase your energy, this is a distortion of the facts.

Energy may be derived from the three major foodstuffs—carbohydrate, fat, and protein. The caloric value of each of these three nutrients may vary somewhat dependent upon the particular structure of the different forms. For example, carbohydrate may exist in several forms, as glucose, sucrose, or starch, and the caloric value of each will differ slightly. In general one gram of each of the three nutrients, measured in a calorimeter, yields the following Calories:

1 gram carbohydrate = 4.30 C
1 gram fat = 9.45 C
1 gram protein = 5.65 C

Unfortunately, or fortunately if one is trying to lose weight, humans do not extract all this energy from the food they eat. The human body is not as efficient as the calorimeter. For one, the body cannot completely absorb all the food eaten. Only about 97 percent of the carbohydrate, 95 percent of the fat, and 92 percent of the protein are absorbed. In addition, a good percentage of the protein is not completely oxidized in the body, with some of the nitrogen waste products being excreted in the urine. In summary, then, the caloric value of food is reduced somewhat in relation to the values given above. Although the following values are not exactly precise, they are approximate enough to be used effectively in the determinaton of the caloric values of the foods we eat. Thus, the following caloric value will be used throughout this text as a practical guide.

1 gram carbohydrate = 4 C
1 gram fat = 9 C
1 gram protein = 4 C

If you study the nutritional labels of most foods purchased today, these values may become second nature to you and it becomes relatively easy to determine the caloric content of many foods, as well as the percentage contribution from each of the three nutrients. If you see a food such as peanut butter, with 6 g of carbohydrate, 9 g of protein, and 16 g of fat per serving, do you realize that about 72 percent of the Calories are derived from fat even though it is only about half the weight? The caloric density of fat is an important consideration for diets and other health aspects.

One other point before we leave this question. Just because fat has more than twice the amount of energy per gram than either carbohydrate or protein does not mean it is a better energy source for the active individual. This important issue will be discussed later when we talk of the efficient utilization of body fuels.

How is energy stored in the body?

The ultimate source of all energy on earth is the sun. Solar energy is harnessed by plants, which take carbon, hydrogen, oxygen, and nitrogen from their environment and manufacture either carbohydrate, fat, or protein. These foods possess stored energy. When we consume these foods, our digestive processes break them down into simple compounds that are absorbed into the body and transported to various cells. One of the basic purposes of body cells is to transform the chemical energy of these simple compounds into forms that may be available for immediate use or other forms that may be available for future use.

Adenosinetriphosphate, (ATP) is the form of energy in the body available for immediate use. It is a complex molecule constructed with high energy bonds, which, when split by enzyme action, can release energy rapidly for a number of body processes, including muscle contraction. It is called a high energy compound and is stored in the tissues in small amounts. Another related high energy phosphate compound, **phosphocreatine (PC)**, is also found in the tissues in small amounts. Although it cannot be used as an immediate source of energy, it can rapidly replenish ATP.

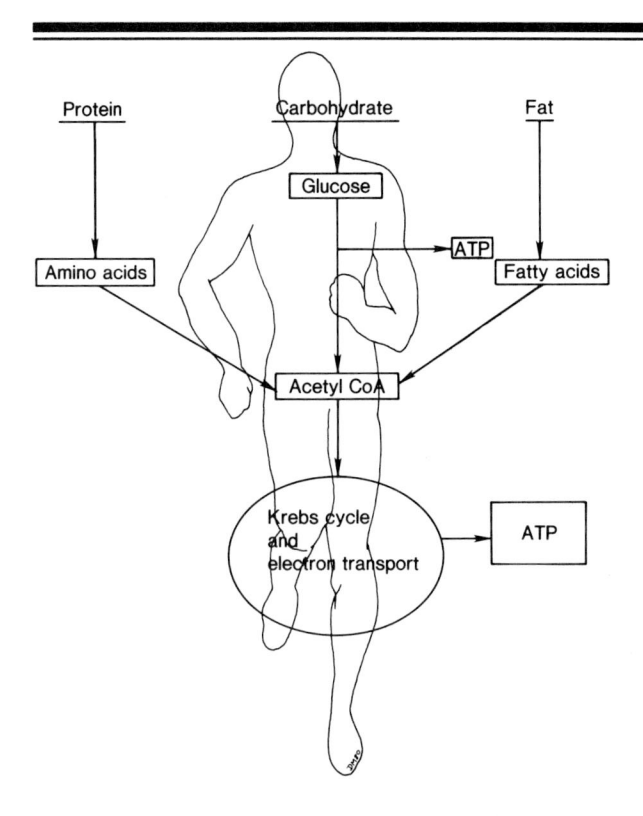

Figure 8.2.
Formation of ATP from carbohydrate, fat, and protein. All three nutrients may be used to form ATP, but carbohydrate and fat are the major sources via aerobic metabolism of the Krebs cycle. Carbohydrate may be used to produce small amounts of ATP under anaerobic conditions, thus providing humans with the ability to produce energy rapidly without oxygen for relatively short periods of time.

ATP may be formed from either carbohydrate, fat, or protein after those nutrients have undergone some complex biochemical changes in the body. Figure 8.2 represents a basic schematic of ATP formation from each of these three nutrients. PC is derived in a similar fashion.

Since ATP and PC are found in very small amounts in the body, and can be used up in a matter of seconds, it is important to have adequate energy stores as a backup system. The digestion and metabolism of carbohydrate, fat, and protein have been discussed in their respective chapters, and it is unnecessary to repeat that full discussion here. However, you may wish to review Figure 2.2 in order to visualize the metabolic interrelationships between the three nutrients in the body. Parts of each of the three nutrients may be used to manufacture the other two. In other words, protein may be converted to fat or carbohydrate, parts of fat may be used to make protein or carbohydrate, and parts of carbohydrate may be used to make fat or protein. These interconversions allow for energy to be stored in the body in all three forms.

Table 8.1 presents a summary of how energy is stored in the human body as carbohydrate, fat, and protein. Carbohydrate is stored in limited amounts as blood glucose and liver and muscle glycogen. Fats are stored as triglycerides in both the muscle tissue and adipose (fat) tissues; free fatty acids (FFA) in the blood are a limited supply. The protein of the body

Table 8.1 Major energy stores in the human body with approximate total caloric value in humans*

Energy source	Major storage mechanism	Total body Calories
Adenosinetriphosphate	In tissues	1
Phosphocreatine	In tissues	4
Carbohydrate	Blood glucose	20
	Liver glycogen	400
	Muscle glycogen	2,000
Fat	FFA and triglyceride	90
	Triglycerides in muscle	2,500
	Triglycerides in adipose tissue	80,000
Protein	Muscle tissue	30,000

*These values may have extreme variations depending on the size of the individual, amount of body fat, physical fitness level, and diet.

tissues, particularly the muscle tissue, is a large reservoir of energy, but is not used under normal circumstances. The role of each of these energy stores during exercise is an important consideration and will be discussed shortly.

What are the human energy systems?

Human energy systems

One need only to watch weekend television programming for several months to realize that a diversity of sports are popular throughout the world. Each of these sports imposes certain requirements on humans if they are to be successful competitors. For some sports, such as weight lifting, the main requirement is brute strength, while for others such as tennis, quick reactions and hand-eye coordination are important. A major consideration in most sports is the production of energy, which can vary from the explosive power needed by a shot-putter to the tremendous endurance capacity of an ultramarathoner. The physical performance demands of various sports require specific sources of energy.

The body stores energy in a variety of ways—ATP, phosphocreatine, muscle glycogen, and so on. In order for this energy to be used to produce muscular contractions and movement, it must undergo certain biochemical reactions in the muscle. These biochemical reactions can serve as a basis for classifying human energy systems. Edward L. Fox, in his excellent book on *Sports Physiology,* has proposed such a classification consisting of three different energy systems. These three systems are: ATP-PC system; Lactic Acid system; and Oxygen system.

The **ATP-PC system** is also known as the phosphogen system because these two compounds, adenosinetriphosphate (ATP) and phosphocreatine (PC) contain phosphates. ATP is the immediate source of energy for

Figure 8.3.
ATP, adenosinetriphosphate. (1) ATP is stored in the muscle in limited amounts. (2) Splitting of a high energy bond releases energy, which (3) can be used for many body processes including muscular contraction. The ATP stores are used for fast, all-out bursts of power that last about one second. ATP must be replenished from other sources in order for muscle contraction to continue.

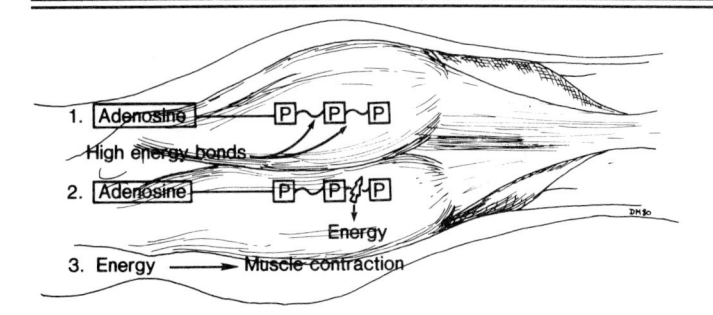

muscle contraction. It is a high energy compound stored in the muscles whose energy is released rapidly when an electrical impulse arrives in the muscle. No matter what you do, scratch your nose or lift 100 pounds, ATP breakdown is responsible for the movement. ATP must be present in order for the muscles to contract. The body has a limited supply of ATP and must replace it rapidly if muscular work is to continue. See Figure 8.3 for a graphical representation of ATP breakdown and resynthesis.

PC is also a high energy compound found in the muscle and can help form ATP rapidly when it is used. PC is also in short supply and needs to be replenished if used. PC breakdown is illustrated in Figure 8.4.

The ATP-PC system is critical to energy production. These phosphogens are in short supply so that any all-out exercise for 5–6 seconds could deplete them in a given muscle. Hence, they must be replaced, and this is the function of the other energy sources. We cannot eat ATP-PC, but we can produce it from the other nutrients stored in our body. We shall not talk about PC replenishment per se, but keep in mind that when ATP is being regenerated, so too is some PC. In summary, the value of the ATP-PC system is its ability to provide energy rapidly.

The **Lactic Acid system** cannot be used directly as a source of energy for muscular contraction, but it can help to replace ATP rapidly when necessary. If you are exercising at a high intensity level, the next best source of energy besides ATP-PC is the muscle glycogen. In order to be used for energy, muscle glycogen must be broken down in a series of reactions to eventually form ATP. This process is called **glycolysis,** which means the breakdown of glycogen. The fate of the muscle glycogen depends upon whether or not enough oxygen is available in the muscle cell. In simple terms, if oxygen is available a large amount of ATP is formed. This is known as **aerobic** glycolysis. If little or no oxygen is available, then few ATP are formed and lactic acid is a by-product. This is known as **anaerobic,** or without oxygen, glycolysis. The Lactic Acid system is diagramed in Figure 8.5.

The Lactic Acid system has the advantage of producing ATP rapidly. Its capacity is limited, for only about 5 percent of the total ATP production from muscle glycogen can be released in comparison to aerobic glycolysis.

Figure 8.4.
Phosphocreatine (PC). (1) PC is stored in the muscle in limited amounts. (2) Splitting of the high energy bond releases energy, which (3) can be used to rapidly synthesize ATP. ATP and PC are called phosphagens and together represent the ATP-PC energy system. This system is utilized for quick, maximal exercises lasting about one to six seconds, such as sprinting.

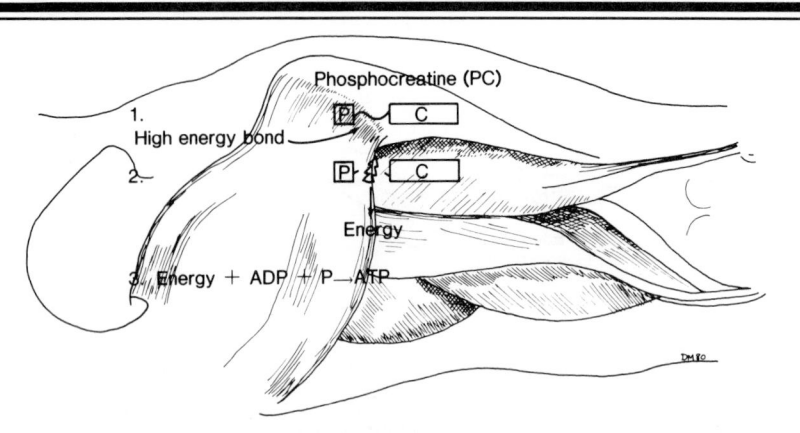

Figure 8.5.
The lactic acid energy system. Muscle glycogen can break down without the utilization of oxygen. This process is called anaerobic glycolysis. ATP is produced rapidly, but lactic acid is the end product. Lactic acid can be a major cause of fatigue in the muscle. The lactic acid system is utilized during exercise bouts of very high intensity, those which are conducted at maximal rates for about one to three minutes.

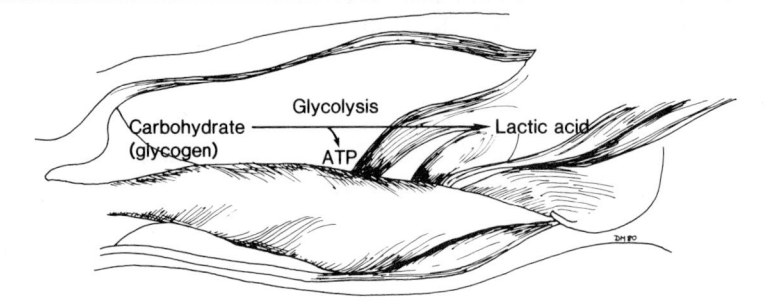

Moreover, the lactic acid produced as a by-product may be involved in the onset of fatigue. The lactic acid increases the acidity within the muscle cell and disturbs the normal cell environment. The processes of energy release and muscle contraction in the muscle cell are conrolled by enzymes, whose functions may be impaired by the increased acidity in the cell.

A term often associated with the lactic acid system is the **Anaerobic threshold.** Although there is some controversy among scientists concerning the measurement of the anaerobic threshold, it is generally defined to be that point where lactic acid accumulates in the blood very rapidly during exercise.

The third system is the **Oxygen system.** It is also known as the aerobics system, a term used by Dr. Kenneth Cooper in 1968 to describe a system of exercising that created an exercise revolution in this country. Aerobic-type exercises will be covered in more detail in Chapter 13.

The Oxygen system, like the Lactic Acid system, cannot be used directly as a source of energy for muscle contraction, but it does produce ATP in rather large quantities from other energy sources in the body. Muscle glycogen, liver glycogen, blood glucose, muscle triglycerides, blood FFA and triglycerides, adipose cell triglycerides, and body protein may all be ultimate sources of energy for ATP production. To do so, they must be oxidized within the muscle cell. These substances enter the muscle cell as

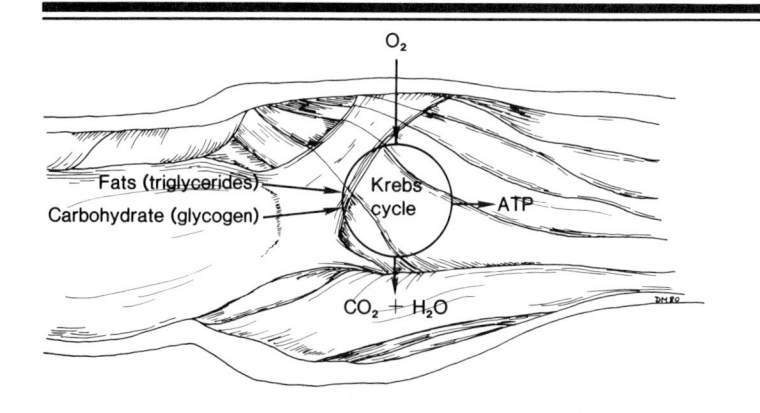

Figure 8.6.
The oxygen system. The muscle stores of glycogen and triglycerides, through complex changes, can enter the Krebs cycle. When they eventually combine with oxygen, large amounts of ATP may be produced. The oxygen system is utilized during endurance-type exercises, those lasting longer than four or five minutes.

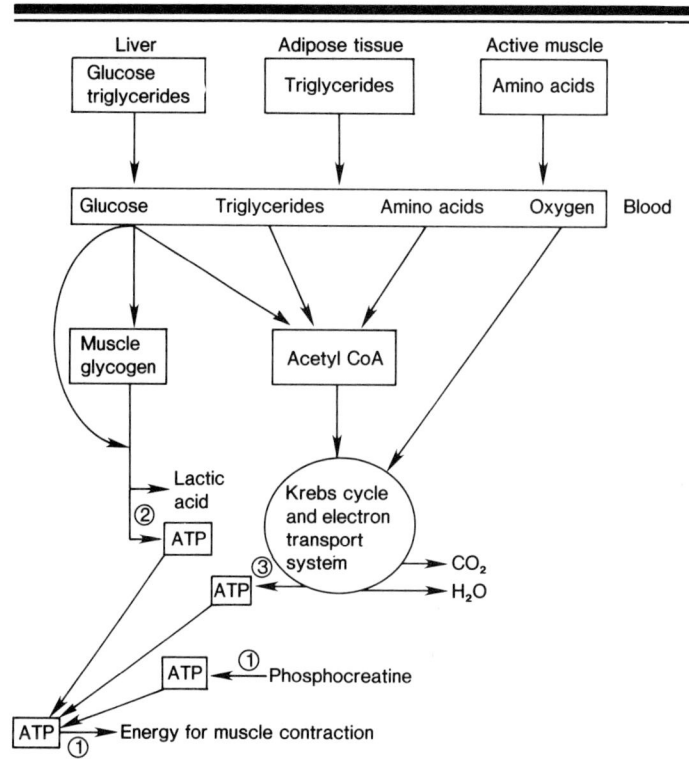

Figure 8.7.
Flow diagram of the three energy systems. Following digestion, the major nutrients and oxygen are transported to the cells for energy production. In the muscles ATP is the immediate source of energy for muscle contraction. The ATP-PC system (1) is represented by muscle stores of ATP and phosphocreatine. Glucose or muscle glycogen can produce ATP rapidly via the lactic acid system (2). The oxygen system (3) can produce large amounts of ATP via the aerobic processes in the Krebs cycle.

glucose, FFA, or amino acids, and through a complex series of reactions combine with oxygen to produce energy, carbon dioxide, and water. These reactions occur in the energy powerhouse of the cell, the mitochondrion. The whole series of events of oxidative energy production is sometimes called the Krebs cycle. The Oxygen system is depicted in Figure 8.6.

The major advantage of the Oxygen system is the production of large amounts of energy in the form of ATP. However, oxygen from the air we breathe must be delivered to the muscle cells deep in the body and enter the mitochondria to be used. This process may be adequate to handle mild and moderate levels of exercise, but may not be able to meet the demand of very strenuous exercise.

Figure 8.7 presents a simplified schematic reviewing the three human energy systems.

What nutrients are necessary for the operation of the human energy systems?

Although the energy for the formation of ATP is derived from the energy stores in carbohydrate and fat, and sometimes protein, this energy transformation and utilization would not occur without the participation of many vitamins and minerals. As you may recall, these two classes of nutrients function very closely with protein in the structure and function of numerous enzymes, many of which are active in the muscle cell energy processes.

Several vitamins are needed in order for energy to be released from the cell sources. Niacin serves an important function in glycolysis, while riboflavin is essential as a coenzyme helping to form ATP through the Krebs cycle and electron transport system. Pantothenic acid is involved in the central role of acetyl CoA. Thiamine is necessary to form acetyl CoA from muscle glycogen. Pyridoxine, folacin, biotin, and vitamin B_{12} are also involved in various facets of energy transformation within the cell.

Minerals too are essential for cellular energy processes. Iron is one of the more critical compounds. Aside from helping to deliver oxygen to the muscle cell, it is also a component of myoglobin and the cytochrome part of the electron transport system. It is needed for proper utilization of oxygen within the cell itself. Other minerals such as zinc, magnesium, potassium, sodium, and calcium are involved in a variety of ways, either as parts of active enzymes, energy storage, or the muscle contraction process.

Proper utilization of body energy sources requires attention not only to the major energy nutrients but also to the regulatory nutrients—vitamins and minerals—as well. A balanced diet is the primary way to see that these nutritional requirements are satisfied.

What energy sources are used during rest?

Energy utilization during rest and exercise

During resting conditions such as sitting and standing, and even during very mild exercise like slow walking, the rate of energy expenditure is relatively low, at least when we compare it to maximal exercise. For the average-sized individual, a total of 75 C might be expended during an hour of sitting, while about 200 C used while walking slowly for the same period of time. The same individual, if well conditioned, might expend up to 1,200 C during an hour of running or other high intensity exercise. From this brief introduction we can see that the main factor influencing energy expenditure appears to be movement caused by increased levels of muscular activity.

As will be noted, the vast majority of the energy consumed during a resting situation is used to drive the automatic physiological processes in the body. Since the rate of energy expenditure by the muscles themselves is low during rest and very light exercise, there is no need to produce ATP rapidly. Hence, the Oxygen system is able to provide the necessary ATP for resting physiological processes.

The Oxygen system can use carbohydrates, fats, and protein as energy sources. However, as noted in Chapter 4, protein is not used as a major energy source under normal dietary conditions. Carbohydrates and fats, when combined with oxygen in the cells, are the major energy substrates during rest. The composition of the diet may influence which of these two nutrients is used. If a high carbohydrate diet is consumed, then the body will use more carbohydrate as an energy source. The opposite is true on a high fat diet as more fat will be used. Other factors may also influence which of the two nutrients is predominantly used but, in general, on a mixed diet of carbohydrate, protein and fat, about 40 percent of the energy expenditure at rest is derived from carbohydrate and about 60 percent comes from fat.

The nervous system under normal circumstances uses only glucose, and nervous tissue is one of the most active during rest. Blood glucose supplies the energy substrate to the nerve cells, and it is replenished by glucose from the liver. The muscle cells, at rest, use very little of their glycogen and rely mainly on triglycerides for energy. That which is used may be replaced by blood glucose and triglycerides.

Since carbohydrate supplies are limited, they may be nearly depleted after a day or so with no carbohydrate intake. In this case, the major energy source is fat. Small amounts of glucose may be produced in the liver from protein in order to supply the nervous system. However, over time the nervous system can adapt to using primarily products of fat metabolism.

What energy sources are used during exercise?

This is a relatively complex question as there are many interacting factors influencing which of the body energy sources or which combination of energy sources are used. Diet, previous training, insulin and other hormones, body energy stores, muscle fiber types, intensity and duration of exercise, oxygen supply, and other factors may influence the answer. In most cases the intensity of the exercise is the key factor that determines which energy source will predominate.

The intensity of an exercise is the rate, speed, or tempo that you pursue a given activity. In general, the faster you do something, the higher your rate of energy expenditure and the more rapidly you must produce ATP for muscular contraction. Very rapid muscular movements are characterized by high rates of power production. If you were asked to run 10 yards as fast as you could, you would exert maximal speed for a short period of time. On the other hand, if you were asked to run 5 miles, you certainly would not

Table 8.2 Major characteristics of the human energy systems*

	ATP-PC	Lactic acid	Oxygen
Main energy source	ATP Phosphocreatine	muscle glycogen	muscle glycogen fats
Intensity level	highest	high	lower
Rate of ATP production	highest	high	lower
Power production	highest	high	lower
Capacity for total ATP production	low	low	high
Endurance capacity	low	low	high
Oxygen needed	no	no	yes
Anaerobic/aerobic	anaerobic	anaerobic	aerobic
Characteristic track event	100-yard dash	440–880 yards	2-mile run
Time factor	1–20 seconds	30–120 seconds	5 minutes or more

*Keep in mind that during most exercises, all three energy systems will be operating to one degree or another. However, one source may predominate, depending primarily on the intensity of the activity. See text for further explanation.

run at the same speed as you would for the 10 yards. In the 10-yard run your energy expenditure would be very rapid, characterized by a high power production. The 5-mile run would be characterized by low power production, or endurance.

The source of energy for exercise is related to a **power-endurance continuum.** On the power end, we have extremely high rates of energy expenditure that a sprinter might use; while on the endurance end, we see lower rates that might be characteristic of a marathon runner. The closer we are to the power end of the continuum, the more rapidly we must produce ATP. As we move towards the endurance end, our *rate* of ATP production does not need to be as great, but we need the *capacity* to produce ATP for a longer time.

It should be noted from the outset that all three energy systems, ATP-PC, Lactic Acid, and Oxygen, are used in one way or another during most athletic activities. However, one system may predominate depending primarily upon the intensity level of the activity. In this regard, the three human energy systems may be ranked according to several characteristics, and these are displayed in Table 8.2.

Both the ATP-PC and the lactic acid systems are able to produce ATP rapidly and are used in events characterized by high intensity levels but for short periods of time since their capacity for total ATP production is rather limited. Since both these systems may function without oxygen, they are called anaerobic. Relative to physical performance, the ATP-PC system predominates in short, powerful bursts of muscular activity such as the short dashes like 100 yards, whereas the lactic acid system begins to

Table 8.3 Percentage contribution of anaerobic and aerobic energy sources during different time periods of maximal work

Time	10 sec	1 min	2 min	4 min	10 min	30 min	60 min	130 min
Anaerobic	85	70	50	30	15	5	2	1
Aerobic	15	30	50	70	85	95	98	99

predominate during the longer sprints and middle distances such as 440 and 880 yards. In any athletic event where maximal power production is about 1–20 seconds, then the ATP-PC system is the major energy source. The lactic acid system begins to predominate in events lasting 30–120 seconds.

The oxygen system possesses a lower rate of ATP production than the other two systems, but its capacity for total ATP production is much greater. Although the intensity level of exercise while using the oxygen system is by necessity lower, this does not necessarily mean that an individual cannot perform at a relatively high speed for a long period of time. The oxygen system can be improved through a physical conditioning program so that ATP production may be able to meet the demands of relatively high intensity exercise. Endurance-type activities, such as those that last 5 minutes or more, are dependent primarily upon the oxygen system.

In summary, we may simplify this discussion by categorizing the energy sources as either aerobic or anaerobic. Anaerobic sources include both the ATP-PC and lactic acid systems while the oxygen system is aerobic. Table 8.3 illustrates the percentage contribution of anaerobic and aerobic energy sources, dependent upon the level of maximal intensity that can be sustained for a given time period. Thus, for a 100-meter dash covered in ten seconds, 85 percent of the energy is derived from anaerobic sources. For a marathoner (26.2 miles), with times approximately 130 minutes in international level competitors, the aerobic energy processes contribute 99 percent. The key point is that the longer you exercise, the less your intensity has to be, and the more you rely on your oxygen system for energy production.

How is the intensity of exercise measured?

There are a number of different ways to measure exercise intensity, and several simple methods will be presented in Chapter 13. For the purpose of this present discussion, it is necessary to introduce the term **maximal oxygen uptake,** or $\dot{V}O_2$ **max.** $\dot{V}O_2$ max represents the highest amount of oxygen that an individual may consume under exercise situations. It is typically measured in a laboratory setting using a treadmill, bicycle, or other exercise mode. In essence, the oxygen uptake of the individual is monitored while the exercise intensity is increased in stages. When the oxygen uptake does not increase with an increase in workload, $\dot{V}O_2$ max has been reached.

What effect does the intensity of exercise have upon the utilization of fat and carbohydrate as energy sources?

As noted in the last question, exercise intensity is the key factor in determining what energy source is used. Now we know that the primary sources of ATP are carbohydrate and fat. The carbohydrate is found as muscle glycogen, liver glycogen, and blood glucose. The fats are found primarily as triglycerides in the muscle and adipose cells. During exercise, all of these sources may be used, but intensity and duration determine which ones.

The human body possesses several different types of muscle fibers, but for simplicity sake we may classify them as white, fast twitch anaerobic fibers or red, slow twitch aerobic fibers, as discussed in Chapter 2. The fast twitch fibers are designed to produce ATP rapidly; they primarily use the lactic acid system, which uses only muscle glycogen as an energy source. The slow twitch fibers produce ATP at a slower rate via the oxygen system, which can use either fats or carbohydrates.

At high intensity levels of anaerobic exercise that are sustained for several minutes, the lactic acid system is the key energy system. Hence, since it uses only muscle glycogen, then carbohydrate is the main fuel used during this type of exercise. However, as noted previously, the duration may be very short as lactic acid may cause fatigue.

With the oxygen system, intensity may also determine whether carbohydrate or fat is used. We can measure the intensity of an exercise in several different ways. The best method is to measure your oxygen uptake level and compare it to your VO_2 max. If you have a VO_2 max of 4 liters, and if you are consuming 2 liters of oxygen you are exercising at 50 percent of your capacity. A second way is to monitor your heart rate (HR) and do the same types of calculations. If you have a maximal HR (HR max) of 200, then an exercise HR of 180 has you at 90 percent of your capacity. There is not an exact correlation between oxygen uptake and HR, but the association is close enough so that our HR can tell us at what intensity we may be working. More will be said about this in Chapters 10 and 13.

Now back to the Oxygen system and the use of carbohydrate and fat. As you do mild to moderate exercise, say up to 50 percent of your capacity, you will use about 50 percent carbohydrate and 50 percent fat. The muscle glycogen and triglycerides in the muscle as well as glucose delivered from the liver and free fatty acids from the adipose tissues are your main sources. As you start to exceed 50 percent of your capacity, that is as you increase your speed or intensity, you begin to rely more and more on carbohydrate as an energy source. Apparently the biochemical processes for fat metabolism are too slow to meet the increased need for faster production of ATP, and carbohydrate utilization increases. The major source of this carbohydrate is the muscle glycogen. At high levels of energy expenditure, 70–80 percent of $\dot{V}O_2$ max, carbohydrates may contribute over 80 percent of the energy sources. This speaks for the need of adequate muscle glycogen stores when this level of exercise is to be sustained for long periods of time, say in events lasting over an hour or more.

Is the utilization of one type of energy source more efficient than others?

If we look at the caloric value of carbohydrate (1 g = 4 C) and fat (1 g = 9 C) we might think that fat is a better source of energy. Indeed, this is so if we just look at Calories per gram. However, more oxygen is needed to metabolize the fat, and if we look at how many Calories we get from one liter of oxygen, we will find that carbohydrate yields about 5.05 and fat gives only 4.69. Thus, carbohydrate appears to be a more efficient fuel than fat, by about 7 percent.

Now this is not to say that fat is not an important source of energy during exercise. It may contribute substantially at moderate levels of intensity and does contribute smaller amounts even at higher intensity levels. In very long distance events, body carbohydrate stores may become depleted and fat will have to serve as the primary energy source. As we shall see later, both physical conditioning and caffeine may help increase fat utilization and possibly help to delay carbohydrate depletion.

As I get in better physical condition through endurance training, do I use different fuels during exercise?

As you begin an exercise program emphasizing endurance-type activities, such as jogging or running long distances, your body undergoes several significant changes that have implications for physical performance and the fuels used. Figure 8.8 schematically represents some of these changes. The following have been noted to occur following several months of endurance training:

1. More glycogen is stored in the muscle. This means you may maintain an optimal speed for a longer period of time.

2. In the muscle cell there is an increase in the enzymes that metabolize both carbohydrates and fats. This makes the energy producing processes in the cell more efficient.

3. More fats begin to be used at a standardized exercise workload. For example suppose you ran an 8-minute mile both before and after a conditioning period and an exercise physiology laboratory assessed your carbohydrate and fat utilization. You would use a greater percentage of fat after training than before. This would help to spare carbohydrate, the muscle glycogen, which could help increase your endurance capacity.

Figure 8.8.
Some of the effects of aerobic or endurance training upon skeletal muscle. Glycogen and triglyceride increases provide a greater energy store, while the increase in mitochondria size and number, myoglobin content, oxidative enzymes, and slow twitch muscle fiber size facilitates the use of oxygen for production of energy.

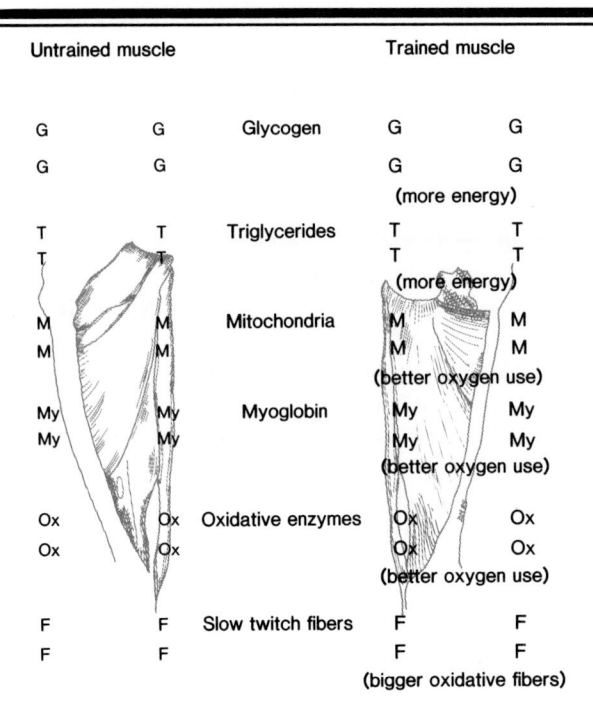

Untrained muscle		Trained muscle	
G G	Glycogen	G G	
G G		G G	
		(more energy)	
T T	Triglycerides	T T	
T T		T T	
		(more energy)	
M M	Mitochondria	M M	
M M		M M	
		(better oxygen use)	
My My	Myoglobin	My My	
My My		My My	
		(better oxygen use)	
Ox Ox	Oxidative enzymes	Ox Ox	
Ox Ox		Ox Ox	
		(better oxygen use)	
F F	Slow twitch fibers	F F	
F F		F F	
		(bigger oxidative fibers)	

4. There would be a greater release of fats from your adipose tissue, which could be delivered to and used by the muscles. This could help in weight reduction programs to lose excess body fat stores.

5. You will increase your $\dot{V}O_2$ max. This will help you deliver more oxygen to the muscle tissues and use it, significantly increasing your endurance capacity.

6. Of equal or greater importance, you will be able to work at a greater percentage of your $\dot{V}O_2$ max without fatigue. At the beginning of your training program you may start producing lactic acid once you get beyond 50 percent of your $\dot{V}O_2$ max, which may cause early fatigue. However, after training, you may be able to perform at 60–70 percent of your capacity without lactic acid production. World class marathoners may operate above 80 percent. What does this mean? You may be able to run a mile in 7 minutes instead of 8, or similar such changes. You can cruise in high gear for longer periods of time without fatigue. You have increased your anaerobic threshold.

Energy requirements of physical exercise

Human beings consume and expend energy, and both the consumption and expenditure can be expressed in Calories. In order to maintain a stable body weight, there must be a balance between the input and output of Calories. During the growth and development years of childhood and adolescence, the input predominates slightly, creating a positive energy balance and a growth of body mass. As the adolescent enters young adulthood, the major growth processes are just about complete, and now dietary input and metabolic output must be equal. If not, an individual will lose weight if output predominates, a condition of negative caloric balance. If the input is greater, a positive caloric balance exists, and the individual will gain weight. For example, the input of an extra doughnut a day (125 Calories), if not balanced by an increased energy expenditure of 125 Calories, can lead to an increase of about 13 pounds body weight in a year. Overweight and obesity can creep up on us.

Weight control is an important issue, and both diet and exercise are important means to reach and maintain an ideal weight. The purpose of this chapter is to discuss the ways whereby humans expend energy, with special consideration to the role of exercise.

What is metabolism?

Human **metabolism** represents the sum total of all physical and chemical changes that take place within the body. The transformation of food to energy, the formation of new compounds such as hormones and enzymes, the growth of bone and muscle tissue, the destruction of body tissues, and a host of other physiological processes are parts of the metabolic process.

Metabolism involves two fundamental processes, anabolism and catabolism. **Anabolism** is a building-up process, or constructive metabolism. Complex body components are synthesized from the basic nutrients. For the active individual, this may mean an increased muscle mass through weight training or an increased amount of cellular enzymes to better use oxygen following endurance-type training. **Catabolism** is the tearing-down process, or destructive metabolism. This involves the disintegration of body compounds into their simpler components. The breakdown of muscle glycogen to glucose and eventually CO_2 and H_2O is an example of a catabolic process.

Metabolism is life. It represents human energy. The **metabolic rate** reflects how rapidly the body is using its energy stores, and this rate can vary tremendously depending upon a number of factors with the most influential one being exercise.

Basal and resting metabolism

What is the basal metabolic rate (BMR) and the resting metabolic rate (RMR)?

The body is constantly using energy to build up and tear down substances within the cells. Certain automatic body functions such as contraction of the heart, breathing, secretion of hormones, and the constant activity of the nervous system are also consuming energy. Energy expenditure in humans may be measured by several means, one of which is the amount of oxygen an individual consumes.

Basal metabolism, or the **basal metabolic rate (BMR)**, represents the energy requirements of the various cellular and tissue processes that are necessary to continuing physiological activities in a resting, postabsorptive state. Other than sleeping, it is the lowest level of energy expenditure. The determination of the BMR is a clinical procedure conducted in a laboratory or hospital setting. The individual fasts for twelve hours. Then while in a lying position, the oxygen consumption and carbon dioxide production are measured. Through proper calculations, the BMR is determined. It is usually expressed as Calories/kg body weight/hr.

The BMR is extremely high during infancy and declines through childhood, adolescence, and adulthood. The decline in BMR in adults may be attributed partially to inactivity and the subsequent loss of active tissue such as muscle. Women have a lower BMR than men, mainly because men have more muscle tissue and less fat. The difference in the BMR between the sexes is about 10–15 percent.

In the average individual, approximately 50 percent of the total daily energy expenditure is accounted for by the BMR. There are individual variations in the BMR and deviations of 10 percent above or below the average are considered normal. If two individuals are about the same size, about equally active, and eat about the same amount of food, the one with the higher BMR will have the advantage in maintaining body weight at a lower level.

The **resting metabolic rate (RMR)** is slightly higher than the BMR. It represents the BMR plus any additional energy expenditure associated with digestion of food, sitting, reading, standing, or other sedentary activities.

How can I estimate my daily BMR?

There are several ways to estimate the BMR, but whichever method is used, keep in mind that the value obtained is an estimate. In order to get a truly accurate value, a standard BMR test would be needed. However, various formula estimates may give you a good approximation of your daily BMR.

Table 9.1 Estimation of the daily basal metabolic rate

Adult male:
BMR estimate = 1 C/kg body weight/hr

Example: 154-lb male
       154 lbs ÷ 2.2 = 70 kg
       70 × 1 C = 70 C/hr
       70 × 24 hours = 1,680 C/day

Rounded BMR estimate: 1,700 C/day

Adult female:
BMR estimate = 0.9 C/kg body weight/hr

       121-lb woman
       121 lbs ÷ 2.2 = 55 kg
       55 × 0.9 C = 49.5 C/hr
       49.5 × 24 hr = 1,188 C/day

Rounded BMR estimate = 1,200 C/day

As noted previously, there are individual variations in the BMR. When the Food and Nutrition Board of the National Research Council establishes the RDA for Calories, they offer a range of caloric values that incorporates about a 10 percent variation above the average value for both men and women.

The most common way to express the BMR is in Calories per unit of body weight. Either pounds or kilograms may be used; recall that 1 kg equals 2.2 lbs. Table 9.1 represents one method for calculating the BMR of adult males and females. It is not appropriate for growing children.

In order to get a range of values, simply add or subtract a normal 10 percent variation to the rounded BMR estimate.

Adult male: 10 percent of 1,700 = 170
Normal range = 1,530–1,870 C/day

Adult female: 10 percent of 1,200 = 120
Normal range = 1,080–1,320 C/day

In addition, the BMR declines with age, about 2 percent per decade. Hence, the estimated BMR should be lowered by 2 percent for those in the 30's, 4 percent for those in the 40's, 6 percent for those in the 50's and so on.

A simpler method has been developed by Ronald Deutsch in his excellent book, *Realities of Nutrition,* and is presented in Table 9.2.

Table 9.2   Simplified method of estimating daily basal metabolic rate

Adult males:
BMR estimate = Add a zero to your weight in pounds
                Add double your weight to this value

   Example: 154-lb male
             1,540 + (2 × 154) = 1,848 C/day

Adult females:
BMR estimate = Add a zero to your weight in pounds
                Add your body weight to this value

   Example: 121-lb woman
             1,210 + 121 = 1,331 C/day

Note that the estimated BMR values obtained by this technique are near the upper range values of the first technique. Other techniques result in estimated BMR values closer to the bottom part of the range. The key point is that no matter which technique you may use, the value obtained is merely an approximation.

The estimated BMR does not represent the amount of Calories you need daily in order to maintain your body weight. It would if you remained in a basal state all day, but you sit, stand, talk, walk and do other activities increasing your metabolic rate above BMR levels. You sleep, which lowers caloric expenditure below the BMR. The sum total of these additional activities increases your need for Calories above the BMR.

Can I change my metabolic rate?

There are several parts to this question, as the metabolic rate may be conveniently subdivided into three components:

Basal metabolic rate (BMR)—energy for the basic life functions.
Resting metabolic rate (RMR)—energy required for normal daily sedentary activities above the BMR.
Exercise metabolic rate (EMR)—energy required for active muscular exercise above the BMR.

A schematic is presented in Figure 9.1.

The BMR may be influenced by several factors such as age, sex, body size and shape, climate, and the food we eat, but essentially the BMR remains relatively stable for any given set of conditions. There is good general knowledge about the effect of some of these factors on the BMR. BMR declines with age; males have a higher BMR than females; the greater the size of the individual, the higher the BMR; lean individuals, because of a greater body surface area ratio to their weight causing more heat radiation, have higher BMR than do stocky individuals. Individuals with greater muscle mass in comparison to body fat have higher BMR; cold climates will increase BMR due to muscular shivering; hot climates will

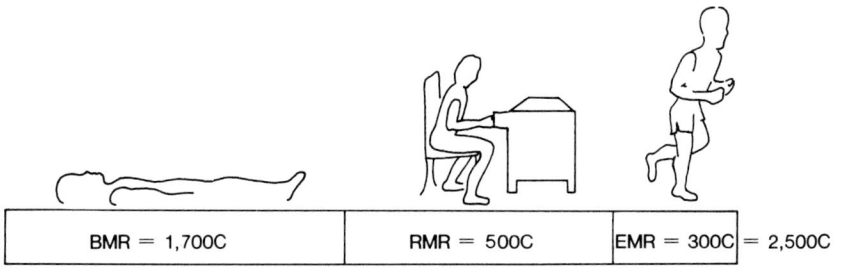

Figure 9.1.
Total daily expenditure for an average sized male (154 pounds). BMR represents basal metabolic rate, RMR is the resting metabolic rate, and EMR is the exercise metabolic rate. EMR could be increased considerably through an expanded exercise program.

BMR = 1,700C   RMR = 500C   EMR = 300C   = 2,500C

increase BMR due to increased cardiovascular demands and sweating, which consumes energy; and, the digestion of food will elevate the BMR, sometimes this effect being called the specific dynamic action (SDA) of food. Some research also indicates that a very low calorie diet (less than 800 C/day) will decrease the BMR, even more than the decrease which would be normally observed with the weight loss of both fat and muscle tissues.

Many factors controlling BMR are, of course, genetically determined, or like climatic conditions, not totally under our control. Of all the factors that influence the BMR, a change in body composition may be one way to alter it. Decreasing the amount of body fat and increasing lean body mass (muscle tissue) may increase the BMR; this effect may be due to the increased activity levels of muscle tissue as compared to fat tissue or the increased ratio of body surface area to body weight. The composition of the diet may also influence BMR, as it takes more energy to digest and metabolize protein than either carbohydrates or fat. Both of these points will be discussed further in several of the following chapters.

The RMR may be increased or decreased depending on your average daily activities. Sitting burns fewer Calories than standing, standing burns fewer than walking, and so on. Simply changing the nature of your daily sedentary activities, like walking to the store rather than driving, may increase the RMR. Unfortunately, most of us are inclined to save energy during most daily activities, and unless conscious effort is made to change them, then the RMR will remain relatively constant as a percentage of our daily energy expenditure. Some research has reported that the RMR accounts for about 30 percent of our caloric expenditure above the BMR. Thus for a BMR of 1,500 Calories, the RMR would add 30 percent of that to the daily caloric needs. Thus, the daily caloric needs would be 1,500 + (.30 × 1,500) = 1,950 Calories Simply increasing the RMR from 450 in this example to 500, an increase of 50 Calories per day, could account for over 5 lbs of body fat in one year.

The **exercise metabolic rate (EMR)** is one directly under our control and probably is the most effective way to affect our over-all metabolic rate. The effect of exercise on the metabolic rate is one of the most important topics to be covered in this book, so several pages will be devoted to this subject.

Table 9.3 Approximate daily energy expenditure in Calories of adult men and women in sedentary occupations

Daily activity	Time (hr)	Man, 70 kg Rate C/min	Man, 70 kg Total Calories	Woman, 58 kg Rate C/min	Woman, 58 kg Total Calories
BMR (sleeping, lying)	8	1.0–1.2	540	0.9–1.1	440
Light RMR (sitting and standing activities)	12	up to 2.5	1,300	up to 2.0	900
Moderate RMR (slow walking, moderately active work while standing)	3	2.5–4.9	600	2.0–3.9	450
Light EMR (walking at good pace, active work such as lifting)	1	5.0–7.4	300	4.0–5.9	240
Moderate to heavy EMR (jogging, walking uphill, heavy labor)	0	7.5–12.0	0	6.0–10.0	0
Totals	24		2,740		2,030

In summary, then, the total metabolic rate is composed of three components, the BMR, RMR, EMR, and the percentage participation of each of these components will vary throughout the day. Table 9.3 represents an example of daily expenditures for adult men and women involved in sedentary occupations. It is a modification of some data provided by the Food and Nutrition Board of the National Research Council. Note that these values are for the average-sized man or woman engaged in a light occupation with no moderate to heavy exercise in their daily activities.

You may be able to adjust your metabolic rate for sixteen of the twenty-four hour day, but for all practical purposes your best bet is to concentrate on the last category, moderate to heavy exercise, and incorporate it daily into your life-style.

What effect does exercise have on the metabolic rate?

Exercise and the metabolic rate

The muscle cell itself is rather a simple machine in design, but extremely complex in function. It is a tube-like structure with various filaments in it that can slide by one another and cause a shortening of the total muscle. The shortening of the muscle moves bones, and hence work is accomplished, be it simply the raising of a barbell as in weight training or moving the whole body as in running. Like most other machines, the muscle cell has the capability of producing work at different rates, ranging from very low levels of energy expenditure during sleep to nearly a fifty-fold increase during maximal anaerobic exercise.

The most important factor affecting the metabolic rate is the intensity or speed of the exercise. In order to move faster, your muscles must contract more rapidly, consuming proportionately more energy. However, the influence of exercise upon the metabolic rate is also dependent upon a number of other factors. First, the nature of the activity is critical; swimming a mile expends more Calories than running the same distance, and running the mile costs more than bicycling. Second, the efficiency of movement in some activities will modify the number of Calories expended; a beginning swimmer wastes a lot of energy, while one who is more accomplished may swim with less effort, saving Calories. Third, the individual with a greater body weight will burn more Calories for any given amount of work where the body has to be moved, as in walking, jogging, or running. It simply costs more energy to move a heavier load. Fourth, a high fat diet may adversely affect efficiency slightly during exercise and cause a greater energy expenditure for a given exercise task. It is not recommended that you become less skilled, gain body weight, or eat a high fat diet in order to burn more Calories during exercise. In fact, the opposite is true, to try to become more efficient so that the exercise task may become more enjoyable.

Exercise not only increases the metabolic rate during exercise but, depending upon the intensity and duration of the activity, will also keep the metabolic rate elevated during the recovery period. The increased body temperature and amount of circulating hormones such as adrenalin will continue to influence some cellular activity, and some other metabolic processes like the circulation and respiration will remain elevated for a limited time. The amount of Calories used during recovery is above and beyond those used during the exercise itself. This process has been labelled the **metabolic aftereffects of exercise** and may have some implications for a weight control program. Controlled research has shown that the RMR after exercise was elevated 7.5–28 percent above normal, and the increase persisted four to six hours. The average amount of additional Calories would be about forty-five to fifty after each exercise session, which could equal a pound a body fat in ten to eleven weeks.

Can I tell what my metabolic rate is during exercise?

The human body is basically a muscle machine designed for movement. Most all of the other body systems serve the muscular system. The nervous system causes the muscles to contract. The digestive system supplies nutrients. The cardiovascular system delivers these nutrients along with oxygen in cooperation with the respiratory system. The endocrine system secretes hormones that affect muscle nutrition. The excretory system removes its waste products. When humans exercise then, almost all body systems increase their activity in order to accommodate the increased energy demands of the muscle cell. In most types of sustained exercises, however, the major demand of the muscle cells is for oxygen.

Figure 9.2.
Relationships between oxygen consumption, heart rate, and respiration responses to increasing exercise rates. In general, as the intensity of exercise continues, there is a rise in oxygen consumption, which is accompanied by proportional increases in heart rate and respiration.

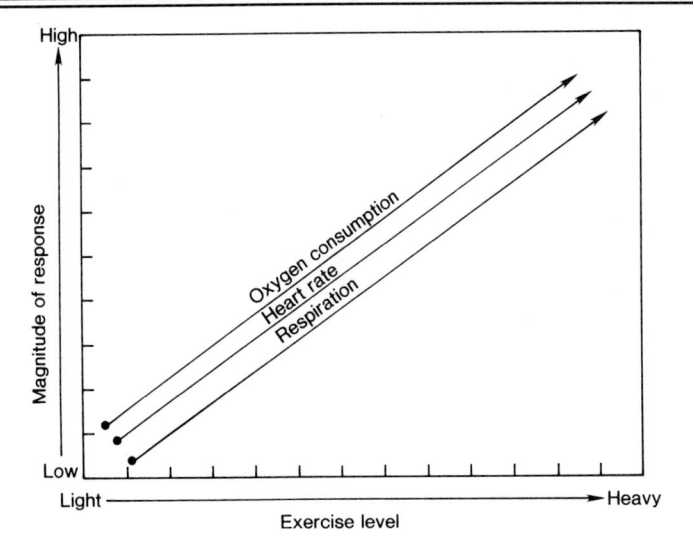

The major technique for evaluating metabolic rate is to measure the oxygen consumption of an individual during exercise. Rather elaborate laboratory equipment is needed for these determinations, but highly accurate measurements of oxygen uptake may be obtained. However, due to some interesting relationships among exercise rate, oxygen consumption, and heart rate, the average individual may be able to get a relative approximation of the metabolic rate during exercise.

There is a rather linear relationship between exercise intensity and oxygen uptake. As the intensity level of work increases, so too does the amount of oxygen consumed. The two systems primarily responsible for delivering the oxygen to the muscles are the cardiovascular and respiratory systems. There is also a rather linear relationship between their responses and oxygen consumption. A simplified schematic is presented in Figure 9.2.

Since the heart rate (HR) generally is linearly related to **oxygen consumption** (the main expression of metabolic rate) and since it is rather easy to measure this physiological response during exercise either at the wrist or neck pulse, it may prove to be a practical guide to your metabolic rate. However, a number of factors may influence your specific heart rate response to exercise, such as your level of physical fitness, sex, age, skill efficiency, percent of body fat, and a number of environmental conditions. It is difficult to predict your exact metabolic rate from your exercise HR, but as we shall see in Chapter 13, the use of HR data during exercise may be used as a basis for establishing a personal fitness program.

How can I calculate the energy expenditure of exercise?

A number of research studies have been conducted in order to determine the caloric cost or energy expenditure of a wide variety of sports and other physical activities. The energy costs have been reported in a variety of ways, including Calories per kg body weight, kilojoules (kj), oxygen uptake, and by **METS,** which represents multiples of the resting metabolic rate. These concepts are, of course, all interrelated, so an exercise can be expressed in any one of the four terms and be converted into the others. For our purposes, we will express energy cost in Calories per unit body weight as that appears to be the most practical method for this book. However, just in case you see the other values in another book or magazine, here is how you make the conversion. We know the following approximate values:

1 C = 4 kj
1 l O_2 = 5 C
1 MET = 3.5 ml O_2/kg/min (amount of oxygen consumed during rest)

These values are needed for the following calculations:

EXAMPLE: Exercise cost = 20 kj/minute
To get Calorie cost, divide kj by the equivalent value for Calories.
20 kj/min ÷ 4 = 5 C/min

EXAMPLE: Exercise cost = 25 l of O_2
To get Calorie cost, multiply liters of O_2 × Calories per liter
Caloric cost = 25 × 5 = 125 C

EXAMPLE: Exercise cost = 20 ml O_2/kg body weight
You need body weight in kg, which is weight in pounds divided by 2.2. For this example 176 lbs = 80 kg. Determine total O_2 cost/min by multiplying body weight times O_2 cost/kg/min
80 × 20 = 1,600 ml O_2
Convert ml to l: 1,600 ml = 1.6 l
Multiply liters O_2 × Calories per liter
Caloric cost = 1.6 × 5 = 8 C/min

EXAMPLE: Exercise cost = 12 METS
You need body weight in kg. For this example, 80 kg. Multiply total METS times O_2 equivalent of 1 MET.
12 × 3.5 ml O_2/kg/min = 42.0 ml O_2/kg/min
Multiply body weight times this result
80 × 42 ml O_2/kg/min = 3,360 ml O_2/min
Convert ml to l: 3,360 ml O_2/min = 3.36 l O_2/min
Multiply liters O_2 × Calories per liter
Caloric cost = 3.36 × 5 = 16.85 C/min

In order to facilitate the determination of the energy cost of a wide variety of physical activities, Appendix C has been developed. This is a composite table of a wide variety of individual reports in the literature. When using this appendix, keep the following points in mind.

1. The figures include the RMR. Thus the total cost of the exercise includes not only the energy expended by the exercise itself, but also the amount you would have used anyway during that same period of time. Suppose you ran for one hour and the calculated energy cost was 800 Calories During that same time at rest you may have expended 75 Calories. The net cost of the exercise is only 725 Calories.
2. The figures in the table are only for the time you are doing the activity. For example, in an hour of basketball you may only exercise strenuously for 35–40 minutes, as you may take timeouts and rest during foul shots. In general, record only the amount of time that you are actually moving during the activity.
3. The figures may give you some guidelines to total energy expenditure, but actual caloric cost might vary somewhat due to such factors as your skill level, running against the wind or up hill, and so forth.
4. Not all body weights could be listed, but you may approximate by going to the closest weight listed.
5. There may be small differences between men and women, but not enough to make a marked difference in the total caloric value for most exercises.

As one example, suppose we calculate the energy expenditure of a 154 pound individual who ran 5 miles in 30 minutes. You must calculate either the minutes per mile or miles per hour (MPH).

1. 30 minutes ÷ 5 miles = 6 min/mile
2. 60 minutes ÷ 6 minutes/mile = 10 MPH

Consult Appendix C and find the caloric value per minute for a body weight of 155 lbs and a running speed of 10 MPH, a value of 18.8 Calories/minute. Multiply this value times the number of minutes of running, and you get the total caloric cost of that exercise. In this example, 30 × 18.8 = 564 total C expended.

If the activity you do does not appear in Appendix C, try to find one you think closely matches the movements found in your activity. Then, check the caloric expenditure relative to the related activity.

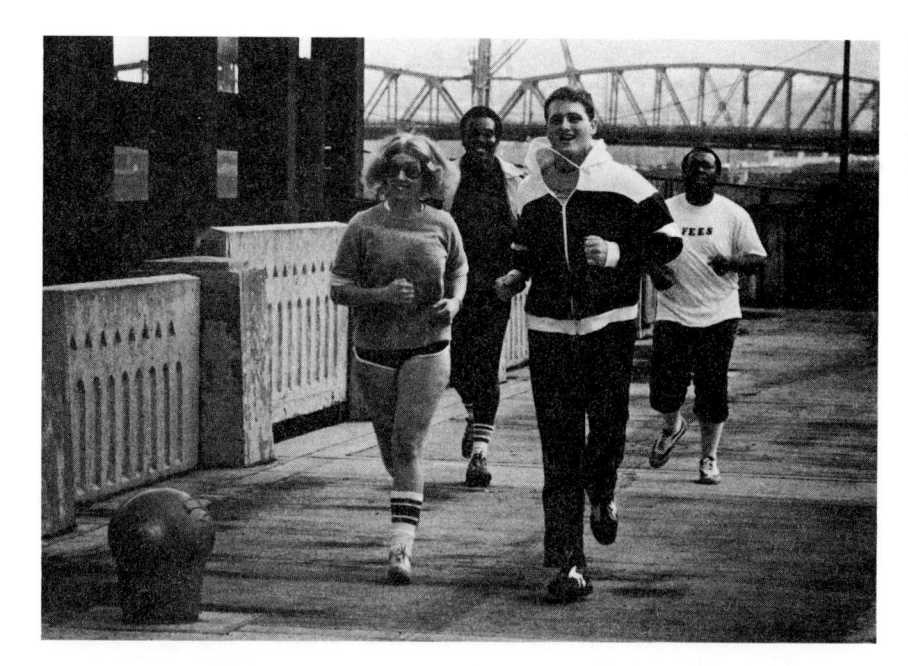

Exercise can be an effective means of increasing energy expenditure and losing excess Calories.
(John Maker/EKM-Nepenthe)

What are the best types of activities to increase energy expenditure?

Activities using the large muscle groups of the body and that are performed in a continuous manner will usually expend the greatest amount of Calories. Intensity and duration are the two key determinants of total energy expenditure. Activities in which you may be able to exercise continuously at a fairly high intensity for a prolonged period of time will maximize your caloric loss. Although this may encompass a wide variety of different physical activities, those which recently have become increasingly popular include walking, jogging, running, swimming, and bicycling. A few general comments would appear to be in order relative to these common modes of exercising.

As a general rule, the caloric cost of running a given distance does not depend on the speed. It will take you a longer time to cover the distance at a slower speed, but the total caloric cost will be similar to that expended at a faster speed. However, walking is more economical than running and hence you generally expend fewer Calories for a given distance walking than you do running. This does not hold true, however, if you walk vigorously at a high speed. At high walking speeds, you may expend more energy than if you jogged at the same speed. Fast, vigorous walking, known as aerobic walking, can be an effective means to expend Calories. Due to water resistance, swimming takes more energy to cover a given distance than does either walking or running. The opposite is true of bicycling.

You may calculate the approximate caloric expenditure for running a given distance by either one of the following formulae:

Caloric cost = 1 C/kg body weight/kilometer
Caloric cost = 0.73 C/pound body weight/mile

If you are an average-sized male of about 154 lbs (70 kg), or an average sized female of about 121 lbs (55 kg), you would burn about the following amounts of Calories for either a kilometer or mile.

	Male (154 lbs, 70 kg)	*Female* (121 lbs, 55 kg)
Kilometer	70 Calories	55 Calories
Mile	112 Calories	88 Calories

Slow leisurely walking would use about half the number of Calories per mile. Rapid aerobic walking would use comparable amounts. Swimming would use approximately four times this amount, while bicycling would be about one-third. High speeds of swimming and bicycling would increase the caloric cost due to increased water and air resistance respectively.

The implications of these types of exercises in weight control programs will be discussed in a later chapter.

Body weight and composition

10

The human body is a remarkable machine. In most cases it may consume nearly a ton of food over a year and not change its body weight a single pound. We are constantly harnessing and expending energy through the intricacies of our bodily metabolism in order to remain in energy balance. To maintain a given body weight, energy input must balance energy output. However, sometimes the energy balance equation becomes unbalanced, and body weight will either increase or decrease.

One of the major health problems in the United States is excessive body weight, or obesity. Several health conditions such as diabetes mellitus, hyperlipidemia, and high blood pressure are known to be related or due to obesity, while others such as coronary heart disease, cirrhosis of the liver, chronic lung disease, and emotional disorders may be aggravated by the condition. Obesity is a complex serious medical, problem which may have many causes, and a full discussion is beyond the scope of this text. However, many of the dietary and exercise principles to be discussed would be effective in the treatment of clinical obesity.

Although obesity may have serious health implications, simply being even a little overweight may prove to be detrimental to physical performance in the active individual. On the other hand increased body mass, provided it is of the right composition, may be advantageous to some athletes. Body weight and body composition represent important considerations for the active individual. The purpose of this chapter is to explore some basic questions relative to these concepts, which will be discussed further in the next three chapters.

What is the ideal body weight?

We have all heard at one time or another that there is an ideal body weight for our particular height. But ideal in terms of what? Health? Appearance? Physical Performance? There does not appear to be any sound evidence to suggest a specific ideal weight for a given individual. However, data collected during the past century, primarily by life insurance companies, have revealed some normal or desirable body weight values for a given height and age.

Tables 10.1 and 10.2 represent the 1959 height-weight charts that have been developed for adults by the Metropolitan Life Insurance Company. Although the Metropolitan Life Insurance Company has recently released new height-weight tables for Americans, the American Heart Association has recommended that we continue to use the 1959 data since the new tables contain much heavier weights for individuals in the lower height classes.

Ideal body weight

Table 10.1 Desirable weights for females age twenty-five and over

Height/Weight female*

Height** In Cm	Small frame Lb	Kg	Medium frame Lb	Kg	Large frame Lb	Kg
6'0"—182.9	138–148	62.6–67.1	144–159	65.3–72.1	153–173	69.4–78.5
5'11"—180.3	134–144	60.8–65.3	140–155	63.5–70.3	149–168	67.6–76.2
5'10"—177.8	130–140	59.0–63.5	136–151	61.7–68.5	145–163	65.8–74.0
5'9"—175.3	126–135	57.2–61.2	132–147	59.9–66.7	141–158	64.0–71.7
5'8"—172.7	121–131	54.9–59.4	128–143	58.1–64.9	137–154	62.1–69.9
5'7"—170.2	118–127	53.5–57.6	124–139	56.2–63.1	133–150	60.3–68.1
5'6"—167.6	114–123	51.7–55.8	120–135	54.4–61.2	129–146	58.5–66.2
5'5"—165.1	111–119	50.3–54.0	116–130	52.6–59.0	125–142	56.7–64.4
5'4"—162.6	108–116	49.0–52.6	113–126	51.3–57.2	121–138	54.9–62.6
5'3"—160.0	105–113	47.6–51.3	110–122	49.9–55.3	118–134	53.5–60.8
5'2"—157.5	102–110	46.3–49.9	107–119	48.5–54.0	115–131	52.2–59.4
5'1"—154.9	99–107	44.9–48.5	104–116	47.2–52.6	112–128	50.8–58.1
5'0"—152.4	96–104	43.6–47.2	101–113	45.8–51.3	109–125	49.4–56.7
4'11"—149.8	94–101	42.6–45.8	98–110	44.4–49.9	106–122	48.1–55.3
4'10"—147.3	92–98	41.7–44.4	96–107	43.5–48.5	104–119	47.2–54.0

*For women between eighteen and twenty-five, subtract one pound for each year under twenty-five.
**With shoes with two-inch heels.

given for three body frames—small, medium, and large. Body frames are usually measured by the width of various body parts like the shoulders and hips. By visually comparing your general body frame with others of your age and sex you may get a general idea how you would be classified. Your shirt or blouse size—small, medium, or large—also may be a useful guide as to your body frame.

Tables 10.1 and 10.2 have been developed for males and females twenty-five years of age and over. For women between the ages of eighteen and twenty-five, one pound should be subtracted for each year under twenty-five. As an example, a 5'8", 20-year-old woman with a medium frame would have a weight range of 123–138, or 5 pounds below the desirable level at age twenty-five. Although different age levels are not built into this scale, the range of values for each height and body frame helps to account for this. In general, as we get older our body weight should decrease slightly, although it usually increases. This may be more relevant to the sedentary individual, who may be developing more body fat and less muscle tissue, than to the active individual who may be maintaining good body composition through training.

Table 10.2 Desirable weights for males age twenty-five and over

Height/Weight male

Height* In Cm	Small frame Lb	Kg	Medium frame Lb	Kg	Large frame Lb	Kg
6'4"—193.0	164-175	74.4-79.4	172-190	78.0-86.2	182-204	82.6-92.6
6'3"—190.5	160-171	72.6-77.6	167-185	75.3-83.9	178-199	80.8-90.3
6'2"—188.0	156-167	70.8-75.8	162-180	73.5-81.7	173-194	78.5-88.0
6'1"—185.4	152-162	69.0-73.5	158-175	71.7-79.4	168-189	76.2-85.8
6'0"—182.9	148-158	67.1-71.7	154-170	69.9-77.1	164-184	74.4-83.5
5'11"—180.3	144-154	65.3-69.9	150-165	68.1-74.9	159-179	72.1-81.2
5'10"—177.8	140-150	63.5-68.1	146-160	66.2-72.6	155-174	70.3-78.9
5'9"—175.3	136-145	61.7-65.8	142-156	64.4-70.3	151-170	68.5-77.1
5'8"—172.7	132-141	59.9-64.0	138-152	62.6-69.0	147-166	66.7-75.3
5'7"—170.2	128-137	58.1-62.1	134-147	60.8-66.7	142-161	64.4-73.0
5'6"—167.6	124-133	56.2-60.3	130-143	59.0-64.9	138-156	62.6-70.8
5'5"—165.1	121-129	54.9-58.5	127-139	57.6-63.1	135-152	61.2-69.0
5'4"—162.6	118-126	53.5-57.2	124-136	56.2-61.7	132-148	59.9-67.1
5'3"—160.0	115-123	52.2-55.8	121-133	54.9-60.3	129-144	58.5-65.3
5'2"—157.5	112-120	50.8-54.4	118-129	53.5-58.5	126-141	57.2-64.0

*With shoes with one-inch heels.

Appendix E contains two tables that represent some average height and weight data for boys and girls age five to nineteen. These tables are more restricted than Tables 10.1 and 10.2 in that no body frame is specified nor is a range of weight values given. Hence, the values in Appendix E should be used only as a rough guide.

What are the values and limitations of height and weight charts?

Height and weight charts are based on measurements obtained from large populations of people. The data obtained is then treated statistically, and the values that tend to cluster towards the midpoint (the mean or median) are considered to be normal, average, or desirable. In relation to determining whether or not an individual possesses normal body weight for a given age and sex, these tables may have value as a screening device. If you are more than 10 percent below the average you may be considered to be underweight. Ten percent over the normal value may be classified as overweight and 20 percent above normal is classified as obese.

However, these tables reveal nothing to us of our body composition. Two individuals may be exactly the same height and weight and hence might be classified as having normal body weight. However, the distribution of their body weight might be so different that one individual could possibly be considered obese while the other might be considered very muscular.

What is the composition of our body?

Body composition and physical performance

The human body has been derived from the elements of the earth, twenty-five of which appear to be essential for normal physiological functioning. About 3–4 percent of our body is composed of various minerals, primarily calcium and phosphorus in the bones, but also including others such as iron, potassium, sodium, chloride, and magnesium. The vast majority of our body consists of four elements—carbon, hydrogen, oxygen, and nitrogen. These elements are the structural basis for body protein, carbohydrate, fats, and water.

The average adult body weight is approximately 60 percent water, the remaining 40 percent consisting of dry weight materials that exist in this internal water environment. Some tissues like the blood have a high water content, while others like bone tissue are relatively low. Under normal conditions the water concentration of a given tissue is regulated quite nicely relative to its needs. When we look at the percent of the body weight that may be attributed to a given body tissue, the weight of that tissue includes its normal water content. For the average adult male and female then, the following values represent approximate percentages of the body weight due to a specific tissue:

	Adult Male		*Adult Female*	
Muscle	43		36	
Bone	15		12	
Total fat	15		26	
Essential fat		3		15
Storage fat		12		11
Other tissues	27		26	
Total	100%		100%	

Body composition may be influenced by a number of factors such as age, sex, diet, and exercise. Age effects are significant during the developmental years as muscle and other body tissues are being formed. Also, during adulthood, muscle mass may decrease, probably due primarily to physical inactivity. There are some minor differences in body composition between boys and girls up to the age of puberty, but at this age the differences become fairly great. In general, the female deposits more fat beginning with puberty, while the male develops more muscle tissue. Diet can affect body composition over the short haul, such as in acute water restriction and starvation, but the main effects are seen over the long haul. For example, chronic overeating may lead to increased body fat stores. Physical activity may also be very influential, with a sound exercise program helping to build muscle and lose fat.

For our purposes, we may condense body composition into two components—body fat and lean body mass. **Total body fat** consists of both essential fat and storage fat. **Essential fat** is necessary in the structure of various cells and also for protection of some internal organs. **Storage fat** is simply a depot for excess energy, and the quantity of body fat in this form may vary considerably. **Lean body mass** consists of those tissues other than body fat. The muscle tissue is the main component of lean body mass, but the heart, liver, kidneys, and other organs are included also.

How can I measure my body composition?

A variety of methods have been developed to assess body composition, some relatively simple and others rather complex. Theoretically, all techniques are designed to measure the amount of body fat in comparison to lean body mass. The simpler techniques usually give you a rough approximation of body fatness while the more sophisticated procedures may give you an accurate body fat percent.

One simple test is to pinch the fat away from the underlying muscle at the back of the upper arm about midway between the shoulder and elbow. Hold this fat between your thumb and forefinger and measure the width of it with a ruler. Normal values are between 0.5 and 1.0 inch.

The ruler test is a second simple test. Lie flat on your back in a relaxed condition. Place a ruler on your stomach parallel with the long axis of the body. The surface of the abdomen between the ribs and the pubic area is normally flat, so the ruler should touch both the ribs and pubic bone.

The circumference test involves measurement of the girth of the chest at the level of the nipples and the girth of the abdomen at the level of the naval. In general, the chest should be larger than the abdomen by several inches. This test is sex biased, of course, for males only.

The above tests are relatively simple, but they do not provide you with an accurate assessment of your body composition as to body fat percentage. They may provide you with an idea that your body composition is not what it should be. In order to obtain a good estimate of your body fat percentage, you would need access to other more sophisticated techniques.

One of the most common techniques is **underwater weighing;** body weights are measured on land and underwater and lung volumes are determined. The technique is based on Archimedes' principle, noting that a body immersed in a fluid is acted upon by a buoyancy force in relation to the amount of fluid the body displaces. Since fat is less dense and muscle

Underwater weighing is one of the more accurate means for determining body composition.
(The Center for Fitness and Sport Research. The University of Michigan)

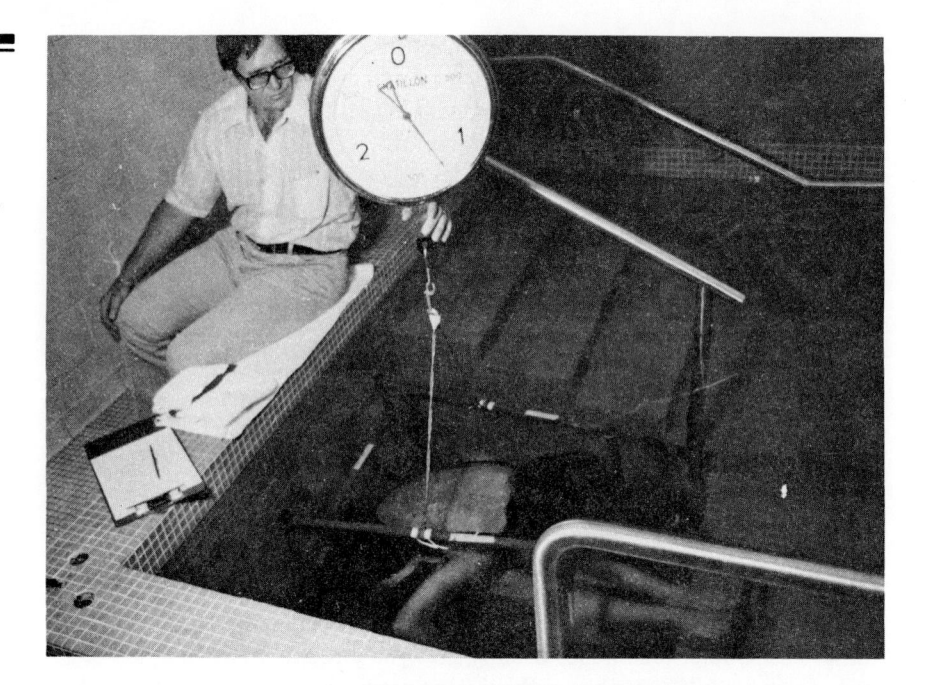

tissue more dense than water, a given weight of fat will displace more water and experience a greater buoyant effect than the corresponding weight of muscle tissue. By using appropriate formulae adjusting for lung volumes, fairly accurate measures of body fat percent may be obtained. Other sophisticated methods for determining body fat percent have been developed but need not be discussed here.

A good compromise between the simple practical tests and the more complex but accurate ones is the **skinfold technique.** Using special calipers, skinfold measurements are made at specific sites of the body depending upon which formula one is to use. A number of different skinfold tests have been developed, but it is beyond the scope of this text to go into detail relative to the merit of each test. If you have access to a skinfold caliper, or any caliper, you may get a simple idea of whether you have too much body fat. Simply measure the skinfold at the back of the arm as in the pinch test explained before, and compare your value with the following expressed in either millimeters or inches.

	Males		*Females*	
	mm	in	mm	in
Leanness	7	.25	10	.40
Acceptable	7–13	.25–.50	10–15	.40–.60
Overfat	13	.50	15	.60

For those who have access to a good skinfold caliper, several general equations for the calculation of body fat may be found in Appendix J.

Most of us do not need a highly accurate assessment of body composition. The critical question probably should be, "How can I tell if I am too fat?" Jean Mayer, the internationally renowned nutritionist, has suggested the use of the mirror test to answer this question. He suggests you look at yourself, nude, in a full length mirror using both a front and side view. This is usually all the evidence we need if we study ourselves objectively.

Does extra body weight have any effects upon physical performance?

In some sports, extra body weight might prove to be an advantage, especially in football, ice hockey, suma wrestling, and other sports where body contact may occur or where maintaining body stability is important. The effect of the extra weight may be neutralized, however, if the individual loses a corresponding amount of speed. Hence, increases in body weight for sports competition should maximize muscle mass and minimize body fat gains.

On the other hand, there are a variety of sports where excess body weight may serve to be a disadvantage. Whenever the body has to be moved rapidly or efficiently, excess weight in the form of body fat only serves as a burden. Take a good look at high jumpers, long jumpers, gymnasts, sprinters, and long distance runners. The amount of musculature may vary in each, but the body fat percentage is extremely low. Research has shown that professional football players also have low percentages of body fat. A high jumper can develop only so much power through muscular force when taking off. According to basic laws of physics, an extra five pounds of body fat would decrease the height to which the body center of gravity could be raised, thus decreasing the height that could probably be cleared. Five extra pounds of weight on a marathoner over a 26.2-mile course could add a considerable energy cost. Recent research has suggested that the loss of 10–12 pounds of fat could save 5–6 minutes in a marathon run. In essence, the body becomes a less efficient machine when it must transport extra weight that has no useful purpose. That extra weight is usually excess body fat.

How much fat should I have?

That is a complex question. There is a need for the essential body fat previously described; however, one can still perform efficiently with relatively low levels of storage fat, most of which is found just under the skin in the subcutaneous tissue.

Normal body fat percentage for men is about 12–15 percent while for women it is about 22–26 percent. This is not to say that amount is desirable. Male wrestlers and gymnasts function effectively at 5–8 percent body fat, while some elite male marathon runners have been reported to have only 2–3 percent. It is recommended that females who compete in sports similar to these have no more than 10 percent body fat. If you compete in a sport where excess body fat may be detrimental to your performance, then it is important to keep the percent low, while still maintaining good strength and cardiovascular endurance levels. For the typical male active individual, the recommended level may be 8–10 percent, while 12–14 percent is a sound level for the active female.

It should be noted that women who lose weight rapidly or who have very low levels of body fat may be more prone to secondary amenorrhea, a cessation of menstrual flow. More will be said about this in Chapter 17.

How many Calories are in a pound of body fat?

Calories and weight control

One pound is equivalent to 454 g. Since we know that 1 g of fat is equal to 9 Calories, it would appear that a pound of body fat would equal 4,086 Calories (9 × 454). However, the fat stored in adipose tissue contains a small amount of water, which reduces the caloric content of one pound of body fat to approximately 3,500 Calories.

Is the caloric concept of weight control valid?

The **caloric concept of weight control** is relatively simple. If you take in more Calories than you expend, you will gain weight. If you expend more than you take in, you lose weight. To maintain your body weight, caloric input and output must be equal. As far as we know, human energy systems are governed by the same laws of physics that rule all energy transformations. The first Law of Thermodynamics is as pertinent to us in the conservation and expenditure of our energy sources as it is to any other machine. Since a Calorie is a unit of energy, and since energy can neither be created nor destroyed, those Calories that we eat must either be expended in some way or conserved in the body. No substantial evidence is available to disprove the caloric theory. It is still the physical basis for body weight control.

Keep in mind, however, that the total body weight is made up of different components, those notable in weight control programs being body water, protein, and fat stores. Changes in these components may bring about body weight fluctuations that would appear to be contrary to the caloric concept. You may lose five pounds in an hour, but it will be water weight. Starvation techniques may lead to rapid weight losses, but a good proportion of the weight loss will be in body protein stores such as muscle mass. In programs to lose body weight, we usually desire to lose excess body fat, and certain dietary and exercise techniques may help to maximize fat losses while minimizing protein losses. The metabolism of human energy sources is complex, and although the caloric theory is valid relative to body weight control, one must be aware that weight changes will not always be in line with caloric input and output and that weight losses may not be due to body fat loss alone. These concepts are explored further in Chapters 12 and 13.

How many Calories do I need per day to maintain my body weight?

This depends upon a number of factors, notably age, body weight, sex, basal metabolic rate (BMR), and physical activity levels. The caloric requirement per kilogram body weight is very high during the early years of life when the child is developing and adding large amounts of body tissue. The Calorie/kilogram requirement decreases throughout the years from birth to old age. Body weight influences the total amount of daily Calories you need, but not the Calorie/kilogram level. The large individual simply needs more total calories to maintain body weight. Up to the age of eleven or twelve, the caloric needs of boys and girls are similar in terms of Calories/kilogram body weight. After puberty, however, males need more Calories/kilogram probably due to their greater percentage of muscle tissue in comparison to females. Individual variations in BMR may either increase or decrease daily caloric needs, depending on whether the BMR is above or below normal. Individual variations may vary 10–20 percent from normal. Physical activity levels above resting may have a very significant impact upon caloric needs, in some cases adding 1,000–1,500 or more Calories to the daily energy requirement. All of these factors make it difficult to make an exact recommendation relative to daily caloric needs. The Food and Nutrition Board of the National Research Council, for example, presents the following range of caloric needs for the average adult male and female aged 23–50: males (2,300–3,100); females (1,600–2,400). Additional ranges for other age levels are presented in Appendix A.

For children involved in normal activities and for adults involved in light work, Table 10.3 presents caloric needs based on body weight, expressed in both kilograms and pounds. To calculate your average caloric needs, simply multiply your body weight by the appropriate figure in the table. For example, a twenty-five-year-old woman who weighed 55 kg or 121 lbs would need approximately 1,980 Calories/day (55 $\times$ 36). Those values are, of course, only estimated averages and may be modified by the factors discussed above, primarily physical activity.

Table 10.3 Approximate daily caloric intake needed to maintain desirable body weight*

Age	Males C/lb	C/kg	Females C/lb	C/kg
11–14	27	60	22	48
15–18	19	42	17	38
19–22	19	41	17	38
23–50	17	38	16	36
51–75	15	34	15	33
76+	13	29	13	29

*These values are based upon the RDA for calories for typical Americans. Increased levels of physical activity will increase these values, while a very sedentary lifestyle will decrease them.

How much weight may I lose safely per week?

If you decide to lose weight without the guidance of a physician, the recommended maximal value is 2 lbs/week. Since there are 3,500 Calories in a pound of body fat, this would necessitate a deficit of 7,000 Calories for the week, or 1,000 Calories/day. For growing children, the general recommendation is only about 1 lb/week, or a daily 500 Calorie deficit.

As we shall see in Chapter 12, weight losses may not parallel the caloric deficit we incur during early stages of a weight reduction program, and the 2 lb limit may be adjusted during that time period. In addition, as mentioned previously, we want our weight loss to be body fat tissue, not lean body mass. A loss of 10 lbs of body weight may help improve physical performance, but if 5 lbs is muscle tissue, then performance could possibly deteriorate.

11
Gaining body weight—diet and exercise

Although most individuals in our society have a body weight problem and desire to lose excess poundage, there are some persons who want to gain weight, either to improve their physical appearance or to have greater body mass for athletic competition. This may be a typical feeling for the male teenage athlete undergoing a significant growth spurt during puberty without the necessary weight gain to fill out his body.

No matter what the reason for gaining body weight, you should be concerned about where the extra pounds will be stored. The energy balance equation works equally as well for gaining weight as it does for losing weight, but excess body fat in general will not improve physical appearance or physical performance. On the contrary, it may detract from both. To put on body weight you have to concentrate on means to increase lean body mass, particularly muscle tissue, with little or no increase in body fat stores. Although gaining weight is difficult for some individuals, this brief chapter will cover the main techniques most commonly recommended.

Why are some individuals underweight?

Basic considerations

Being significantly under your normal body weight may be due to several factors. Heredity may be an important factor, as your parents' genetic material may have predisposed their children toward leanness. For example, a high basal metabolic rate may have been acquired through your parents. Medical problems could adversely affect food intake and digestion, so a physician should be consulted to rule out nutritional problems caused by organic diseases, hormonal imbalance, chronic diarrhea, or inadequate absorption of nutrients. Social pressures, such as the strong desire of a teenage girl to have a very slender body, could lead to undernutrition; an extreme example is anorexia nervosa, a severe restriction in food intake primarily in females between the ages of twelve and twenty-one. Emotional problems may also affect food intake. In many cases, food intake is increased during periods of emotional crisis, but the appetite may also be depressed in some individuals for long periods of time.

Extreme underweight may be considered to be a symptom of malnutrition or undernutrition. It is important to determine the cause before prescribing a treatment. Our concern is with the individual who does not have any of these problems, medical or otherwise, but who simply is expending more calories than are being consumed. Input has to be increased, and the output has to be modified somewhat.

How can I gain lean body mass but not body fat?

When you initiate a program to gain body weight, the following guidelines may help to maximize your gains in muscle mass and keep body fat increases relatively low.

1. Set a reasonable goal within a certain time period. In general, about one to two pounds per week is a sound approach.

2. Calculate your average energy needs daily. Use Table 10.3 on page 160 to determine how many Calories you need just to maintain body weight.

3. In conjunction with the above point, check your living habits. Do you get enough rest and sleep? If not, you are burning more energy than the estimate obtained here. Get enough sleep and rest.

4. Keep a three to four day record of what you normally eat, recording your caloric intake from nutritional labels on the foods you eat or from values presented in Appendix B. See page 182 for additional guidelines. From this data, determine your average daily caloric intake. If this value is below your energy needs calculated under item two above, then this may be a reason why you are not gaining weight.

5. Use a good cloth or steel tape to take body measurements. Be sure you take them at the same points about once a week. Those body parts measured should include the neck, upper and lower arm, chest, abdomen, thigh and calf. This is to insure that body weight gains are proportionately distributed. You should look for good gains in the chest and limbs; the abdominal girth increase should be kept low because that is where the fat will increase the most.

6. Increase your caloric intake. It is not known exactly how many additional Calories are necessary to form one pound of muscle tissue in human beings, nor is it known in what form these Calories have to be consumed. However, the general recommendation is to increase your caloric intake approximately 350–700 Calories above your daily energy needs. The 2500–5000 extra Calories per week should be more than sufficient to help synthesize the 1–2 lbs of muscle mass. Muscle tissue consists of about 70 percent water, 22 percent protein, and the remainder in fat and carbohydrate. The total caloric value is only about 700–800 per pound of muscle tissue, but extra energy is needed to help synthesize the muscle tissue.

7. Start a weight training exercise program. This type of exercise program will serve as a stimulus to build muscle tissue.

In summary, adequate rest, increased caloric intake, and a proper weight training program may be very effective as a means to gain the right kind of body weight.

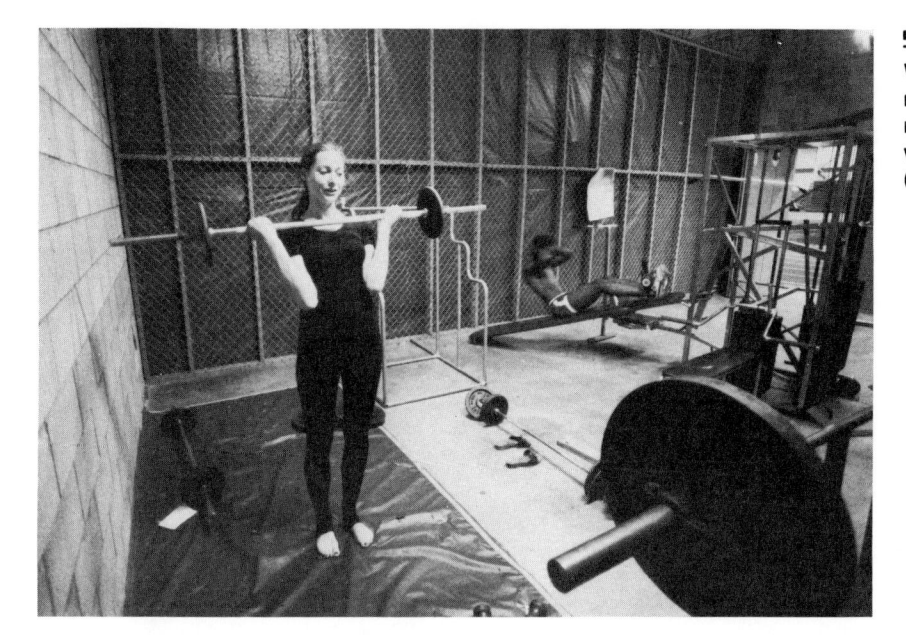

Weight training exercises may help an individual gain muscle mass and body weight.
(Robert Eckert/EKM-Nepenthe)

What is an example of a weight training program which may help me to gain weight?

The **overload principle** is the basis for all weight training programs. The use of weights places a stress on the muscle cell that is greater than it usually meets in normal activities. This overload stress stimulates the muscle to grow, to become stronger in order to more effectively overcome the increased resistance imposed by the weights. As the muscle continues to get stronger during your training program, you must increase the amount of resistance, the overload, in order to continue to get the proper stimulus for muscle growth. This is known as **progressive resistance** and is another basic principle of weight training.

Weight lifting is usually done in sets and repetitions. Although there is no single one best combination of sets and repetitions, usually two to three sets with six to ten repetitions will provide an adequate stimulus for muscle growth. A recommended combination for beginners is three sets with six repetitions in each set. The first step for each individual exercise is to determine the amount of weight that you can lift only for six repetitions. If you can do more than six repetitions, the weight is too light and you need to add more poundage. As you get stronger during the succeeding weeks, you will be able to lift the original weight more easily. When you can perform ten repetitions, add more weight to force you back down to six repetitions; this is the progressive resistance principle. Over the months, the weight will probably need to be increased several times as you continue to get stronger.

Exercise principles

Gaining body weight—diet and exercise

Table 11.1 Major muscle groups and common exercises for each

Body area	Muscle	Exercise	Description
Neck (3)*	Neck muscle group	Isometric neck exercise	Place heel of your hand on forehead. Push back with hand while trying to move head forward and down. Do also from back and both sides, resisting force of the hand.
Shoulder (9)	Deltoid	Dumbbell side raise	Standing with dumbbells in hands. Raise arms sideways to shoulder level.
Front of upper arm (4)	Biceps	Biceps curl	Standing with weight held in front of the body. Bend the elbows and bring the weight to the chest.
Back of upper arm (5)	Triceps	Triceps extension	Sitting with weight held behind head near neck, hands are close together, elbows bent. Straighten elbows and press weight over head to full extension.
Forearms (11)	Forearm muscle group	Wrist curl	Sitting, back of forearm resting on thighs, weight in hands with wrist just past the knees. Curl the weight towards the body, just moving the hands and wrist.
Chest (2)	Pectoralis Major	Bench press	Lying on back on a bench, weight held on chest, elbow bent. Press weight to full extension straight up.
Stomach (8)	Abdominal muscle group	Sit up	Lying on back, bent knees, hands behind head. Sit up and touch one elbow to opposite knee; do opposite elbow on alternate sit ups; use weight held behind head for additional resistance.
Upper back (7)	Trapezius	Shoulder shrug	Standing, weight held at arms length in front of body at waist level. Keep arms straight, hunch shoulders up towards ears.
Sides and middle back (1)	Latissimus dorsi	Pull up	Use pull up bar from full hang position; pull up until chin is over bar. Use weights hung from a special belt around your waist for additional resistance.
Front of thigh (6)	Quadriceps muscle group	Half squat	Standing with weight on shoulders (padded). Bend at knees until buttocks touches a chair placed behind you; do not sit on chair, just touch it lightly; return to standing position.

Table 11.1 *Continued*

Body area	Muscle	Exercise	Description
Back of thigh (6)	Hamstring muscle group	Half squat	Same as above.
Back of lower leg (10)	Calf muscle group	Heel raises	Sitting with weights across knees (padded), feet flat on floor. Raise up on toes bringing heel up as high as possible with toes still on the floor.

*Numbers correspond to body areas in Figure 11.1.

There are many different weight training routines to use, and a full discussion is beyond the scope of this book. However, one sound technique involves a **sequence of exercises** so that different muscles are overloaded in a logical order. For example, the first exercise in a sequence might stress the biceps muscle, the second the abdominals, the third the quadriceps of the thigh, and so forth. If you had ten exercises in your routine, they would be arranged in a sequence so that fatigue would not limit your lifting ability. After you perform one set of all ten exercises, you would then do a complete second set followed by the third set.

There are a number of different weight training apparatus available, such as Nautilus, Universal Gym, and other similar machines. They are effective for increasing strength and body weight; however, they are relatively expensive. Moreover, research has shown that they are no more effective than regular barbells and dumbbells, so called free weights, for strength and weight gains. These free weights are relatively inexpensive and can be utilized for a wide variety of exercises. They may also be constructed at home, using pipe or solid broomstick handles for the bar and different sized tin cans filled with cement for the weights.

In order to maximize lean body mass weight gains, all major muscle groups should be exercised. Table 11.1 presents the major muscle groups and a common exercise for each. Other exercises, if desired, may be obtained from books on weight training, but those in table 11.1 will provide you with a sound basic weight training program. Figure 11.1 depicts the areas to be stressed in sequence.

If exercise burns Calories, won't I lose weight on a weight training program?

Although exercise does cost Calories, the amount expended during weight training is relatively small. In any weight training workout, the amount of time actually spent lifting the weights is not great enough to use substantial amounts of Calories. For example, in an hour workout, only about ten minutes may be involved in actual exercise, the remainder being recovery

Figure 11.1.
Major muscle groups and sequence of exercises. The muscles should be exercised in the numerical sequence listed. Table 11.1 provides an appropriate exercise for each. *Legend:* 1—latissimus dorsi; 2—pectoralis major; 3—neck muscles; 4—biceps; 5—triceps; 6—quadriceps (front), hamstrings (back); 7—trapezius; 8—rectus abdominis; 9—deltoid; 10—gastrocnemius (calf); 11—forearm muscle group.

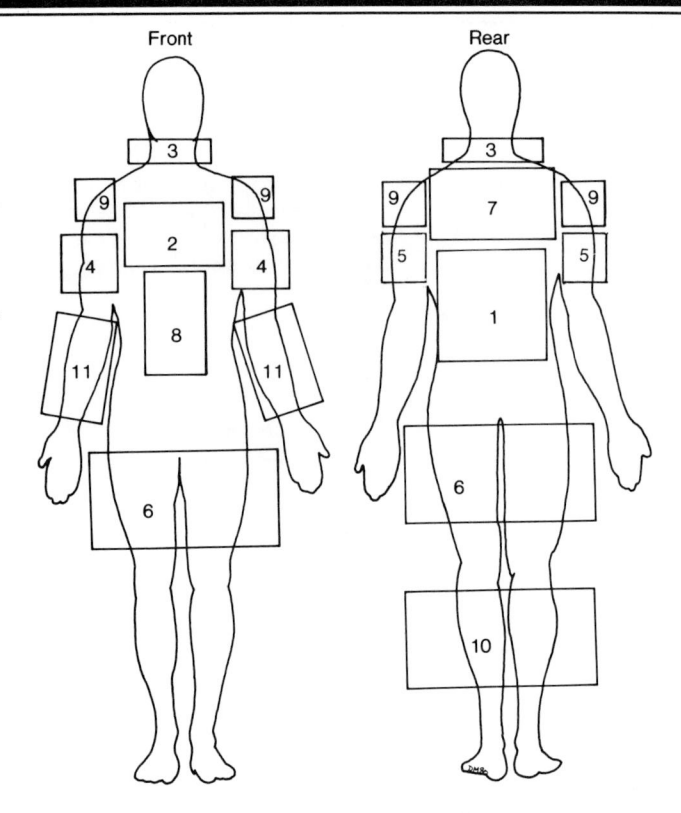

during each exercise. Although weight training can be a high intensity exercise, the duration is usually too short, therefore limiting the number of calories used. Research has shown that about 200–300 calories may be expended in a typical one-hour workout.

Should I do other exercises besides weight training during a weight gaining program?

Although weight training exercises are highly recommended if you are on a weight gaining program, you should not neglect exercises that will condition your cardiovascular system. These exercise programs do consume more Calories, so you would have to balance the expenditure with increased food intake. However, the expenditure does not need to be excessive in order to get a training effect. For example, running two miles a day would provide you with an adequate training effect for your heart, but it would only cost you about 200 C. This 200 C expenditure could be replaced easily by consuming two glasses of orange juice or similar small amounts of food. More will be said about this topic in Chapter 13.

What is an example of a balanced diet that will help me gain weight?

Nutritional principles

An individual on a weight gaining program should follow the same dietary principles advocated for those who are maintaining or even trying to lose body weight. The dietary intake should be selected from the Basic Four Food Groups, the major difference being that greater amounts of these foods need to be consumed in order to gain weight. In addition to the basic nutrition principles presented in Chapter 1, the following suggestions may be helpful for those trying to gain weight.

1. Decrease the intake of bulky foods that are filling yet contain few calories, such as bran and grain products, low-calorie vegetables, and foods with high water content. High calorie fruits and vegetables can provide adequate amounts of fiber.

2. Increase the intake of foods high in both nutrient and caloric content. Lean meats and poultry, milk, high caloric vegetables like corn, peas, and French fried potatoes, orange juice, dried fruit like dates, and similar types of foods are recommended.

3. Although the amount of saturated fat and simple sugars will normally increase in this type of diet, try to keep the intake of these types of foods to a minimum. Use vegetables fats and oils rather than animal fat substituting, for example, polyunsaturated margarine for butter.

4. Eat three balanced meals per day supplemented with two or three snacks. Some of the high-Calorie high-nutrient liquid meals on the market make good snacks; although convenient, they are relatively expensive.

5. There are many foods high in Calories and nutrients, and the costs may vary considerably. Gaining weight may be expensive, but wise selection of high energy content foods may help keep food costs down.

Table 11.2 presents an example of a high calorie diet plan based upon the Basic Four Food Group concept. It consists of three main meals and two snacks and totals 4500 C. Alternate foods may be substituted from the food exchange list presented in Appendix B.

This suggested diet would provide the necessary nutrients, calories, and protein essential to increased development of body mass. The total number of calories could be adjusted to meet individual needs as suggested earlier in this chapter.

Table 11.2 A high-Calorie diet based on the four food group concept

	Calories	Totals
Breakfast		
1 glass orange juice	110	
2 scrambled eggs with milk	220	
2 pieces whole wheat toast	140	
2 pats margarine	70	
2 tablespoons jelly	100	
1 glass milk	<u>160</u>	
		800
Mid-morning snack		
1 glass apricot nectar	140	
2 large figs	<u>120</u>	
		260
Lunch		
4 ounces lean sandwich meat	270	
2 slices whole wheat bread	140	
1 tablespoon mayonnaise	100	
1 large order french fried potatoes	300	
1 vegetable salad with 2 tablespoons french dressing	180	
3 granola cookies	150	
1 glass milk	<u>160</u>	
		1,300
Dinner		
1 cup cream of chicken soup	180	
5 ounces baked chicken breast	300	
1 sweet potato, candied	300	
1 cup of peas	160	
2 dinner rolls	170	
2 pats margarine	70	
1 piece apple pie	350	
1 glass milk	<u>160</u>	
		1,690
Evening snack		
½ cup dried peaches	210	
1 glass malted milk	<u>240</u>	
		450
Total Calories		4,500

Would such a high-Calorie diet be ill-advised for some individuals?

If there is a history of heart disease in the family or if an individual is known to have high blood lipid levels, this diet could be potentially harmful. The high fat content, even though primarily vegetable fat, could aggravate lipid metabolism in the body and possibly contribute in some way to the problems associated with coronary heart disease (CHD). Although being underweight is considered to lower one of the risk factors associated with CHD, any person initiating such a weight gaining program as advised here should be aware of his or her medical history.

Is protein supplementation necessary during a weight gaining program?

If we mean supplementation by expensive protein powders or pills, the answer is no. The average American diet provides sufficient protein to meet the needs of a weight gaining program, even more so if a high-Calorie diet is used as recommended above. A brief review of some mathematics presented in Chapter 4 on page 67 may help to substantiate the above statement. Although the daily RDA for protein is about 1 g/kg body weight, some authorities in sports nutrition have recommended 2.0–2.5 g/kg for the athlete who is training to increase muscle mass. The average weight for a male between the ages of 15–18 approximates 60–70 kg, or 132–154 lbs. Let's suppose we have a 16-year-old boy who weighs 132 lbs and wants to gain weight. His average caloric intake is 3,000 Calories. If the protein content of his diet is normal, about 15 percent, then 450 Calories would be derived from protein sources. Since 1 g protein is equal to 4 Calories, this would represent about 110 g protein. The 60-kg boy would receive about 1.8 g protein/kg (110/60). As an athlete in training, his caloric intake might approximate 4,000 Calories, resulting in a protein level of 2.5 g/kg. If he was on a diet similar to the one recommended earlier with 4,500 Calories, he would receive a whopping 2.8 g/kg. His protein needs would be met through a balanced diet. Expensive supplements as advertised in many sports magazines are unnecessary.

Looking at it another way, how much additional protein would you need to add 1 lb of muscle tissue per week? One pound of muscle is equal to 454 g, but only about 22 percent of this tissue, or about 100 g, is protein; the remainder is primarily water with a small amount of lipids. If we divide 100 g by 7 days, we would need approximately 14 g of protein per day above our normal protein requirements if we are in protein balance. However, the average American diet already contains extra protein, and this need is probably satisfied. Incidentally, 14 g of protein could be obtained in such small amounts of food as 1½ glasses of milk, 2 ounces of cheese, 2 scrambled eggs, or about 2 ounces of meat, fish, or poultry.

What about the use of drugs to increase body weight?

Certain drugs have been utilized by some athletes because of their potential to increase muscle mass. The synthetic **anabolic steroids,** patterned after the male sex hormone testosterone, may effectively increase muscle mass if used in conjunction with a weight training program and increased caloric intake. However, they are not recommended for the developing adolescent or young athlete as there are some possible inherent medical risks associated with their use. They may be used in some special cases, but only under the guidance of an experienced physician.

Losing body weight—dieting

Special diets may be designed by nutritionalists and dieticians for a variety of reasons. Certain nutrients in the diet may have an adverse effect on the health status of individuals with metabolic disorders. Persons with diabetes, high blood pressure, gout, and atherosclerosis are among those who need to restrict the intake of specific nutrients in their diets. However, when the average individual talks of dieting it is usually related to losing body weight.

As you are probably aware, there are literally hundreds of different diet plans available to help you lose weight. Hardly a month goes by without a new miracle diet being revealed in a leading magazine or Sunday newspaper supplement. No detailed analysis of the various published diets will be presented here. The interested reader is referred to the recent edition of *Rating The Diets* by the editors of Consumer Guide. Their book is well grounded in nutritional principles and evaluates the vast majority of the popular diets.

For the normal healthy individual attempting to lose weight, the principles of dieting are rather basic. One must reduce caloric intake in order to create a negative caloric balance. At the same time, the intake of essential nutrients must be assured. Body weight may also be lost by increased caloric output, such as by exercise, and this topic will be covered in the next chapter. This chapter centers upon some basic questions relative to the construction, implementation, and maintenance of a dietary program. The principles and suggestions advanced here apply to the overweight individual who wants to lose excess body fat, and also the person with normal body weight who may want to lose additional poundage in order to participate in a particular sport such as wrestling or long distance running.

Clinical obesity, or exteme overweight, is believed to be caused by a multitude of factors, paramount of which is the genetic background you obtain from your parents. If you are unfortunate enough to have the innate predisposition to store body fat more readily than others, your condition may merit medical supervision in order to effectively reduce excess body fat. The etiology and treatment of clinical obesity are complex and beyond the scope of this text. Nevertheless, the principles relative to reduced food intake and increased physical activity are still basic to any weight reduction program.

A comprehensive weight control program involves three components—diet, exercise and behavior modification.

Predicting body weight loss

How does the human body normally control its own weight?

A properly functioning human body is amazing. It can consume over a ton of food in a year and yet not gain one additional pound of body weight. In order to do this the body must possess an intricate regulatory system that helps to balance energy intake and output. At the present time we do not appear to know the exact physiological mechanisms whereby body weight is maintained relatively constant over long periods of time. Appetite regulation in relation to energy needs involves a complex interaction of numerous physiological factors including the appetite centers in the brain, feedback from peripheral centers outside the brain, metabolism of ingested food, and hormone action. Cultural background also influences food intake. These factors may interact to regulate the appetite on a short-term basis (daily basis), or on a long-term basis as in keeping the body weight constant for a year. However, although a great deal of research has been conducted relative to the regulation of food intake, a variety of theories currently exist. Let us try to summarize briefly the available evidence.

The control of appetite appears to be centered in the **hypothalamus,** a small center in the brain responsible for regulating many diverse automatic processes in the body. Two small subcenters affecting appetite exist in the hypothalamus. A **feeding center,** when activated, stimulates eating behavior. The **satiety center,** when stimulated, will inhibit the feeding center. Now what causes stimulation of these centers is where we are still involved in theories. The following may be involved in one way or another:

1. Stimulation of several senses like taste and smell. We are all aware of how these factors may stimulate or depress our appetites.

2. An empty or full stomach. An empty stomach may stimulate the feeding center by various neural pathways, whereas a full stomach may stimulate the satiety center.

3. Receptors in the hypothalamus, liver or elsewhere that may be able to monitor blood levels of various nutrients. In regards to this, three theories have been proposed centered around the three energy nutrients. The **glucostatic theory** suggests that food intake is related to changes in the levels of blood glucose. A fall will stimulate appetite whereas an increased blood glucose level would decrease appetite. The **lipostatic theory** suggests a similar mechanism for fats as does the **aminostatic theory** for amino acids, or protein.

4. A thermostat in the hypothalamus may respond to an increase in body temperature and inhibit the feeding center.

5. A number of different hormones in the body have been shown to affect feeding behavior, including insulin and thyroxine among several others.

Although all of the above may be involved in the physiological regulation of food intake, the ultimate control of body weight appears to be intimately involved with a balance of energy. Energy input and output, in the form of Calories, is responsible for the control of body weight on a long-term basis.

Is it a good idea to count Calories when attempting to lose body weight?

There are both pros and cons to counting Calories. On the con side, counting Calories may not be practical for many who are too busy to plan a daily menu centered around a caloric limit. How many Calories are in the lunch or dinner you eat out daily? Also, it is difficult to get an exact amount of Calories consumed, as the caloric content in foods may vary somewhat. For example, a large orange may contain twice the Calories of a small one. Certain slices of bread are larger than others and may have a correspondingly higher caloric content. And how about serving sizes? Can you picture three ounces of roast beef or an ounce of cheese? Moreover, some evidence suggests that not all Calories are the same. The caloric value of protein is the same as carbohydrate. However, the metabolism of protein in the body is more complex than carbohydrate and costs more energy. Protein metabolism may raise the metabolic rate, the so-called **specific dynamic action (SDA)** of protein, and increase the expenditure of Calories. Based upon these general statements, Calorie counting has not been highly recommended by some authors in the field of nutrition.

On the pro side, a low-Calorie diet, if designed properly, may serve as a guide to a balanced meal pattern containing all the essential nutrients. A 1,200 Calorie diet could be constructed so as to include low-Calorie foods from across the Basic Four Food Groups. Knowledge of food exchange lists, to be discussed later, will enable you to substitute one low-Calorie food for another in your daily menu. As you become familiar with the caloric content of various foods it becomes easier to select those which are low in Calories, but high in nutrient value, and to avoid those foods just the opposite, high in Calories and low in nutrients. It will require a little effort in the beginning phases of a diet to learn the Calories in a given quantity of a certain food, but once learned and incorporated into your life-style it is a valuable asset to possess when trying to lose weight. Knowledge, however, is not the total answer; your behavior should reflect your knowledge. For example, you may know that regular milk contains about eighty more Calories per glass than skim milk, but if you cannot develop a taste for skim milk then the advantage of your knowledge is lost in this instance.

Counting Calories may be useful during the early stages of a diet. You should study the Basic Four Food Groups and find those foods in each group low and high in Calories. Learn to estimate portion sizes. As you incorporate low-Calorie–high-nutrient foods into your diet, it will eventually become second nature to you, and you may eliminate the need to count Calories.

Once you have attained your desired weight, a good set of scales would be most helpful. Keeping track of your weight on a day-to-day basis will enable you to decrease your caloric intake for several days once you notice your weight beginning to increase again. Short-term prevention is more effective than long-term treatment. The dietary habits you acquire during the Calorie counting phase of your diet will help you during these short-term prevention periods.

How can you predict body weight loss through dieting?

As mentioned in Chapter 10, the human body is composed of different compounds, most commonly compartmentalized into body fat and lean body mass. Because of this fact, it is difficult to predict *exactly* how much body weight one will lose on any given diet, but an approximate value may be obtained. Remember, on a dietary program, weight loss may reflect decreases in body fat, body water, or muscle mass.

For our purposes, we will use the value of 3,500 Calorie to represent one pound of body fat, or body weight, loss. In order to lose one pound of body fat, you must create a 3,500 Calorie deficit. Thus, you must be aware of both your caloric intake and your caloric expenditure. The caloric intake reflects your dietary restrictions, while your caloric expenditure involves your basal metabolic rate and your normal daily activities. To calculate your daily energy expenditure, refer to Table 10.3 on page 160 to determine how many Calories per day you need to maintain your body weight. Once you calculate this value, subtract your dietary Calories from it; the result will be your daily **caloric deficit.** The number of days it takes for this daily deficit to reach 3,500 is how long it will take you to lose one pound. An example is presented below:

EXAMPLE: 35-year-old woman, weighs 140 pounds

1. From Table 10.3, Calories/lb needed to maintain body weight.
   16

2. Predicted total number of Calories to maintain body weight.
   16 × 140 = 2,240 Calories/day

3. Suggested diet = 1,240 Calories/day

4. Predicted caloric deficit
   2,240–1,240 = 1,000 Calories/day

Table 12.1   Approximate number of days required to lose weight for a given caloric deficit

Daily caloric deficit	To lose 5 pounds	To lose 10 pounds	To lose 15 pounds	To lose 20 pounds	To lose 25 pounds
100	175	350	525	700	875
200	87	175	262	350	438
300	58	116	175	232	292
400	44	88	131	176	219
500	35	70	105	140	175
600	29	58	87	116	146
700	25	50	75	100	125
800	22	44	66	88	109
900	19	39	58	78	97
1,000	17	35	52	70	88
1,250	14	28	42	56	70
1,500	12	23	35	46	58

See text for explanation.

5. Calories in one pound of fat = 3,500

6. Days to lose one pound of fat
   3,500 ÷ 1,000 = 3.5 days

The key point is the caloric deficit. You can approximate yours by following the example above for your own age, sex, body weight, and the number of Calories you select in your diet. Some suggestions relative to low-Calorie diets are presented later in this chapter.

Table 12.1 illustrates the importance of the caloric deficit in determining the rapidity of weight loss by dieting. The higher the deficit, the faster you lose weight. However, rapid weight loss programs are not usually desirable, and the dieter should realize a moderate caloric deficit, say 500 Calories/day, may effectively reduce weight in time and yet provide a satisfying diet.

This table is based upon the value of 3,500 Calories for a pound of body fat. There is one precaution, however. Once you lose five pounds, and every succeeding five pounds thereafter, you must adjust the number of Calories it takes to maintain your body weight, for now you are five pounds lighter. In our example above, the woman would need to reduce about 80 Calories (5 × 16 = 80 Calories) from her diet in order to keep the caloric deficit at 1,000 Calories/day.

Although these prediction methods are good for the long run, daily body weight changes may not coincide with daily caloric deficits.

Rapid and slow weight losses

Why does a person usually lose the most amount of weight during the first week on a reducing diet?

If you start a diet with a significant caloric deficit, say 1,000 Calories/day, it would normally take you about 3.5 days to lose one pound of body fat. However, body weight loss would be more rapid than this during the first several days, possibly totalling as much as 3–4 lbs. A large percentage of this weight loss would be due to a decrease in body carbohydrate and water stores. When you restrict your food intake, the body would then draw on its reserves to meet its energy needs. These reserves consist of both fat and carbohydrate stores, but much of the carbohydrate, stored as liver and muscle glycogen, could be used up in a day or so. Since 1 g of glycogen is stored with about 3 g of water, a significant weight loss could occur. For example, 300 g of glycogen, along with 900 g of water stored with it, would account for a loss of 1,200 g, or 1.2 kg; this would equal over 2.5 lbs alone. About 70 percent of the weight loss during the first few days of a reduced Calorie diet is due to body water losses. About 25 percent comes from body fat stores and 5 percent from protein tissue. It should be noted that loss of body protein is also accompanied by body water losses.

If you desired to lose a maximal amount of weight during a two to three day period, water restriction would increase weight loss even greater. However, this practice is not recommended as you would only be decreasing body water levels. They would return to normal when you returned to normal water intake. There is one additional point relative to body water. At the conclusion of your diet, if you return to a normal caloric diet to maintain your new body weight, you may experience a rapid weight gain of two or three pounds. This may represent a replenishment of your body glycogen stores with the accompanying water weight. It is important to keep in mind that rather large fluctuations in daily body weight, say in the order of two to three pounds, are not due to rapid changes in body fat or lean body mass; these fluctuations are due primarily to body water changes accompanying carbohydrate and protein losses.

Why does it become more difficult to lose weight after several weeks or months on a diet program?

Weight loss is rapid during the first few days on a diet, primarily due to water loss. Since water has no Calories, our caloric loss does not need to total 3,500 in order to lose one pound of weight. We may lose one pound of body weight with a deficit of only about 1,200 Calories, since 70 percent of the weight loss is water. The 1,200 Calories is mostly from carbohydrate and fat with a small amount of protein. However, by the end of the second week of dieting, water loss may account for only about 20 percent of body weight loss; one pound of weight loss will now cost us approximately 2,800 Calories. At the end of the third week, water losses are minimal. The energy deficit to lose one pound of body weight is now 3,500 Calories, the caloric value of one pound of body fat. In essence, as you continue your diet, weight losses cost you more Calories since less body water is being lost. At the end of three weeks, you can still be losing weight, but at a much slower rate than during the early stages.

Another factor also slows down the rate of weight loss. As you lose weight, you need fewer Calories to maintain your new body weight. Let's take an example. Suppose you weighed 200 lbs and from Table 10.3 you see that you need 17 Calories/pound body weight to maintain your weight. At 200 lbs this would represent 3,400 Calories/day (200 × 17). However, if your weight drops to 180 lbs after dieting for two months, you now need only 3,060 Calories, a difference of 340 Calories per day.

If you want to continue to have a standard caloric deficit, then you will have to adjust your caloric intake as you lose weight. Suppose our 200-pounder wanted to have a daily caloric deficit of 1,000 Calories. His diet should then contain about 2,400 Calories/day (3,400 − 1,000). However, once he is down to 180 lbs, his diet should now include only 2,060 Calories/day (3,060 − 1,000). If he did not adjust his diet from 2,400 Calories, then the daily deficit would only be 660 Calories/day, not the standard 1,000 he wanted. Weight loss would continue, but at a slower rate.

You should realize that the rate of weight loss will decrease as a natural consequence of your diet, but the weight you are losing at that point is primarily body fat. To keep a standard caloric deficit may also require an additional reduction in caloric intake as you progress on your diet. Knowledge of these factors may help you through the latter stages of a diet designed to attain a set weight goal.

How can I determine the number of Calories I eat daily?

Simply keep an accurate daily record of what you eat and then approximate the caloric value from Appendix B. Food intake should be recorded over a seven-day period, as one single day may give a biased value. Experiments have shown that this method may provide relatively accurate accounts of caloric intake if the amounts of food ingested are measured accurately. The main problem for most people is determining what and how much has been eaten. An eight-ounce glass of skim milk is easy to record, and the caloric value in Appendix B is rather precise. However, how many Calories are in a slice of pizza at your favorite Italian restaurant? How big was the piece? What is the caloric content of the cheese, green peppers, pepperoni and mushrooms? When we deal with complex food combinations such as this, our estimates of caloric content are not as precise, but we can get an approximate value.

Strategies to lose body weight

Although you may wish to use a ruler, a small measuring scale, and a measuring cup at home to accurately record the amount of food you eat, they are not practical for many dining situations. The following may serve as guidelines for you to record the type and amount of food you eat:

1. Keep a small notepad with you. Record the foods you have eaten as soon as possible, noting the kind of food and the amount.

2. Check the labels of the foods you eat. Most commercial products today have nutritional information listed, including the number of Calories per serving. Record this data when available.

3. You may wish to purchase one of the brand name calorie books available in many drugstores and supermarkets, although these are becoming obsolete with the current practice of nutritional labelling.

4. Calories for most fluids are given in relationship to ounces. For fluids remember that one cup or regular glass is about eight ounces. A regular canned drink is twelve ounces.

5. Calories for meat, poultry, fish and other related products are usually given by ounces. To get an idea of how many ounces are in these products, you could purchase a set weight of meat, say sixteen ounces, and cut it into four equal pieces. Each would weigh approximately four ounces. Get a mental picture of this size and use it as a guide to portion sizes.

6. For fruits and vegetables the caloric values are usually expressed relative to one-half cup or a small piece. At home, measure one-half cup of vegetables or fruit and place it in a bowl or on a plate. Again, make a mental picture of this serving size and use it as a reference. You are probably aware of the small size of most fruits and vegetables. Simply add about one-half the Calories for a medium piece and double the value for a large one.

7. For grain products, the Calories are most often expressed per serving, such as a slice of bread, a dinner roll, or a piece of pie. In these cases it is relatively easy to determine quantity. However, in some cases measurements are given, such as 1/12 of a ten-inch diameter cake. These are normal serving sizes, but you might make a mental image of a ruler and practice estimating sizes. Also, measure the length of your hand or your fingers. If the distance from your wrist to the end of your middle finger is seven inches, you have a handy (no pun intended) measuring device with you at all times. For dry cereals, the measure is usually 3/4 cup. Rice and pasta servings are 1/2 cup. Use the mental picture concept again to estimate quantities.

8. For substances such as jams, jellies, peanut butter, sugar, nondairy creamers, and related products, make a mental picture of a teaspoon and tablespoon. These are common means whereby Calories are given.

9. If a complex food, such as a special homemade casserole, is not included in Appendix B, try to find a food similar in nature to it in order to get an approximation of caloric content. Caloric values for many fast food restaurant items may be found in Appendix F.

10. Some specific examples of caloric values are presented in Appendix B.

Through experience you should be able to readily identify, within a small error range, the quantities of food you eat. This is helpful not only for determining your caloric intake, but may also serve as a motivational device to restrict portion sizes when you are on a weight loss diet.

The following represents an example of how you might record one meal and calculate the caloric intake from Appendix B.

BREAKFAST

Food	Quantity	Calories
Milk, skim	1 glass, 8 ounces	80
Eggs	2, poached	160
Toast, whole wheat	2 slices	140
with butter	2 pats	90
with jelly	1 tablespoon	50
Orange juice, frozen diluted with water	1 glass, 6 ounces	80
Coffee	1 cup, 8 ounces	0
with sugar	1 teaspoon	20
	TOTAL	620

Computer programs are available to calculate caloric intake as well as a number of nutrients. Local hospitals and/or universities should be able to direct you to a source. Moreover, nutritional analysis software programs are available for personal home computers.

Aside from determining my caloric intake, is there anything else I can do to assess my eating habits?

Although not all weight control experts recommend that you keep a diary of your daily activities, some suggest it may help you to identify some **behavioral patterns** that may contribute to overeating and extra body weight. The following are some of the factors that might be recorded each time you eat, along with a brief explanation of their possible importance.

1. Type of food and amount. This may be related to the other factors. For example, do you eat a specific type of food during your snacks?

2. Meal or snack. You may find yourself snacking four or five times a day.

Losing body weight—dieting

3. Time of day. Do you eat at regular hours or have a full meal just before retiring at night?

4. Degree of hunger. How hungry were you when you ate—very hungry or not hungry at all? You may be snacking when not hungry.

5. Activity. What were you doing while eating? You may find TV watching and eating snack foods are related.

6. Location. Where do you eat? The office cafeteria may be the place you eat a high-Calorie meal.

7. Persons involved. Who do you eat with? Do you eat more when alone or with others? Being with certain people may trigger overeating.

8. Emotional feelings. How do you feel when eating? You might eat more when depressed than when happy, or vice versa.

Recording this information may make you aware of the circumstances under which you tend to overeat. This awareness may be useful to help implement behavioral changes that may make dieting easier.

Other than changing my diet are there other strategies I could use to help lose body weight?

Changing dietary habits ofttimes involves a significant change in behavior, and many different techniques ranging from the bizarre to the pragmatic have been utilized in attempts to modify eating behavior. In general, these techniques have centered around the elimination of cues that stimulate eating, the substitution of some other activity for eating, or the development of self-discipline. These techniques are often referred to as *behavior modification* strategies.

Although we may be unaware of it, many cues in our life-style may trigger an eating response. Keeping a diary of your eating behavior as suggested above may give you some insight relative to situations in which you normally eat. For example, TV commercials may be associated with a rush to the refrigerator for a quick snack. By eliminating tempting cues, food intake may be decreased. The following are a few suggestions:

1. Keep food out of sight. Put it in sealed containers or cupboards. A bowl of peanuts sitting on a table is hard to bypass without taking a handful. If snacks are a part of your daily meal plan, have low-Calorie vegetables like celery and carrots available.

2. If possible, do your food shopping when you are not hungry. Plan what you are going to eat and prepare a shopping list. Do not deviate from this list. If you do not buy the high-Calorie food, you will not eat it.

3. Have a designated eating space such as the kitchen table. Do not eat anywhere in the house except there.

4. Change the act of eating. Eat slowly. Do not do anything else when you are eating, such as reading the paper or watching TV. Enjoy what you eat.

5. Substitute behaviors can help reduce eating. If you feel yourself getting hungry do something physical like a brief walk. If possible, exercise before eating a meal as it may help to curb your appetite. Get involved in various activities that will keep you active with other people and away from a sedentary night routine.

When breaking any well-established habit, self-discipline or will power is the key. We are constantly bombarded with food stimuli from TV, other advertising media, and our family and friends which may make it difficult to adhere to a weight reduction diet. You must be convinced that reduced body weight will enhance your self-concept, and you must establish this as a high priority in your life. If you do, the will power to refuse unnecessary food intake should be a natural consequence. Weighing yourself every morning may provide you with a positive stimulus to help reinforce your will power. If you need moral support, join Weight Watchers International or a similar organization.

How may I modify my diet to lose weight?

As you probably know by now, you will have to reduce the total number of Calories you ingest. There are literally hundreds of diets available to help you cut Calorie intake, some may be potentially hazardous to your health while others are highly recommended. For example, the high-fat/high-protein diets may help you lose weight but may contribute to cardiovascular disease problems in certain individuals due to high fat and cholesterol content. One-food diets such as the rice diet or the bananas-and-milk diet may be deficient in certain key nutrients. On the other hand, highly recommended diets are based upon sound nutritional principles and are also designed to satisfy the individual's personal food tastes.

Dietary modifications

Research with dieters has shown that any weight reduction diet, to be effective, should adhere to the following principles.

1. It should be low in Calories and yet supply all nutrients essential to normal body functions.

2. It should contain foods that appeal to your taste and help to prevent hunger sensations between meals.

3. It should be able to be accommodated within your current life-style, being easily obtainable whether you eat most of your meals at home or you dine out frequently.

4. It should be a life-long diet, one which will satisfy the above three principles once you attain your desired weight.

A key dietary principle is to select foods high in nutrients but low in Calories.
(David Corona)

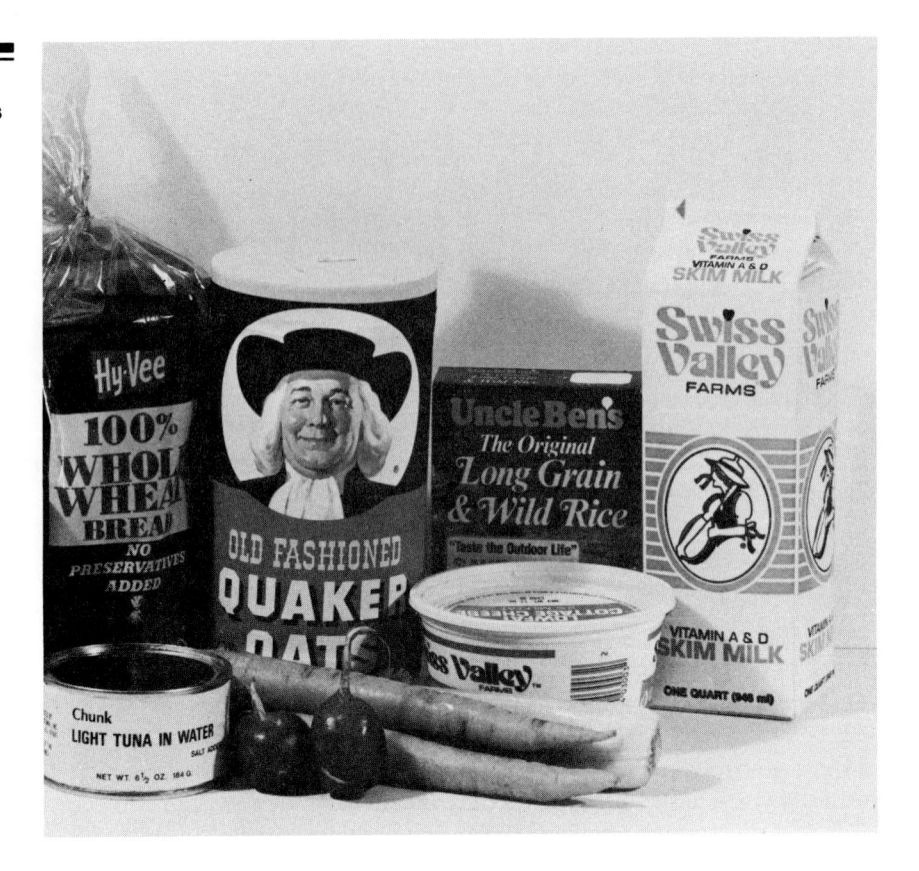

As for the diet itself, there are a variety of helpful suggestions in the battle against Calories.

1. The key principle is to select low-Calorie/high-nutrient foods from across the Basic Four Food Groups—milk, meat, fruits and vegetables, and breads and cereals. Avoid refined processed foods as much as possible and include more natural unrefined products in your diet.

2. Milk group products are excellent sources of protein but may contain excessive Calories unless the fat is removed. Use skim milk, low-fat cottage cheese, low-fat yogurt, and nonfat dried milk instead of their high fat counterparts like whole milk, sour cream, and powdered creamers.

3. The meat group products are also sources of protein and many other nutrients, but also may contain excessive fat Calories. Use leaner cuts of meat, and also trim away excess fat; broil or bake your meats. Fish, chicken, and eggs are excellent low-Calorie substitutes.

4. Fruits and vegetables may provide many of the necessary vitamins and minerals. They may provide bulk to the diet and a sensation of fullness without excessive amounts of Calories. Low-Calorie items like carrots, radishes, and celery are highly nutritious snacks for munching.

5. The grain products are also high in vitamins and minerals. Use whole grain breads, cereals, brown rice, oatmeal, beans, and bran products for dietary fiber.

6. Fluid intake should remain high, especially on high-protein diets as the water is necessary to eliminate protein waste products from the body. Water is the recommended fluid, although diet drinks and unsweetened coffee and tea may be used.

7. Salt intake should be limited to that which occurs naturally in our foods. Try to use dry herbs, spices, and other nonsalt seasonings as substitutes to flavor your food.

8. Avoid high-Calorie foods like salad dressings, butter, margarine, and cooking oil. Substitute low-Calorie dietary versions instead.

9. Avoid alcohol as much as possible. It is high in Calories and zero in nutrient value. One gram of alcohol is equal to seven Calories, almost twice the value of protein and carbohydrate.

10. Instead of two or three large meals a day, eat five or six smaller ones. Research has shown that this may help in the fight against obesity and help to control sensations of hunger between meals.

11. Another approach is to cut the size of the portion you eat. Cook only half of an eight-ounce steak rather than the whole piece.

12. Learn what foods are low in Calories in each of the four food groups and incorporate those palatable to you in your diet. The key to a lifelong weight maintenance diet is your knowledge of sound nutritional principles and the application of this knowledge to the design of your personal diet. Study and learn the approximate caloric values of the foods in the exchange lists in Appendix B.

What is an example of a nutritionally balanced low-Calorie diet?

As mentioned above, low-Calorie foods must be selected wisely from among the Basic Four Food Groups. For our purposes here six different classifications will be used. This conforms to the common food exchange systems designed by such organizations as the Mayo Clinic and the American Dietetic Association. In essence, fruit and vegetables are listed separately and a fat group has been added.

A food exchange list may be found in Appendix B. If you study this list carefully, you will begin to get an appreciation for the amount of Calories in the foods you eat. In ascending order, the caloric content of one serving from each of the six groups is as follows:

1 vegetable exchange	= 25 Calories
1 fruit exchange	= 40 Calories
1 fat exchange	= 45 Calories
1 meat exchange	= 55 Calories
1 bread exchange	= 70 Calories
1 milk exchange	= 80 Calories

Table 12.2 presents a suggested meal pattern as developed by the Committee on Dietetics of the Mayo Clinic. The total caloric values are close approximations for a three-meal pattern. If you decide to include snacks in your diet, such as a fruit or vegetable, then remove it from one of the main meals. The beverages, other than milk, should contain no Calories. Note that under the total exchange system, starchy vegetables such as potatoes are included in the bread group because their caloric content is similar. If you need a diet higher than 1,400 Calories do a little addition or multiplication. For example, if you double the portions in the 800 diet you will have 1,600 Calories. Adding the 800 and 1,000 calorie diets will give you 1,800 Calories, and so on.

Appropriate food exchanges for each of the six classifications are presented in Appendix B. Take a few minutes and construct a diet for yourself from this list. Use the following as a guideline and do your calculations below.

Personal Diet

1. Calculate the number of Calories you want per day. See page 156 for guidelines.

2. Use Table 12.2 to determine how many servings you need from each group. For example, if you want 2,400 Calories per day, you can multiply the number of servings in the 800 Calorie diet by a factor of 3, or those in the 1,200 Calorie diet by 2. The results will not be identical but will provide you with adequate nutrition.

3. Multiply the number of servings by the Calories per serving in order to get the total Calories. Add the total Calories column to get total daily intake.

4. Select appropriate foods from the exchange list in Appendix B.

5. If you would prefer to use a Calorie restricted diet based upon the food exchange lists, Appendix I presents balanced diets of 1,000, 1,200, 1,500, 2,000, 2,200, 2,500, and 3,000 Calories.

Table 12.2 Suggested meal pattern based on the food exchange list

	800 Calorie diet	1,000 Calorie diet	1,200 Calorie diet	1,400 Calorie diet
Breakfast				
Milk	--	--	--	1
Meat	1	1	1	1
Fruit	1	1	1	1
Vegetable	--	--	--	--
Bread	1	1	1	1
Fat	--	1	1	1
Beverage	1	1	1	1
Lunch				
Milk	1	1	1	1
Meat	2	3	3	3
Fruit	1	1	1	1
Vegetable	1	1	1	1
Bread	--	--	1	2
Fat	--	--	1	1
Beverage	1	1	1	1
Dinner				
Milk	1	1	1	1
Meat	3	3	3	4
Fruit	1	1	1	1
Vegetable	1	1	1	1
Bread	--	1	2	2
Fat	--	--	1	1
Beverage	--	--	1	1

See Appendix B for food exchange lists. Note that some starchy vegetables are included in the bread list. Beverages should contain no Calories. Foods should not be fried or prepared in fat products unless it is counted as the fat group. Low-Calorie vegetables like lettuce and radishes may be used as salads to complement the meals.

Personal Diet

CALORIES _____

Food Group	Number of servings	Calories per serving	Total Calories	Foods selected
Breakfast				
Milk		80		
Meat		55		
Fruit		40		
Vegetable		25		
Bread		70		
Fat		45		
Beverage		0		
Lunch				
Milk		80		
Meat		55		
Fruit		40		
Vegetable		25		
Bread		70		
Fat		45		
Beverage		0		
Dinner				
Milk		80		
Meat		55		
Fruit		40		
Vegetable		25		
Bread		70		
Fat		45		
Beverage		0		

Although most simple foods may be accounted for by use of the exchange lists, mixed-food groups like macaroni and cheese pose a small problem. Although it takes a little effort, you may consult a table of the nutritive value of foods found in most basic nutrition books and get a breakdown of the caloric, protein, carbohydrate, and fat content and then categorize it as one or several of the exchange foods.

Table 12.3 presents a breakdown of the carbohydrate, fat, protein, and caloric content of each food exchange. From a nutritive value of food table we find that one cup of macaroni and cheese contains 40 g of carbohydrate, 22 g of fat, and 17 g of protein for a total of 430 Calories. We know macaroni is in the bread group, so 40 g would be about 2.5 bread exchanges (40 g carbohydrate divided by 15 g in one bread exchange). Cheddar cheese is a high fat meat exchange and so our 17 g would account for about two meat plus 2 fat exchanges. Butter or margarine in the macaroni and

Table 12.3 Carbohydrate, fat, protein, and Calories in the six food exchanges

Food exchange	Carbohydrate	Fat	Protein	Calories
Vegetables	5	0	2	25
Fruits	10	0	0	40
Fat	0	5	0	45
Meat	0	3	7	55
Bread	15	0	2	70
Milk	12	0	8	80

Carbohydrate, fat, and protein in grams.
1 g carbohydrate   = 4 Calories
1 g fat   = 9 Calories
1 g protein   = 4 Calories

cheese would account for the remaining two fat exchanges. In total, we could approximate the macaroni and cheese as containing two and one-half bread exchanges, two meat exchanges, and four fat exchanges. If you carry out the mathematics, this would equal about 38 g carbohydrate, 19 g protein, and 16 g fat.

This would be a tedious process to use for all the complex foods we eat. If you simply know the high protein foods belong to the meat and milk groups, high fat foods belong to the fat and meat groups, and that high carbohydrate foods are in the fruit, vegetable, bread, and milk groups, you should be able to make a fair guess as to which food exchange a given product belongs.

Is fasting an effective and desirable means to lose body weight?

Although complete **fasting,** or starvation, may cause a rather rapid initial decrease in body weight, it is not a recommended long-range dietary program for the average individual. Much of this early weight loss is due primarily to water depletion and some significant decreases in lean body mass. It has been theorized that since the lean tissues of the body use fat as an energy source, these decreases in lean tissue actually may decrease somewhat the ability to use body fat stores. Moreover, diets with less than 800 Calories per day may lower the BMR. A better compromise for the healthy individual who wants to lose weight is to consume a low-Calorie balanced diet (minimum of 1200 Calories/day) and to exercise the major muscles of the body. This technique will help to prevent significant losses of lean body mass, particularly muscle tissue.

While fasting is not recommended as a long-term diet program for the slightly overweight individual, it has been shown to be an effective technique with very obese patients who are under medical supervision. It is recommended that any individual contemplating a long-range fasting program should consult their physician, as certain medical conditions may be aggravated during starvation. Liver and kidney functions may be impaired, while gouty arthritis, anemia, hypoglycemia, and low blood pressure may possibly develop in some individuals.

There apparently is no harm caused by a one- or two-day fast for healthy individuals, although it may cause some drop in blood sugar and some sensation of fatigue. The loss of body fluids and minerals may also contribute to decreased endurance capacity. Research has shown that healthy individuals appear to be weak physically and are apathetic towards exercise following a period of starvation. Their responses to physical work tasks exhibit some decreases in anaerobic capacity. However, as the individual becomes familiar with repeated one- to two-day fasts, the body begins to make more favorable physiological adaptations. Moreover, even small amounts of Calories, about 450–500 Calories/day, along with vitamin and mineral supplements have been shown to help prevent significant decreases in physical performance during ten days of starvation. Nevertheless, low body water levels and loss of body protein did occur.

Starvation techniques, along with water deprivation, have been utilized by athletes who are involved in sports where a lower body weight might confer a slight advantage or enable them to compete in a given weight class. Wrestling, boxing, gymnastics, lightweight football, and crew are prime examples. Although these weight reduction techniques for young boys and girls have been denounced by many sports medicine authorities, the practices still exist and probably will continue until practical and enforcable weight control standards for such sports are available. Further discussion of this topic is presented in Chapter 17.

Losing body weight—exercise

13

Humans are meticulously designed for physical activity, and yet our modern mechanical age has eliminated many of the opportunities we once had to incorporate moderate physical activity as a natural part of our lives. The regulation of food intake was never designed, through the evolutionary process, to adapt to the highly mechanized conditions in today's society. Hence, the combination of overeating and inactivity has led to increasing levels of overweight and obesity, one of the major health problems in the United States today. Dr. Jean Mayer, an international authority on weight control, has reported that no single factor is more frequently responsible for the development of obesity than lack of physical exercise.

A large body of knowledge substantiates the point that exercise can help to reduce and control body weight. In addition, recent national surveys have indicated that when people want to become more physically fit, they also have become more conscious of their nutritional practices. A proper exercise program may be an effective means to reduce excess body fat, and the purpose of this chapter is to explore the role exercise may play in this regard.

What role does exercise play in weight reduction?

Simply put, exercise raises the levels of energy expenditure and may help unbalance the caloric equation so that energy output is greater than energy input. Over time, the individual will lose excess body fat. As mentioned in chapter 9, the metabolic rate may be increased tremendously during exercise. For example, while the average person may expend only about 60–70 Calories per hour during rest, this value may approach 1,000 Calories per hour during a sustained high level activity such as running, swimming, or bicycling. Fat is mobilized from the body's fat cells in order to supply energy to the muscle cells. Hence, body fat stores are reduced.

The role of exercise

A major misconception exists that may deter one from initiating an exercise program for weight control. Many individuals believe that exercise is a poor means to lose body weight because it expends so few Calories. For example, they have heard that you have to jog about thirty-five miles to lose a pound of body fat. Since the average person uses approximately 100 C per mile, and since one pound of body fat contains about 3,500 C, there is some truth to that statement. However, you must look at the **long haul concept** of weight control. Jogging about two miles a day will expend about 6,000 C in a month, accounting for almost two pounds of body fat. Over six to eight months or longer, the weight loss may be substantial.

Figure 13.1.
Effect of speed (mph) and gross body weight (lb) on energy expenditure (Calories/minutes) of **walking.** The heavier the individual, the greater the expenditure of Calories for any given speed of walking. The same would be true for running and other physical activities in which the body must be moved by foot. (From *Textbook of Work Physiology* by P. O. Astrand and K. Rodahl. Copyright © 1977, by McGraw-Hill, Inc. Used with permission of McGraw-Hill Book Company.)

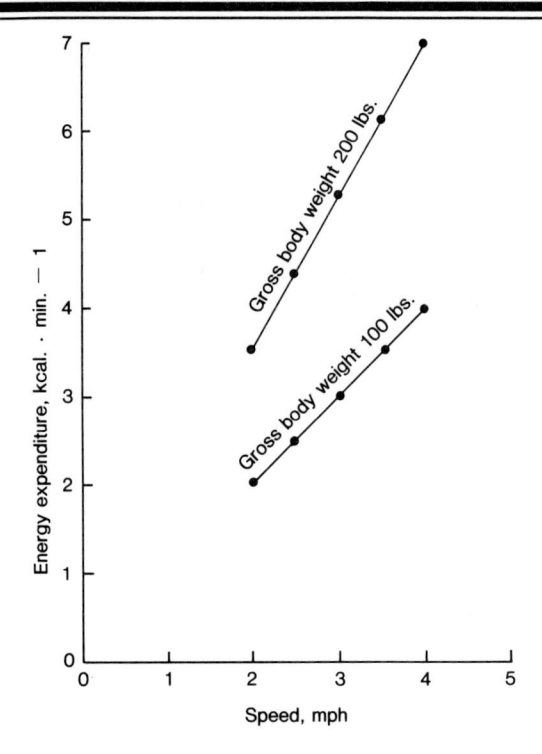

Besides the direct effect of increased energy output during exercise, research has shown that the metabolic rate also may remain elevated for several hours after exercise, especially if the exercise session had been strenuous. The increased body temperature and adrenalin levels may produce these **metabolic aftereffects of exercise,** which may account for about a total of 50 Calories more than what would normally be expended at rest. Exercising on a daily basis, this could account for about an extra half pound of body fat per month.

If you are overweight, the same amount of exercise will cost you more Calories than your leaner counterpart. Since you have more weight to move, it will cost you more energy and will result in a greater loss of body fat in the long run. Based on information provided on page 132, the energy cost of jogging one mile would be 70 Calories for the 100-pound individual and 140 for someone twice that weight. Figure 13.1 depicts this concept graphically for one type of exercise—walking.

It is generally recognized that prevention of obesity or excess body weight is more effective than treatment. Most people do not become overweight overnight, but rather accumulate an extra 75–150 Calories per day, which over time will lead to excess fat tissue. A daily exercise program could easily counteract the effect of these additional Calories.

Properly designed and executed, an exercise regimen can be a very effective means to control body weight. Other fringe benefits, such as a reduction in some coronary heart disease risk factors, may also accrue to the physically fit individual.

Does exercise affect the appetite?

In the long run, in general, increased energy expenditure through exercise is counterbalanced by an increased food intake. This is one of the major mechanisms whereby normal body weight is controlled in the average individual. However, this may not be universally true for sedentary individuals or those who are obese. Research has shown that sedentary persons who begin an exercise program do not increase food consumption above normal. The same has been shown for obese individuals, the appetite actually decreasing in some cases.

An important concern for the active individual is the fact that the appetite may not normally decrease with a decreased activity level. If you are physically active, but then must curtail your activity for an injury or some other reason, the appetite may remain elevated above what you need to maintain body weight at your reduced energy levels. Body fat will increase. Hence, you must reduce your food intake in order to balance the caloric equation or suffer the consequences.

As shall be discussed later, a combined diet and exercise program would be most effective as a means to body weight control. In this regard, exercise may be used to curb the appetite at an appropriate time. Exercise will raise the body temperature and also stimulate the secretion of several hormones in the body, notably adrenalin, both of which have been hypothesized to depress the appetite. If you exercise before a meal, your food intake may be reduced considerably. Try it and see if it works for you. If you have the facilities available, a good half-hour of exercise may be an effective substitute for a large lunch. You may lose Calories two ways, expending them through exercise and replacing the large lunch with a low-Calorie nutritious snack.

What types of exercise programs are most effective for losing body fat?

As you are probably well aware, there are a number of different exercise programs available to lose body weight. Perusal of the daily newspaper reveals numerous advertisements for weight reduction programs sponsored by various commercial physical fitness businesses. Weight training with sophisticated equipment, slimnastics exercises, aerobic dancing, and special exercise apparatus are a few of the approaches often advertised as the best means to lose body fat fast. The truth is that you do not need any special apparatus or any specially designed program. You can design your own once you know a few basic principles about exercise and energy expenditure.

The key points to any exercise program to lose body fat are as follows:

1. It must involve large muscle groups. The muscles of the legs comprise a good portion of the total body mass, as do the muscles of the arms. Many people do not realize that the major muscles in the chest and back are attached to the upper arm and are actively involved in almost all arm movements. Running and bicycling primarily involve the legs while swimming primarily stresses the arms. These are good large muscle activities, although there are a host of others.

2. The second factor is the intensity level. The higher the **exercise intensity,** the more Calories you expend. Per unit of time, walking uses less Calories than jogging, which uses less Calories than fast running. Simply put, it costs you more energy to move your body weight at a faster pace. However, there is an optimal intensity level for each person depending on how long the exercise will last. You can run at a very high intensity for fifty yards, but you certainly could not maintain that same fast pace for two miles. Intensity and duration are interrelated.

   To get an idea of exercises with high intensity, check Appendix C relative to your body weight. Listing those activities with higher caloric expenditure per minute may suggest several that you could blend into your life-style.

3. Probably the most important factor in energy expenditure is the duration of the exercise. In swimming, bicycling, running, or walking, distance is the key. For example, running a mile will cost the average-sized individual about 100 Calories. Five miles would approximate 500 Calories. Running one mile a day would take over one month to lose one pound of fat, whereas five miles a day would shorten the time span to about one week. Thus, if the purpose of the exercise program is to lose weight, the individual should stress the duration concept.

   One of the key points about the **duration concept** is the notion of distance traveled rather than time. For example, an hour of tennis and running are both good exercises. However, the runner will expend considerably more calories due to the fact that the activity is continuous. The tennis player has a number of rest periods in which the energy expenditure is lower. Consequently, at the end of an hour's activity, the runner may have expended two to three times more Calories than the tennis player

4. **Exercise frequency** complements duration and intensity. Frequency of exercise refers to how often each week you participate. As would appear obvious, the more often you exercise, the greater the total weekly caloric expenditure. In general, three to four times per week would be satisfactory, provided duration and intensity were adequate, but six to seven times would just about double your caloric output. A daily exercise program is recommended.

5. An important factor is enjoyment of the exercise. To be effective in the long run, you should select an activity that you enjoy, yet will help expend Calories because it has a recommended intensity level and/or can be performed for a long time. For example, you may not enjoy jogging or running, but other activities may be substituted. Fast walking with a vigorous arm action, swimming, bicycling, tennis, handball, racquetball, and a variety of activities may produce a greater feeling of enjoyment and still burn a considerable number of Calories. Enjoy your exercise. Try to make it a life-long habit.

6. Practicality is another important factor. You may enjoy swimming, tennis, racquetball, and a variety of other sports, but lack of facilities, poor weather conditions, or high costs may limit your ability to participate. For the active person who travels, this may be a major concern.

You have probably noticed by now that there exists an underlying bias towards running throughout this book. It is probably because, to me, it satisfies all the previously mentioned criteria necessary to maintain proper body weight. Moreover, it is very practical. All you need is a good pair of shoes and proper clothes for the weather and nothing short of an injury should deter you from your daily exercise routine, be it fast walking, jogging, or running. You may not learn to enjoy jogging, but it can be a very practical substitute on those days when you cannot participate in your regular physical activity.

If I am inactive now, are there any precautions of which I should be aware before beginning an exercise program for weight reduction?

Before initiating any exercise program, you should be aware of any personal medical problems that could possibly be aggravated. This is especially important in weight reduction exercise programs where the main stress is placed on the heart and blood vessels, the cardiovascular (CV) system. As diseases of the CV system are age related, individuals over the age of thirty-five are advised to have a medical checkup prior to initiating such a program.

Designing your own exercise program

Your initial level of physical fitness is an important determinant of the intensity of exercise during the early stages of the program. If completely unconditioned, you may desire to start at a lower intensity level, such as walking before you jog. A gradual progression is the key point. Examples are presented later.

Other general precautions involve safety factors, timing of meals, environmental hazards, and equipment. The individual should adhere to safety principles for the activity selected, particularly swimming, bicycling, and pedestrian safety. Strenuous exercise should not be undertaken within two or three hours of a heavy meal, but may be done earlier with a light meal or just liquids. A hot environment poses the most serious threat to the person in training. Be aware of signs of heat exposure such as dizziness, nausea, and weakness. If these occur, stop exercising and find a means to help cool the body. Proper equipment should be selected for the chosen activity. For example, of critical importance to the jogger or walker is a well-designed pair of shoes. They may help prevent certain medical problems such as tendonitis and shin splints, which often occur during early stages of training.

What is the general design of exercise programs for weight reduction?

In essence, exercise programs to lose body fat or help to maintain an optimal weight are based on the same principles that underlie exercise programs to improve the efficiency of the cardiovascular system. The total exercise program is based on a balance of exercise intensity, duration, and frequency. However, each daily exercise bout is usually subdivided into three phases—the warm-up, stimulus, and cool-down—in that order.

The **warm-up** precedes the stimulus period and may be done in a variety of ways. It usually is five to ten minutes long. It may consist of general calisthenics, stretching-type exercises, or a lower intensity level of the actual exercise to be done. The goals of the warm-up phase are to gradually increase the response of the CV system and/or to loosen up the muscles as a possible preventive measure against injury.

The **cool-down** phase follows the stimulus period and is designed primarily to help restore the CV system to normal. If one stops exercising abruptly, then blood may possibly pool in the exercised body parts, thereby decreasing return of blood to the heart. With less blood to the heart, less will be pumped to the brain and hence dizziness may result. By gradually cooling down after strenuous exercise, such as walking or jogging after a strenuous run, the muscles help massage the blood through the veins back to the heart.

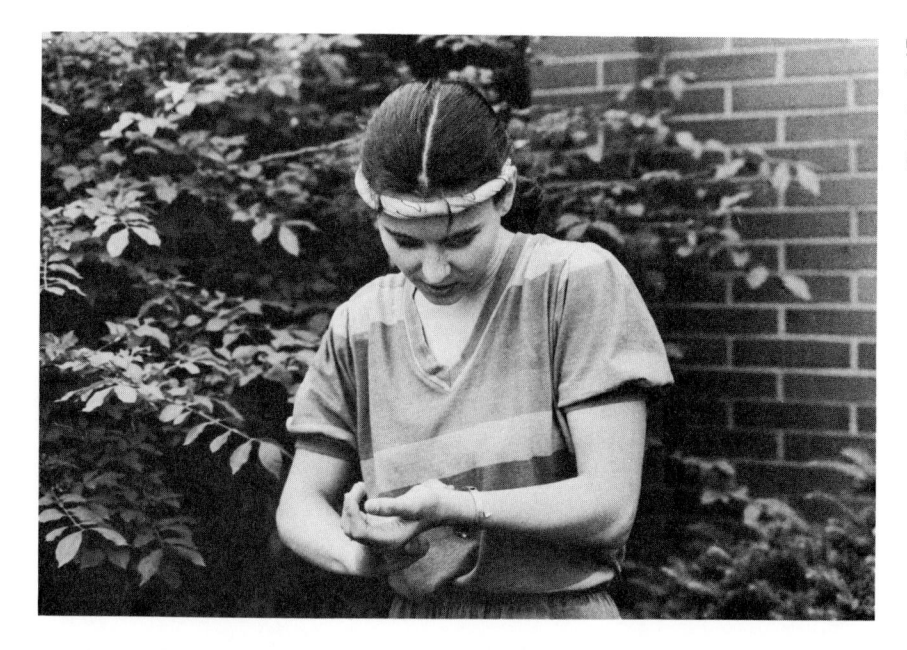

The heart rate may be an excellent indicator of exercise intensity.
(David Corona)

The most important phase is the stimulus period. By modifying the intensity of the exercise, the individual achieves the level of stimulus necessary to elicit a conditioning effect. For the average individual, the heart rate (HR) is the most practical method to gauge stimulus intensity.

How can I determine an appropriate exercise intensity level?

As the HR is obtained easily and parallels increases in oxygen uptake, it is a practical measure of exercise intensity. To obtain pulse rate, which is the same as the HR in most individuals, press lightly with the index and middle fingers at the carotid artery, which is located just under the jawbone and aside the Adam's apple. The radial artery pulse may be obtained by placing all four fingers on the inside of the wrist on the thumb side. These are the two most common locations for monitoring pulse rate, but other locations such as the temple, inside the upper arm, and just over the heart may be used.

To obtain the HR/minute, simply count the pulse rate for ten seconds and multiply by six. Resting and recovery heart rates are easily obtainable since they may be taken while the individual is motionless. It is difficult to manually monitor the HR while exercising. However, research has shown that the exercise HR is correlated very highly with the HR during the early stages of recovery. Hence, to monitor exercise HR, secure the pulse immediately upon cessation of exercise and count the beats in ten seconds. This will provide a reliable measure of exercise HR.

An associated measure of stimulus intensity is the **rating of perceived exertion (RPE)**. The individual simply rates the perceived strenuousness of the exercise according to the following scale:

6
7   very, very light
8
9   very light
10
11 fairly light
12
13 somewhat hard
14
15 hard
16
17 very hard
18
19 very, very hard
20

This scale was designed originally to reflect HR response; adding a zero to the rating should approximate the HR response. As noted below, the RPE may be used as a guide to appropriate exercise intensity.

In order to obtain a conditioning effect, there is rather widespread general agreement that the HR response should be in the range of 60–90 percent of the **maximal heart rate reserve**, which is defined as the difference between the resting HR and the **maximal heart rate (HR max)**. Although there are some individual variations, a general guide for the prediction of the HR max is 220 minus your age. Thus, a forty-year-old individual would have a predicted HR max of 180. Keep in mind, however, that there is considerable individual variation relative to predicted HR max. For example, a forty-year-old man may predict a HR max of 180, yet it may be 200, 160, or even much lower if he was a victim of coronary heart disease.

Continuing with our example of the forty-year-old man, we can calculate the HR range needed to elicit a training effect; this is called the **target range,** or **target HR.** In order to do the calculations, we need to know the age-predicted HR max and the resting HR (RHR), which should be determined under relaxed circumstances. The formula for the 60 percent level is: 0.6 (HR max − RHR) + RHR = 60% target HR. If we assume a RHR of 70, then 0.6(180 − 70) + 70 = 136. The formula for the 90 percent level is: 0.9(HR max − RHR) + RHR = 90% target HR. For this example, 0.9(180 − 70) + 70 = 169. Thus, in order to get a training effect, our forty-year-old man needs to train within a target HR range of 136–169. Table 13.1 provides some ranges for different age groups.

Table 13.1 Age predicted HR max and 60–90 percent target heart rate

Age	HR max	60–90% Target HR	Age	HR max	60–90% Target HR
10	210	154–196	50	170	130–160
15	205	151–191	55	165	127–155
20	200	148–187	60	160	124–151
25	195	145–182	65	155	121–146
30	190	142–178	70	150	118–142
35	185	139–173			
40	180	136–169			
45	175	133–164			

For this example, assume a resting HR of 70 for all age groups.

Although the target HR approach is a sound means to monitor your exercise intensity, you may also wish to use the RPE scale. As you exercise and monitor your HR, also assess the difficulty of the exercise by the RPE scale. You may possibly learn to estimate your HR response by your RPE score.

To determine the exercise intensity necessary to elicit this HR response, use a stopwatch. Where distances are involved such as running, swimming, or cycling, an accurate measure is needed. An ideal situation would be a one-quarter mile high school or college track.

A steady-state HR response may be obtained in three to five minutes of evenly paced activity. A sound method for walking, jogging, or running follows, but this system may be adapted easily to other activities such as swimming, cycling, calisthenics, and others:

> Mark a one-half mile course. Two laps on a quarter-mile track would be ideal, but it may be paced on the sidewalks near your home. Measure your resting HR. Walk until you have an even pace and then time yourself for the one-half mile. Immediately record your HR at the conclusion of the exercise. During your walk, mentally record the RPE. Did you reach the target HR? Was your RPE related to your HR? If the HR response is in the target range or the RPE was not too strenuous, you are at a level to begin your training program. If they were not, rest until your HR returns close to normal and then take the test at a faster pace. Repeat this procedure until you have a plot of the HR, RPE, and time for the one-half mile. Keep a record of this as it will be useful in evaluating the effects of your conditioning program.

For example, suppose you recorded the following data on the one-half mile test on four trials.

Test	Time	RPE	HR
1	8:00	10	102
2	7:20	12	119
3	6:30	14	142
4	6:00	17	172

As your speed increases, both RPE and HR naturally increase. If your predicted HR max is 185, and your resting HR is 70, the 60–90 percent target range approximates 139–173. Tests 1 and 2 do not provide adequate stimulus intensity, but 3 and 4 do. You should do your training at those paces. The RPE may offer a means of judging the intensity of the exercise when you do not have a set distance and watch.

To expand on this system, your speed for the half-mile test may be obtained. Simply double the time for the half-mile and you have the time needed to run one mile. In the example above, the speed for test 1 would be a 16:00 minute mile; the speeds for succeeding tests would be 14:40, 13:00 and 12:00 minutes per mile.

After determining the speed, the Calorie expenditure per minute may be approximated from Appendix C. If other activities besides running are desired, the appropriate caloric level may be used as a guideline for their selection from Appendix C.

How may I design my own exercise program?

Once you determine the intensity of exercise necessary to achieve the target HR, it becomes a relatively simple matter to individualize the exercise program. Other than the intensity of the exercise, the two other important components are duration and frequency.

The intensity of the exercise necessary to elicit the target HR may be too severe for some beginners. For a forty-year-old, the target HR might be in the range of 136–169. As is obvious, the intensity of exercise to produce a HR of 136 will be much less than that needed for a HR of 169. During the earlier stages of training the 136 HR may be tolerated easily while 169 HR may produce a rapid onset of fatigue or intolerance. The intensity of the exercise may be regulated towards the lower end of the target range during the early weeks of training, gradually increasing so that the HR begins to approach the upper limits of the target range. A modified interval training program, as the jog-walk-jog program, may be advisable to produce a varying HR response during the exercise period. For example,

Table 13.2 Example of a jog-walk exercise program

Step	Jog	Walk	Load	Approximate distance jogged
1	Jog 110 yd.	Walk 55 yd.	Start with 8 sets; then in each succeeding workout try to add a set until you can complete 12 sets in succession for 2 days; then go on to the next step.	1/2 to 3/4 mile
2	Jog 220 yd.	Walk 55 yd.	Start with 6 sets; then in each succeeding workout try to add a set until you can complete 12 sets in succession for 2 days; then go on to the next step.	3/4 to 1 1/2 miles
3	Jog 440 yd.	Walk 55 yd.	Start with 6 sets; then in each succeeding workout try to add a set until you can complete 10 sets in succession for 2 days; then go on to the next step.	1 1/2 to 2 1/2 miles
4	Jog 880 yd.	Walk 110 yd.	Start with 4 sets; then in each succeeding workout try to add a set until you can complete 6 sets in succession for 2 days; then go on to the next step.	2 to 3 miles
5	Jog 1 mile	Walk 220 yd.	Start with 2 sets; then in each succeeding workout try to add a set until you can complete 4 sets in succession for 2 days; then go on to the next step.	2 to 4 miles
6	Jog 1 1/2 miles	Walk 2–3 min.	After you jog the first 1 1/2 mile and walk, try to jog another 1 1/2 miles or you may wish to jog only 880-yd segments alternated with walking. When you are able to jog a second 1 1/2 miles continuously, go to the next step, continuous jogging.	3 miles or more
7	Continuous jogging; jog 2 to 4 miles.	Cool down; walking.		2 to 4 miles

From Getchell, Bud. *Physical Fitness: A Way of Life.* New York: John Wiley and Sons, 1979. Reprinted with permission from John Wiley and Sons.

the individual may walk at a pace to achieve a HR of 136 or so for several minutes, then increase the intensity by jogging to achieve a HR of 169 for several minutes, then walk again to reduce the heart rate to the lower levels of the target range. By alternating intensity levels, the HR can be made to vary from the lower to upper levels of the target HR range. Let your RPE also serve as a guide to exercise intensity. An example of a jog-walk program is presented in Table 13.2.

Table 13.3 A twelve-week cardiovascular conditioning program

Week	Target HR percent HR reserve	Duration of exercise	Frequency	Remarks
1	50–60	10 minutes	3/week	During the first weeks, the exercise intensity may have to be adjusted with alternate periods of resting, walking, and jogging. The duration of exercise is the number of minutes that the target HR should be achieved. Rest interval time should not be included
2	50–60	12 minutes	4/week	
3	50–60	15 minutes	5/week	
4	60–70	10 minutes	3/week	
5	60–70	12 minutes	4/week	
6	60–70	15 minutes	5/week	
7	70–80	10 minutes	4/week	
8	70–80	12 minutes	4/week	Learn to associate a given RPE with a HR response.
9	70–80	15 minutes	4/week	
10	70–80	15 minutes	2/week	If the progressive increase in exercise intensity appears too rapid, then train another week at a comfortable intensity level. Instead of twelve weeks it may take fourteen to eighteen or more to reach the maintenance level.
	80–90	10 minutes	2/week	
11	70–80	15 minutes	2/week	
	80–90	12 minutes	3/week	
12	70–80	15 minutes	3/week	
	80–90	15 minutes	3/week	

The duration of the stimulus period should be fifteen to thirty minutes. The target HR should be maintained for fifteen to thirty minutes. This may be continuous or intermittant. If fifteen minutes is the allotted time period, the target HR should be achieved for fifteen continuous minutes or three five-minute intervals of exercise with several minutes of rest in between.

The frequency of exercise should be daily or at least three to four times per week. There are a number of studies available to support a frequency level of at least three times per week as being necessary to develop and maintain CV health. During the early stages, however, it may be advisable to exercise daily in order to form sound habits. The exercise intensity at this time may not be too severe, and hence daily exercise bouts may be undertaken without serious muscle soreness or related injury patterns.

The twelve-week training program in Table 13.3 based on HR response to exercise should serve as a basic program for the unconditioned beginner to achieve a good level of cardiovascular conditioning. The intensity of the exercise should be regulated to achieve the percentage of HR reserve indicated. However, if the RPE for the activity appears to be too intense, especially during the early weeks, then decrease the intensity level slightly so that the exercise is comfortable, say to an RPE of 11–13. Consult Table 13.1 for predicted HR reserve. The target HR ranges there are for 60–90 percent of the HR reserve. For the first several weeks of the beginning program, the percentage of HR reserve is lower than the generally recommended target HR range in order to gradually accustom the individual to the muscular demands of the exercise.

There are a number of other excellent conditioning programs available for the unconditioned individual. Probably the most popular is the aerobics program developed by Dr. Kenneth Cooper. His program is based on a point system. Point values are assigned to various exercises dependent upon their intensity and duration. A progressive program, twelve to sixteen weeks long depending upon the age of the individual, leads to a level of training whereby thirty or more points are earned per week. His most recent programs may be found in *The Aerobics Program for Total Well Being,* a highly recommended paperback found in most bookstores.

From what parts of the body does the weight loss occur during an exercise weight reduction program?

As mentioned previously, weight loss may come from any one of three body sources—body water, lean tissue such as muscle, and body fat stores. A diet program, especially one very low in Calories, will cause a rapid weight loss due to decreases in body water and lean tissue. Body fat losses are minimal at first, but may increase in later stages of the diet. On the other hand, weight losses through an exercise program alone occur at a much slower rate. Body water levels remain relatively normal after replacement of water lost through exercise. The lean tissues, particularly muscle, might actually increase in amount. Since a good proportion of the energy demands for exercise comes from the oxidation of fat, most of the body weight reduction comes from the body fat stores.

Whether or not you can reduce fat from a specific body site, say the stomach, thighs, or back of the arm, is questionable. **Spot reducing** uses local exercises in an attempt to deplete local fat depots. An example would be sit-ups for the abdominal area. The results from a number of earlier studies were conflicting, but recent evidence from a well-controlled study using biopsies of fat tissues did not support spot reducing techniques. The current viewpoint suggests that the reduction of fat in body areas is most likely to occur where fat deposits are the most conspicuous, regardless of the exercise format. Although both large muscle activities and local isolated muscle exercises may both be beneficial in reducing fat stores, the former is recommended because the total caloric expenditure will be larger.

Body weight losses

Is it possible to exercise and still not lose body weight?

Many individuals are disappointed during the early stages of an exercise program because they do not lose weight very rapidly. Unless they understand what is happening in their body, the results on the scale may convince them that exercise is not an effective means to reduce weight, and they may quit exercising altogether. There are several reasons why an individual may not lose weight during the early stages of a weight reduction program and also why it becomes more difficult after weight loss has occurred.

When a sedentary individual begins a daily exercise program, the body reacts to the exercise stress and changes so it can more easily handle the demands of exercise. The bone density will increase. The muscles may increase in size. Certain structures within the muscle cell that process oxygen, along with numerous enzymes involved in oxygen use, will increase in quantity. Energy substances in the cell will increase, particularly glycogen, which binds water. The connective tissue will toughen and thicken. The total blood volume may increase. At the same time, body fat stores will begin to diminish somewhat as fat is used as a source of energy for exercise. Overall, there is an increase in the lean body mass, particularly the muscle tissues, and a decrease in body fat. These changes may counterbalance each other, and the individual may not lose any weight. However, although little or no weight is lost during these early phases, the body composition changes are favorable. Body fat is being lost.

Once these adaptive changes have occurred, which may take about a month, body weight should decrease in relationship to the number of Calories lost through exercise. Keep in mind that weight loss will be slow on an exercise program, but if you can build up to an exercise energy expenditure of above 300 Calories per day, then about three pounds per month will be exercised away.

After several months you may begin to notice that your body weight has stabilized even though you continue to exercise and have not reached your weight goal. Part of the reason may be due to your lower body weight. If you look at Appendix C, you can see that the less you weigh, the fewer Calories you burn for any given exercise. If you have been doing the same amount of exercise all along, you may now be at the body weight where your energy output is matched by your energy input in food and your body weight has stabilized. In addition you may become more skilled, and hence more efficient, in your physical activity. Fewer Calories may then be expended for any given amount of time. However, this is usually only true of activities that involve a skill factor. It can be highly significant in swimming, but not as great in jogging.

In summary, your body weight may not change during the early stages of an exercise program, it may then begin to drop during a second stage, and then plateau at the third stage. If you are aware of these possible stages your adherence to an exercise program may be enhanced. Also, during the third stage, if you desire to lose more weight by exercise, then the amount of exercise will need to be increased.

What about the five or six pounds a person may lose during an hour of exercise?

A rapid weight loss may occur during exercise. Some individuals have lost as much as 10–12 pounds in an hour or so. As you probably suspect, this weight loss may be attributed to body water losses. This is particularly evident while exercising in warm or hot weather. The weight loss is temporary, and under normal food and water intake the body water content will return to normal. Each pound of weight lost this way is one pint of fluid, or 16 ounces. A 2.2 pound weight loss would be the equivalent of one liter.

In the heat of summer, you may occasionally see an individual training with heavy sweat clothes or a rubberized suit. The reason often given is to lose more body weight. They will lose more body weight, but again it will be body water, which will be regained as soon as they drink fluids. In this regard, the technique is worthless. Moreover, it may predispose the individual to an unusually high heat stress causing severe medical problems.

Any water lost through dehydration should be replaced before the next exercise session, especially when exercising in warm environments. The importance of rehydration and problems associated with exercise in the heat will be discussed in the next chapter.

Which is more effective for weight control—diet or exercise?

Dieting alone and exercise alone may be effective means to reduce body fat. The advantages and possible disadvantages of dieting were covered in the last chapter, while the beneficial role of exercise and associated problems were treated in this chapter. It appears that the advantages of one technique help to counterbalance the disadvantages of the other so that a weight reduction program involving both a dietary and an exercise regimen is recommended. Dieting will contribute to a negative caloric balance and may help bring about a rapid weight reduction early in the program. Exercise will help to develop and maintain the lean body mass, which otherwise might be partially lost during a diet program. Very low calorie diets (less than 800 calories/day), although not recommended, may actually lead to a decrease in BMR and partially counteract the purpose of the diet; exercise may help to prevent the decrease in the BMR. In addition, a properly designed diet and exercise program may help in the elimination of risk factors associated with coronary heart disease.

Diet versus exercise

A dietary reduction of 500 Calories per day, along with an exercise energy expenditure of 500 Calories per day could lead to approximately two pounds of weight loss per week, about the maximal amount recommended unless under medical supervision. The removal of 500 Calories from the diet could be done immediately, but it may take a month or more before you may be able to exercise enough to use 500 Calories daily. By following the progressive plan outlined earlier in this chapter you should be able to reach that level safely.

Changing your diet by reducing Calories, saturated fats, and cholesterol, and eating more nutritious foods, along with initiating and continuing a good endurance-type exercise program are considered to be two steps toward positive health and the possible prevention of certain medical problems. These two life-style changes complement each other nicely. Research has shown that when people want to be physically fit they become more concerned with what they eat. A recent Harris survey has shown that almost 60 percent of adult Americans engage in some type of physical activity. However, only those who spend about 300 minutes a week exercising, which is about 15 percent of the population, make any appreciable changes in their diets. This averages to about forty-five minutes a day, which is a serious commitment to exercise. If you recognize exercise as a valuable means to help preserve your health and deter some of the adverse physiological effects of the aging process, then you need to make a serious time commitment to it. Forty-five minutes to an hour of daily, continuous-type endurance exercise will not only directly benefit your body physiologically and psychologically, but it may also help you commit to a general life-style geared toward positive health maintenance. Sound nutritional habits may be a natural spinoff of a commitment to exercise.

Although both dieting and exercise may be effective in the short-term reduction of body weight, it should be noted that weight loss through exercise produces more tissue fat loss compared with dieting. However, a combined diet-exercise program, along with behavior modification, is probably the best approach, and it is hoped that they become a lifelong process.

Exercise in the heat

14

Of all the factors that may influence physical performance on any given day, the one major concern to the active individual is the temperature. Anyone who is physically active for prolonged periods of time is probably aware of the effect that temperature changes have upon performance ability. Unless it is extremely cold, performance is not usually affected by low temperatures. However, as temperature increases, the combination of the environmental heat and the increased body heat from exercise metabolism may bring about bodily adjustments, which at the least may prove detrimental to endurance capacity and at the extreme may have fatal consequences. Given the seriousness of this topic, this chapter will discuss those problems that may confront you when exercising in the heat and how you may prevent or correct them.

What is the normal body temperature?

The temperature of different body parts may vary considerably. The skin may be very cold but your body internally is much warmer. When we speak of body temperature, we mean the internal, or **core temperature,** and not the external **shell temperature.**

Body temperature regulation

In humans, normal body temperature is approximately 98.6° F (37° C). This core temperature may be measured in a variety of ways, but the two most common methods are orally and rectally. Normal body temperature is relatively constant and may range from 97–99° F (36.1–37.2° C). On the other hand, shell temperature, which represents the temperature of the skin and the tissues directly under it, varies considerably depending upon the surrounding environmental temperature.

Humans can survive a wide range of core temperatures for a short period of time but optimal physiological functioning usually occurs within a range of 97–104° F (36.1–40.0° C). A variety of factors may affect the body temperature, but of importance to us is the effect exercise has upon the core temperature and how our body adjusts in order to help maintain heat balance.

What are the major factors that influence body temperature?

Humans are warm-blooded animals and are able to maintain a constant body temperature under varying environmental temperatures. In order to do this the body must constantly make adjustments to either gain or lose heat.

Humans are heat producing machines. The resting, or basal, heat production is provided through normal burning (oxidation) of the three basic foodstuffs in the body—carbohydrate, fat, and protein. A higher basal metabolic rate, infectious diseases, shivering, and exercise are several factors that might increase heat production.

Heat loss is governed by four physical means—conduction, convection, radiation, and evaporation:

Conduction—Heat is transferred from the body by direct physical contact, as when you sit on a cold seat.
Convection—Heat is transferred by movement of air or water over the body.
Radiation—Heat energy radiates from the body into space.
Evaporation—Heat is lost from the body when it is used to convert sweat to a vapor.

Under normal environmental temperatures, the body heat is transported from the core to the shell by way of conduction and convection, the blood being the main carrier of the heat. The vast majority of the heat radiates from the body, with a smaller amount being carried away by the evaporation of insensible perspiration. A cooler environment, increased air movement, increased blood circulation, or increased radiation surface would facilitate heat loss. However, when the environmental temperature exceeds the skin temperature of 92° F (33.3° C) the radiation process may reverse with the body gaining, rather than losing, heat by this means.

The well-known **heat balance equation** may be used to illustrate these interrelationships.

$$H = M \pm W \pm C \pm R - E \quad \text{where}$$

H = Heat balance
M = Resting metabolic rate
W = Work done (exercise)
C = Conduction and convection
R = Radiation
E = Evaporation

If any of these factors governing heat production or heat loss are not balanced by an opposite reaction, then heat balance will be lost and the body will deviate from its normal value. During exercise, W increases heat production. Hence, compensating adjustments in C, R, and E must be made.

How does the body regulate its own temperature?

In the brain is an important structure called the hypothalamus, which is involved in the control of a wide variety of physiological functions including body temperature. The hypothalamus functions pretty much like a thermostat in your house. If your house gets too cold, the heat comes on; if it gets too warm the air conditioning system starts. The human body makes similar adjustments.

The thermostat in your hypothalamus receives input from several sources. First, there are receptors in the skin that can detect temperature changes and send impulses to the hypothalamus. Secondly, the temperature of the blood can directly affect the hypothalamus as it flows through that structure.

In general, if the skin receptors detect a warmer temperature and/or the blood temperature rises, then the body will make adjustments in an attempt to lose heat. Two major adjustments may occur. First, the blood will be channeled closer to the skin so that the heat from within may get closer to the outside and radiate away more easily. Secondly, sweating will begin and evaporation of the sweat will carry away heat from the body.

If the skin receptors detect a colder temperature and/or the blood temperature is lowered, then the body will attempt to conserve heat or increase heat production. First, the blood will be shunted away from the skin to the central core part of the body. This decreases heat loss by radiation and helps keep the vital organs at the proper temperature. Secondly, shivering may begin. Shivering is nothing more than the contraction of muscles, which produces extra heat by increasing the metabolic rate. Figure 14.1 is a simplified schematic of temperature control.

What effect does exercise have upon body temperature?

Exercise effects on the body temperature

As noted in Chapter 9, exercise increases the metabolic rate and the production of energy. Under a normal efficiency rate of 20–25 percent, the remaining 75–80 percent of energy is released as heat. The total amount of heat released from the body is dependent upon the intensity and duration of the exercise. The more intense and longer the exercise, the greater the heat production. Whether or not heat balance is maintained is dependent upon the effectiveness of the body cooling mechanisms. Let us look at a typical example.

A physically conditioned person may be able to perform in a steady state for prolonged periods of time. If a normal sized male, 154 lbs or 70 kg, were to jog for about an hour, he could expend approximately 900 C. Assuming a mechanical efficiency rate of 20 percent, then 80 percent, or 720 C would be released in the body as heat. Since the **specific heat** of the

Figure 14.1.
Simplified schematic of body temperature control. The temperature of the blood returning from the muscles and the skin stimulates the temperature regulation center in the hypothalamus, as do nerve impulses from the warmth and cold receptors in the skin. An overall cold effect will elicit a constriction of the blood vessels near the body surface and muscular shivering, thus helping to conserve body heat. An overall warmth effect will elicit a dilation of blood vessels near the skin and sweating, thus increasing the loss of body heat.

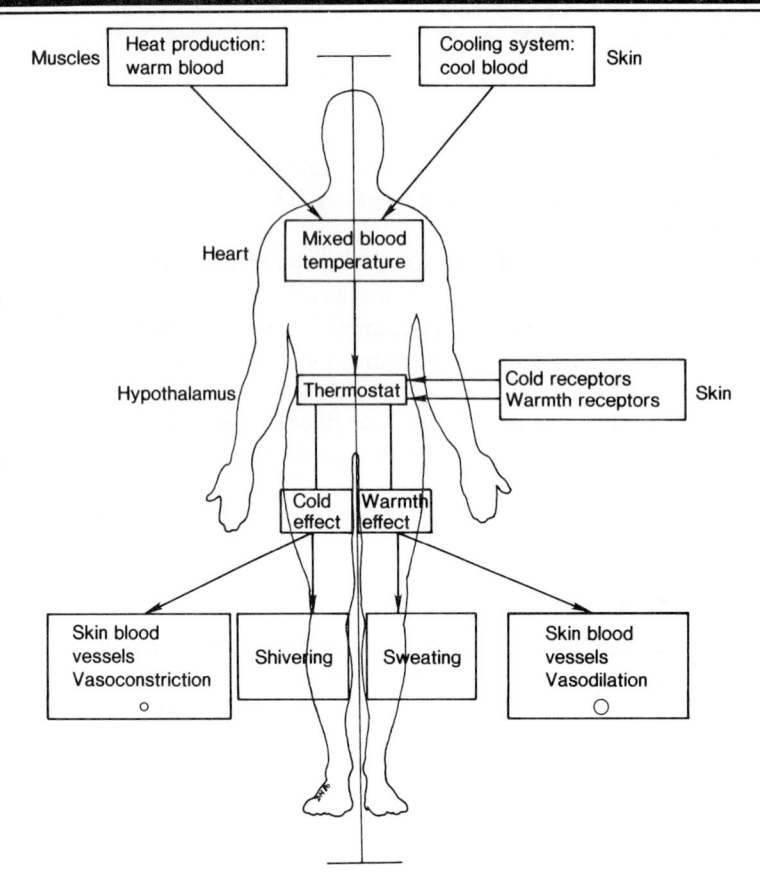

body is 0.83 (0.83 C will raise 1 kg of the body 1° C) then 58 C (70 kg × 0.83) would raise the body temperature 1° C in this person. Thus, unless this excess heat was dissipated, his body temperature would increase over 12.4° C (720 ÷ 58), or over 22° F, a fatal condition. Although the core temperature does rise during exercise, it rarely hits these extreme levels. The average core temperature during exercise, even during moderately warm temperatures, rises to about only 102.2–104.9° F (39–40.5° C). The reason is because of the body's cooling system.

In a cold or cool environment, the air movement around the body, along with some evaporation of sweat, may effectively maintain heat balance. However, when the environmental temperature rises, then the evaporation of sweat becomes the main means of controlling an excessive rise in the core temperature. One liter of sweat, if perfectly evaporated, will dissipate 580 C. In our example above, the evaporation of 1.24 l of sweat (720 ÷ 580) would prevent a rise in the core temperature. However, the evaporation of sweat from the body is not perfect, as sweat can drip off the body and not carry away body heat, so more than 1.24 l may be lost. If we assume that 2.0 l were lost, then this individual would have lost 4.4 lbs of body fluids during the one-hour run; 1 l of sweat weighs 1 kg or 2.2 lbs.

Under normal environmental circumstances, the evaporative mechanisms are able to keep the exercise body temperature in a normal range of 101–104° F.

What environmental conditions are likely to impose a heat stress on the active individual?

The interaction of four environmental factors are important determinants of the heat stress imposed on an individual:

1. Air temperature—Caution should be advised when the regular dry bulb thermometer is 80° F (27° C) or above.

2. Relative humidity—As the water content in the air increases, the relative humidity will rise. The increased humidity will impair the ability of the body sweat to evaporate and thus may restrict the effectiveness of the body's main cooling system. Caution should be used when the relative humidity exceeds 50–60 percent, especially with warmer temperatures.

3. Air movement—Still air limits heat carried away by convection. Even a small breeze may help keep body temperature near normal by helping to evaporate sweat.

4. Radiation—Radiant heat from the sun may add an additional heat load.

Some useful guidelines have been developed taking these four factors into consideration. The wet bulb globe thermometer (WBGT), illustrated in Figure 14.2, measures all four. The dry bulb thermometer (DB) measures air temperature, the globe thermometer (G) measures radiant heat, and the wet bulb thermometer (WB) evaluates relative humidity and air movement as they influence air temperature. The **WBGT Index** is computed as 0.7 WB + 0.2 G + 0.1 DB. For example, if the WB reads 70, the G is 100,

Figure 14.2.
A typical setup for measurement of the wet bulb globe temperature index (WBGT). The dry bulb measures air temperature, the wet bulb indirectly measures humidity, and the black bulb measures the radiant heat from the sun.

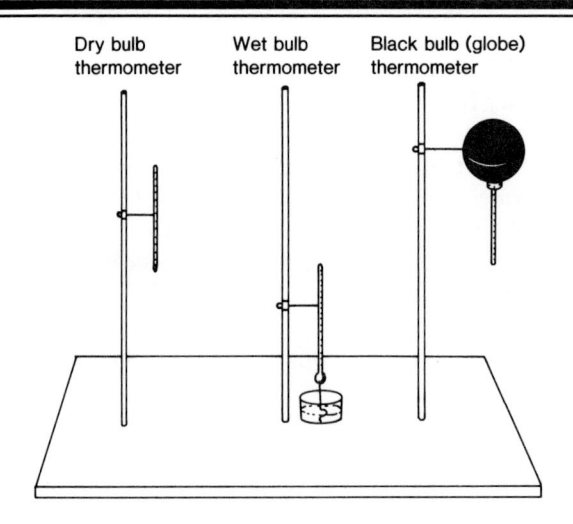

and the DB is 80, then the WBGT = (0.7 × 70) + (0.2 × 100) + (0.1 × 80) = 77° F. Precautions based on the WBGT are noted below:

WBGT	Precautions for Runners
Below 18 C (64 F)	Low risk. Heat injury can still occur, so caution is needed.
18–23 C (64–73 F)	Moderate risk. Athletes should monitor themselves for signs of impending heat injury and decrease exercise rate if necessary.
23–28 C (73–82 F)	High risk. Athlete must decrease exercise pace and be very alert to signs of impending heat injury. Unfit and unacclimatized individuals should be especially careful.
Above 28 C (82 F)	Performance will be hindered even when exercise intensity is reduced. Race directors should seriously consider cancelling races under such conditions.

These precautions should be noted not only by the active individual for safety, but also by those who conduct physical training sessions or athletic competition for others. Commercially available devices are available to readily measure the WBGT.

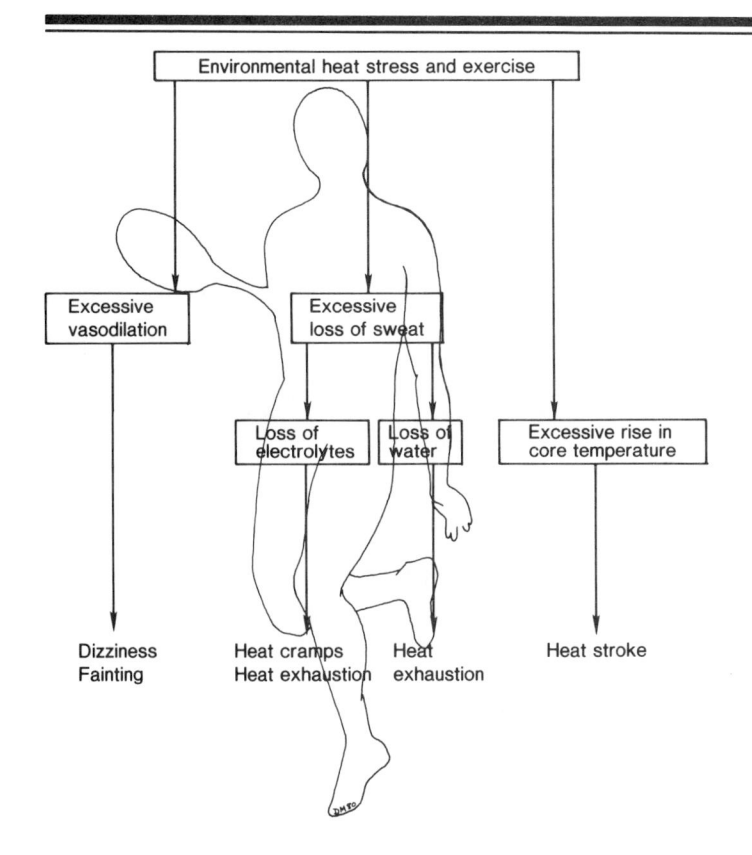

Figure 14.3.
Basic flow chart for heat illnesses. The combination of environmental heat and exercise may cause an excessive vasodilation or pooling of blood, which may decrease blood return to the heart and brain resulting in dizziness and fainting. Excessive loss of sweat may cause significant losses of body water and electrolytes resulting in various heat illnesses. See text for details.

What are the potential health hazards of excessive heat stress imposed on the body?

The individual who exercises unwisely under conditions of environmental heat stress may experience one or several of a variety of heat illnesses, or heat injuries. Three factors may contribute to these illnesses: increased core temperature, loss of body fluids, and loss of electrolytes.

Figure 14.3 represents a simple flow chart of heat disorders. When a combination of exercise and environmental heat stress is imposed on the body, vasodilation and sweating increase in an attempt to cool the body. When these two adjustments begin to falter, problems develop. In addition, if the exercise metabolic load is very great, heat illnesses may develop independent of circulatory and sweating inadequacies.

Preventing heat illnesses

Heat stroke may be caused by exercising in the heat without taking proper precautions.
(Wide World Photos, Inc.)

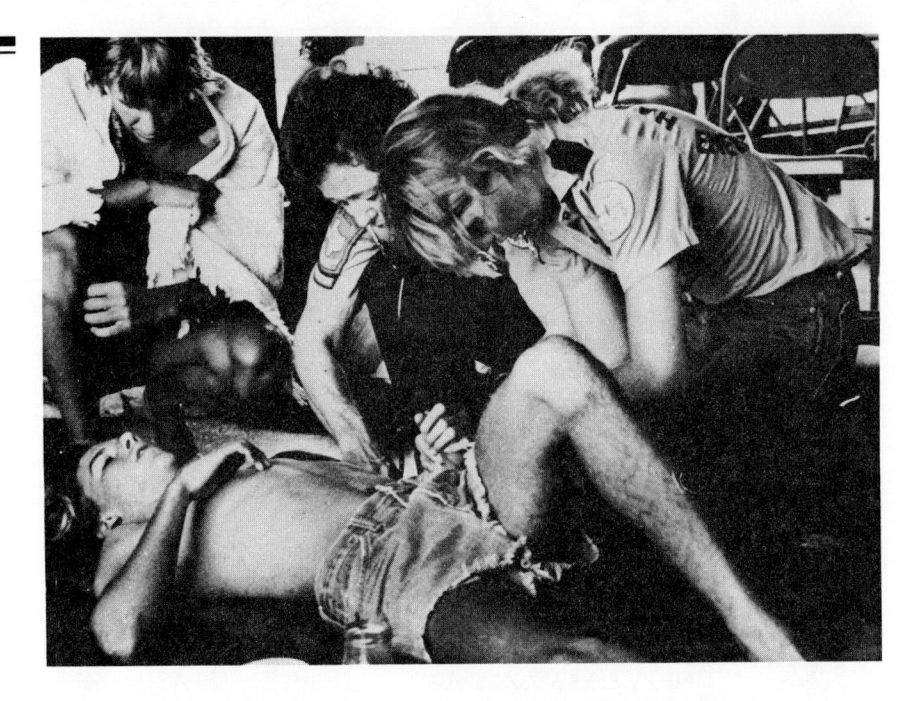

Excessive vasodilation may contribute to circulatory instability. The blood vessels expand and have a much greater capacity. Due to a decreased relative blood volume, dizziness and fainting may occur. This condition is called **heat syncope.**

Although no conclusive evidence is available, **heat cramps** may be caused by excessive loss of body salt through profuse sweating. They usually appear late in the day following ingestion of large amounts of plain water and usually result in severe muscle cramps in the calf of the leg and/or the abdomen.

Salt depletion heat exhaustion occurs most frequently in individuals who are not acclimatized to work in the heat and do not replace the salt they have lost over a period of several days. Fatigue is common, and cramps may develop.

Water depletion heat exhaustion resembles fainting and is caused by inadequate circulation to the brain. Fatigue and nausea are common symptoms, and the individual is usually conscious in the lying position. The skin is usually pale, cool, and covered with sweat. Heat exhaustion may incapacitate the individual for a few hours, but is usually responsive to body cooling treatments. It is the most common heat illness.

Heat stroke is the most dangerous heat illness, as it may be fatal. It may be caused by too great an exercise work load under heat stress conditions without dehydration, or it can occur after excessive loss of body water. It is usually preceded by mental changes ranging from disorientation or unconsciousness. The skin is usually warm and red, and sweating may or may not be present. A rectal temperature over 105.8° F (41° C) is a characteristic sign.

Table 14.1 Heat illnesses: causes, clinical findings, and treatment

Heat illnesses	Cause	Clinical findings	Treatment
Heat syncope	Excessive vasodilation; pooling of blood in skin	Fainting Weakness Fatigue	Place on back in cool environment; give cool fluids
Heat cramps	Excessive loss of electrolytes in sweat, inadequate salt intake	Cramps	Rest in cool environment; oral ingestion of salt drinks; salt foods daily; medical treatment in severe cases
Salt depletion heat exhaustion	Same as *heat cramps*	Nausea Fatigue Fainting Cramps	Rest in cool environment; replace fluids and salt by mouth; medical treatment in severe cases
Water depletion heat exhaustion	Excessive loss of sweat; inadequate fluid intake	Fatigue Nausea Cool pale skin Active sweating Rectal temperature lower than 104° F	Rest in cool environment; drink cool fluids; cool body with water; medical treatment if serious
Heat stroke	Excessive body temperature	Headache Disorientation Unconsciousness Rectal temperature greater than 105.8° F	Cool body immediately to 102° F (38.9° C) with ice packs, cold water; give cool drinks with glucose if conscious; get medical help immediately

What are some of the symptoms of heat illnesses and how are they treated?

Table 14.1 presents the major heat illnesses along with primary causes, clinical findings, and treatment.

Do some individuals have problems tolerating exercise in the heat?

There are always individual differences influencing the response any given person has to a particular situation. For example, one individual may have a greater amount of blood and more sweat glands than another and thus may have a greater capacity to tolerate exercise in the heat. Through experience, you may learn your capacity to deal with environmental heat stress.

Some older research has revealed that females do not have as great a tolerance to exercise in the heat as males, a finding that may have been related to the fact that, in general, the males were in better physical condition than the females. However, some more recent research has revealed that female responses to heat stress are similar to those found in males. The key point appears to be the physical fitness level of the individual. The better the fitness level, the better tolerance to a given heat stress.

Obese and aged individuals appear to be prone to heat illnesses. The obese person, due to larger amounts of fat and the greater amount of heat generated during exercise in conjunction with a usually low level of fitness, is more susceptible to heat illnesses. Age alone does not appear to be a limiting factor in mild or moderate heat stress, but at high levels of heat stress, tolerance to the heat is decreased in older individuals. This may also be related to fitness levels, and as more and more individuals become and remain physically active throughout middle age and advanced years, we may see the older person tolerating exercise in the heat as well as their younger counterparts. The American Academy of Pediatrics also cautions that young children are more prone to heat stress than adults when air temperature exceeds skin temperature.

How can you reduce the potential health hazards associated with exercise in a hot environment?

The following list represents a number of guidelines, which, if followed, will reduce considerably your chances of suffering any of the heat illnesses.

1. Check the temperature and humidity conditions before exercising. Adjust your tempo as needed. Hot humid conditions will cause fatigue sooner, so slow your pace or decrease the time of your activity.

2. Exercise in the cool of the morning or evening in order to avoid the heat of the day.

3. Exercise in the shade, if possible, in order to avoid radiation from the sun.

4. Wear as little clothing as possible. That which is worn should be loose to allow air circulation, white to reflect radiant heat, and porous to permit evaporation to occur.

5. Drink fluids periodically. If on a long training run, have your route planned so you know where some watering holes may be, like gas stations or other sources of water. Take frequent water breaks, consuming about 6–8 ounces of water ever 15 minutes or so. During exercise, thirst is not an adequate stimulus to replace water losses, so you should drink before you get thirsty. Pour water over your head and chest for psychological relief.

6. Replenish your water daily. Keep a record of your body weight. For each pound you lose, drink one pint of fluid. Your body weight should be back to normal before your next exercise workout.

7. Hyperhydrate if you plan to perform prolonged strenuous exercise in the heat. This topic will be covered later in this chapter but, in essence, drink about 16–32 ounces of fluid from 30–60 minutes prior to exercising.

8. Replenish lost electrolytes (salt) if you have sweated excessively. In essence, a balanced diet will maintain electrolyte balance, but you may wish to put a little extra salt on your meals and eat foods high in potassium, such as bananas and citrus fruits. Additional information on this topic is presented later.

9. Avoid excessive intake of protein, as extra heat is produced in the body when protein is metabolized. This may contribute slightly to the heat stress.

10. Minimize the intake of alcohol and caffeine. Both are diuretics which will increase body water losses. Caffeine will also increase the metabolic rate and heat production.

11. If you are sedentary, overweight or aged, you are less likely to tolerate exercise in the heat and should therefore use extra caution.

12. Be aware of the signs and symptoms of heat exhaustion and heat stroke, as well as the treatment for each. Dizziness, weakness, fatigue, mental disorientation, nausea, and headaches are some symptoms that may signify the onset of heat illness. Stop activity, get to a cool place, and consume some cool fluids.

13. If you are going to compete in a sport held under hot environmental conditions, then you must become acclimatized to exercise in the heat.

How can I become acclimatized to exercise in the heat?

It is a well-established fact that **acclimatization** to the heat will help increase performance in comparison to an unacclimatized state. Physical training, in and by itself, will provide some advantage to exercising in the heat. Simply living in a hot environment also confers a certain measure of acclimatization. However, neither of these two adjustments, either singly or collectively, is able to prevent the deterioration of performance in the heat by an unacclimatized individual. Thus, a period of acclimatization is necessary prior to competition in the heat.

The technique of acclimatization is relatively simple. One simply cuts back on the intensity and/or duration of their normal activity. When the hot weather begins, moderate your activity. Do not avoid exercise in the heat completely, but after an initial reduction in your activity level increase it gradually. For example, if you were running five miles a day, cut your distance back to two to three miles in the heat; if you need to do five a day, do the remaining miles in the evening. Eventually build up to three, four, and five miles. The acclimatization process usually takes about two weeks to complete. However, even when acclimatized, endurance capacity in the heat will still be less than under cooler conditions.

If you are monitoring your HR as a guide to your training intensity, you will probably note that you will have a higher exercise HR at a lower exercise intensity while performing in the heat. The need to channel blood to both your muscles and skin (for cooling purposes) imposes an additional workload on the heart. Consequently, exercise intensity will need to be reduced somewhat in order not to excessively exceed the recommended target HR range.

If you live in a cool climate, like New England, and want to compete in the Miami marathon, how do you become acclimatized? Partial acclimatization may occur if you exercise with extra clothes and insulation. These extra layers of clothes can help prevent evaporation and build a hot humid microclimate around your body. Research has shown that this technique can provide a degree of acclimatization. However, this is advisable only in cool weather and should not be attempted under hot conditions. Wearing a sweat suit or rubberized suit while exercising in the heat may precipatate heat illnesses.

The body makes several important adjustments following acclimatization to the heat. The total blood volume increases. The circulatory system makes more efficient use of its blood supply and less becomes channeled to the skin and more to the muscles. This helps to maintain a better supply of oxygen to the muscle and helps to improve endurance capacity. In addition, the efficiency of the evaporative cooling system increases. The acclimatized individual begins to sweat earlier at a lower core temperature and also sweats at a greater rate. Less salt is lost in sweat, increasing the evaporation rate. All these changes help to increase evaporative cooling.

In summary, the acclimatized person may perform a given exercise task with less heat stress than when unacclimatized. The heart rate will be lower, the core temperature will not rise as high, and the performance capacity will be improved significantly.

What is the composition of sweat?

Fluid and electrolyte losses

The composition of sweat may vary somewhat from individual to individual and will even be different in the same individual when acclimatized to the heat as contrasted to the unacclimatized state. The major differences are the concentration of the solid matter in the sweat, the electrolytes or salts.

Sweat is primarily water, but a number of major electrolytes and other nutrients may be found in varying amounts. Sweat is hypotonic in comparison to the fluids in the body. This means that the concentration of electrolytes is lower in sweat than in the body fluids.

The major electrolytes found in sweat are sodium (Na^+), chloride (Cl^-), potassium (K^+), magnesium (Mg^{++}), and calcium (Ca^{++}). Trace minerals lost in small amounts include iron (Fe^{++}), copper (Cu^{++}), and zinc

(Zn^{++}). Small quantities of nitrogen (N) and some of the water soluble vitamins are also present. Although all of these nutrients have been found in sweat, the vast majority consists of the Na^+ and Cl^- ions.

How does the excessive loss of body fluids adversely affect physical performance?

Although the exact cause is not known, dehydration, or excessive loss of body water, has been shown to reduce the amount of time a person can exercise at high levels of energy expenditure. The major physiological measure of endurance, maximal oxygen uptake, is not changed following dehydration, but work time to exhaustion is severely curtailed. In practical terms, one study found that dehydration prior to a 10 kilometer run resulted in a race time nearly 2½ minutes slower. The explanation is probably due to changes at the cell level. Dehydration may disturb the fluid and electrolyte balance within the cell and thus may affect adversely muscular contraction. In addition, water losses as little as 2 percent of the body weight may impair circulatory functions and possibly contribute to a disturbed heat balance. The rising body temperature could hinder performance capacity.

Is excessive sweating likely to create an electrolyte deficiency?

There are two ways to look at this question. What happens to electrolyte balance during exercise and what happens following the exercise period?

The concentration of electrolytes in the blood following excessive sweating has been studied under laboratory conditions as well as immediately after a marathon run. In general, exercise causes an increased concentration of several electrolytes in the blood. Na^+ and K^+ concentrations are elevated; the Na^+ increase may be due to greater body water loss than Na^+ loss and the K^+ may leak from the muscle to the blood therefore increasing the blood concentration of this ion. Mg^{++} levels usually fall, probably due to the fact that the active muscle cells need this ion during exercise and it passes from the blood into the tissues. Cl^- and Ca^{++} ion concentrations remain relatively unchanged during exercise. During acute prolonged bouts of exercise then, even in marathon running, it appears that an electrolyte deficiency will not occur.

This is not to say that electrolyte replacement is not important. What happens during the recovery period after excessive sweating may contribute to an electrolyte deficiency. Prolonged sweating has been shown to decrease the body content of Na^+ and Cl^- by 5–7 percent, while K^+ and Mg^{++} levels dropped only about 1 percent. If these electrolytes are not replaced, then an electrolyte deficiency could occur. However, it should be noted that the body possesses a rather effective mechanism to conserve its mineral resources. If body levels of Na^+ and K^+ begin to decrease, the kidney begins to reabsorb more of these minerals and less are excreted in the urine. Under normal dietary circumstances, it is difficult to create a Na^+ or K^+ deficiency.

How should I replace lost fluids and electrolytes?

Fluid and electrolyte replacement

There is little need to replace electrolytes during exercise itself as the concentration in the body is actually increasing rather than decreasing. The key point is to replace lost body water. Even during strenuous prolonged exercise like marathon running with high levels of sweat losses, several studies have indicated that water alone is the recommended fluid replacement. However, as mentioned in Chapter 2, small amounts of glucose may be helpful during prolonged exercise.

If not adequately replaced, an electrolyte deficit may possibly occur over four to seven days of hard training, especially in hot environmental conditions where fluid losses will tend to be high. However, research has shown that water alone, in combination with a balanced diet, will adequately maintain proper electrolyte levels in the body. A little extra table salt added to the daily meals, along with the selection of high potassium foods such as bananas and citrus fruits, should help to maintain Na^+ and K^+ balance. For example, a large glass of orange juice will replace the K^+ lost in 2 l of sweat. Other nutrients lost in sweat are of such a low magnitude that dietary modifications are usually not necessary. A balanced diet, including foods high in iron content, should provide more than an ample supply to replace the small amounts lost.

Are salt tablets necessary?

Although salt tablets used in moderation to replace lost electrolytes may not do harm, they are probably unnecessary. The common salt tablet contains only Na^+ and Cl^-. Although the concentrations of Na^+ in sweat may vary, some common figures used are 1.8 g of Na^+/quart of sweat in the unacclimatized person and 1.1 g Na^+/quart of sweat in the acclimatized individual. If you would lose 12 lbs of body fluids during an exercise period, a total of 6 quarts of fluid would be lost, since a quart weights 2 lbs. Six quarts of sweat would contain, at the most, 10.8 g of Na^+ in the unacclimatized man. The average American consumes 4–6 g of Na^+ per day. However the average meal contains about 3–4 g Na^+ if well-salted, so three meals a day would offer 9–12 g, about enough to just cover the losses in the sweat. The acclimatized individual would lose less Na^+ and hence need less replacement.

Salt tablets are not necessary to replace lost Na^+, but may be recommended for those who cannot replace the Na^+ through normal dietary means. They should be taken only if you need to drink more than 4 quarts of fluid per day to replace that lost during sweating, that is, an 8-lb weight loss. This is important primarily during the early stages of training while unacclimatized. So checking your body weight before and after exercise will give you a fairly exact measure of your body water losses. The general rule is to take 1 g of salt with each *additional* quart of fluid beyond the 4 quarts. This would be two normal salt tablets, since the average tablet has one-half gram of Na^+. Another way to look at it is to take one pint of water with every salt tablet. The additional sodium may also be obtained by salting your meals; one half teaspoon of salt is about 1 g of Na^+.

Keep in mind the fact that diets high in Na^+ have been associated with high blood pressure. Excessive intakes, if not used to restore losses, may possibly contribute to this condition in susceptible individuals. The RDA for moderately active individuals, in the absence of active sweating, is only 1.1–3.3 g/day. If you do not experience any problems while training, you are most probably in sodium balance. The human body has a very effective control system for Na^+ and K^+ balance.

What is the composition of the various sport drinks or thirst quenchers?

In the past decade a number of commercial preparations have been marketed with the advertised value of replacing sweat losses with fluids of similar electrolyte composition. Glucose has also been added to many of these solutions in order to help replenish energy stores such as blood glucose and muscle glycogen. They are commonly known as **glucose-electrolyte replacement solutions,** or GES for short. Common brands include Gatorade®, Body Punch®, ERG®, Brake Time®, and Quickick®.

Other than water the major ingredients in these solutions are carbohydrates in the form of glucose and/or sucrose and some of the major electrolytes. The glucose/sucrose content varies with the different brands ranging from about 1 percent to over 10 percent. The caloric values range from 1–13.5 per ounce. The major electrolytes include sodium, chloride, potassium, and phosphorus. These ions also are found in varying amounts in different brands.

Some brands also include some of the following: magnesium, calcium, citric acid, sodium citrate, vitamin C, saccharin, sodium bicarbonate, and artificial coloring and flavoring.

Are these sport drink solutions necessary to replace lost fluids, electrolytes, or glucose?

This question is best answered in relation to each of the major components of the GES solutions—fluids, electrolytes, and glucose.

As mentioned previously, water is the essential nutrient that needs to be replenished during prolonged exercise in the heat, for it will help deter some of the adverse responses to dehydration. There is no substantial evidence to indicate that GES solutions will help replenish body water during exercise more effectively than just plain water. During recovery after exercise, any normal fluid can be used to replenish body water.

Electrolytes do not need to be replenished during exercise, as discussed earlier. There is no available evidence that electrolyte replacement will benefit performance in most athletic events. However, in very prolonged bouts of activity, such as in a tennis tournament where one might play off and on all day, prompt electrolyte replacement may be a sound practice. In this case, the GES solutions may be helpful, but balanced eating may be all that is necessary. During repeated days of heavy sweating, a balanced diet with adequate water intake is all that is necessary to maintain electrolyte balance.

Glucose content in GES solutions may be an advantage in some situations and disadvantages in others. As noted in Chapter 2, glucose intake during prolonged exercise may serve as an energy source and may also help prevent hypoglycemia. In this regard, solutions with high concentrations of glucose of 10 percent or more may be helpful. Keep in mind that this type of solution generally may be useful only in prolonged activity, conditions where one is exercising at a high level of intensity for an hour or more. In addition, a high glucose content may be recommended only during performance in a cold environment where fluid losses will not be too great. When exercising in a hot environment with heavy sweat losses, GES solutions with high glucose content are not recommended. The high glucose content will slow down the absorption of water, which is the key substance needed. The glucose content should not exceed 2.5 percent. Many of the commercial GES solutions are 5 percent or more, although several are only 1–2 percent. Check the labels of each brand.

It should be noted that a number of sportsmedicine investigators have compared GES solutions with water and other such compounds to see if there was any particular benefit relative to exercise under heat stress conditions. These investigators concluded that although several GES solutions do offer a scientifically sound means of replenishing body fluids lost through exercise in the heat, they do not appear to help increase performance capacity. Moreover, some GES solutions have a high concentration of sugar and may actually retard the absorption of water from the gastrointestinal tract.

What fluids should I drink during exercise?

During periods of heavy sweating, it is almost impossible to consume enough fluids to replace those lost. The sweating rate is simply greater than the ability of the stomach to empty the fluid into the small intestine for absorption to occur. Nevertheless, any fluid that is absorbed may help to maintain circulatory stability and heat balance and thus prevent a marked deterioration in endurance capacity.

Research has revealed several factors affecting the usefulness of a given fluid to an individual who is exercising at a fairly high intensity. Based on current available evidence, the following solution would be suitable as fluid replacement during exercise in the heat.

1. Contains less than 2.5 g of glucose in 100 ml of water. This is less than 25 g/quart, or 1.5 rounded tablespoons of sugar.

2. Contains little, if any, electrolytes. Less than 0.20 g of sodium chloride and less than 0.20 g of potassium per quart if included.

3. Should be cold, 40–50° F (4.4–10° C).

4. About 3–6 ounces should be consumed during exercise at 10–15 minute intervals.

For some common beverages, the following modifications are recommended, if you can adjust to the taste. These modifications should help to speed up fluid absorption, which is more critical under hot weather conditions as compared to cold ones.

Water, ERG®, Body Punch®	Use as is
Other GES solutions	Check sugar content; dilute with water to less than 25 g glucose/quart
Fruit juices	Dilute with 5 parts water
Colas, sodas, sweetened	Dilute with 3 parts water

What is hyperhydration and what application does it have for the active individual?

Hyperhydration, also known as superhydration, is simply an increase in body fluids by the voluntary ingestion of water or other beverages. It is an attempt to assure that the body water level is high before exercising in a hot environment. This extra water supply can delay the effects of dehydration and help to prolong endurance capacity. The research conducted with hyperhydration before exercise has revealed that it may effectively reduce the effects of heat stress on the core temperature and the cardiovascular system, but is not as effective as rehydration during exercise.

The American College of Sports Medicine recommends that hyperhydration be used prior to exercise in heat stress environments. If you plan to compete in the heat, or do any prolonged exercise, it may be wise for you to hyperhydrate. All you need to do is consume about a pint (16 ounces) of cold fluid about 15–30 minutes prior to exercising. With experience, you may be able to tolerate larger amounts, although the diuretic effect should be kept in mind if you are to be involved in competition.

15

The drug foods—alcohol and caffeine

Alcohol and caffeine are both legally classified as drugs. However, both are so often consumed as components of various beverages served with meals that they ofttimes may be considered as foods.

Alcohol is consumed by the majority of the adult population throughout the world. Although the vast majority are social drinkers, many abuse alcohol. Alcohol is the number one drug problem in the United States in both adults and teenagers. The chronic ingestion of alcohol leading to addiction and alcoholism is a significant problem, with implications for physical fitness and human performance. That topic falls outside the scope of this book.

Some have contended that athletes and physically active persons should avoid alcohol altogether if they want to maximize their physical performance potential. It has been reported that alcohol ingestion will sap energy and greatly increase fatigue. On the other hand, some have contended that alcohol may exert a beneficial effect, a so-called ergogenic effect, upon some types of athletic performance. For example, one current recommendation has been to drink one beer for every six miles in a marathon run.

Caffeine is also consumed by numerous individuals as it is a natural ingredient in coffee, tea, and cola-type sodas. A popular contemporary diet plan suggests that caffeine may be detrimental to health and recommends the complete elimination of caffeine-containing products from the diet. On the other hand, a number of epidemiological reports have not identified coffee or other caffeine beverages as posing any health hazard when consumed in moderation. Athletes have been advised to abstain from caffeine because it could cause an upset stomach or excessive "jitters" before competition. On the contrary, some recent research has suggested that two cups of coffee prior to long endurance-type activities could significantly increase performance capacity.

The purpose of this chapter is to cover briefly the physiological effects of alcohol and caffeine in the human body, with particular attention to the effects during exercise. Whether or not alcohol or caffeine will increase or decrease physical performance or have no effect may be dependent upon the particular type of activity the individual is doing.

Alcohol products may add a considerable number of Calories to the daily intake. (James Ballard)

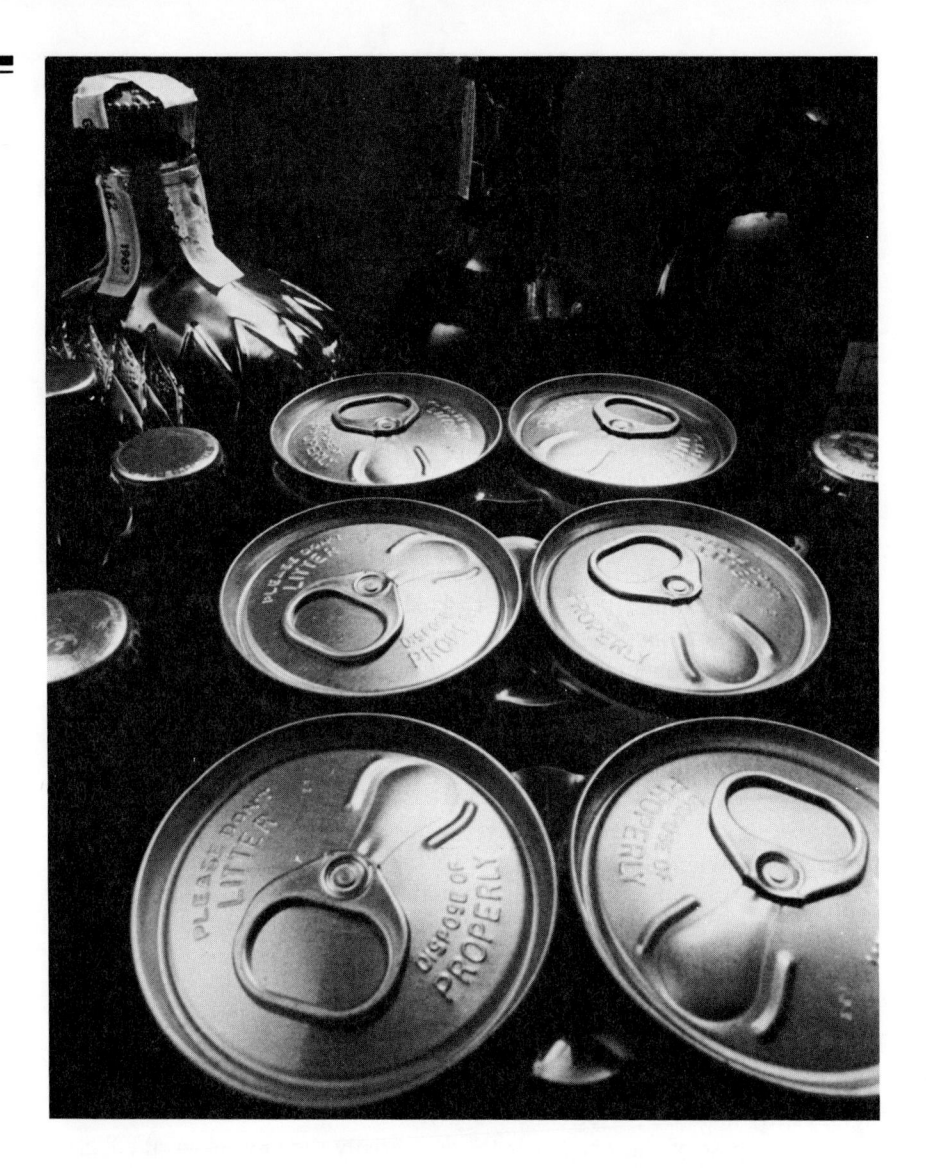

Alcohol nutrition and metabolism

What is alcohol?

Alcohol is a transparent, colorless liquid derived as a waste product from the fermentation of sugars in fruits, vegetables, and grains. It is an organic compound having a general formula of C_2H_5OH. Alcohol is found in a variety of forms and has many uses in medicine and industry as a solvent and preservative. The alcohol designed for human consumption is **ethyl alcohol,** also known as **ethanol.** Ethanol, although classified legally as a drug, is a component of many beverages served throughout the world.

Table 15.1 Energy content of typical alcoholic beverages

Beverage	Amount	Carbohydrate Grams	Carbohydrate Calories	Alcohol Grams	Alcohol Calories	Total Calories
Beer	12 ounces	14	56	13	91	150
Wine, table	4 ounces	4	16	12	84	100
Liquor (80 proof)	1.5 ounces	0	0	14	98	100

The small discrepancies in the calculation of total Calories for beer and liquor may be attributed to a small protein content in beer, with some energy value, and trace amounts of carbohydrate in liquor.

In the United States, alcohol is consumed mainly as a natural ingredient of beer, wine, and liquor. The alcohol content may vary in different types of beer, wine, and liquor, but in general beer is about 4–5 percent alcohol, wine is 12–14 percent, and liquor is 40–45 percent. The alcohol content in liquor is expressed as **proof,** which is double the percentage content. An 80-proof bottle of gin is 40 percent alcohol. The following amounts of these three beverages contain approximately equal amounts of alcohol, about 13 g.

12 ounces of beer	—one bottle
4 ounces of wine	—one wine glass
1.5 ounces of liquor	—one jigger or shot glass

Does alcohol have food value?

The purposes of food are to supply energy, to build and repair body tissues, and to regulate body processes. In this sense, alcohol could be construed to possess food value as it is a concentrated source of energy. Alcohol contains about 7 Calories/g, which is almost twice the value of an equal amount of carbohydrate or protein. Beer and wine also contain carbohydrates that may be an additional source of energy, but liquors such as gin, rum, vodka, and whiskey do not. Light beers have less carbohydrate and alcohol. Table 15.1 represents an approximate breakdown for the energy content found in a typical beverage serving.

In general, the calories found in beer, wine, and liquor are empty calories. They do not provide substantial amounts of any nutrient. A 12-ounce bottle of beer does contain about 1 g of protein, about one-tenth the daily RDA for niacin, folacin and B_6, smaller amounts of vitamins B_1 and B_2, some calcium, magnesium and potassium. Wine contains trace amounts of protein, niacin, vitamins B_1 and B_2, calcium, and iron. Liquor is void of any other nutrients. The nutrient content of beer and wine is considered to be low and will not make any significant contribution to the diet since the vitamins and minerals found in these beverages are distributed widely in other foods.

Alcohol Calories can displace high nutrient Calories, especially when consumed in excess amounts. For 100 Calories in a shot of gin you receive zero nutrient value, but for the same amount of Calories in approximately three ounces of chicken breast you get over one-third your daily RDA in protein plus substantial amounts of niacin, iron, and some other vitamins. Although alcohol may have a certain value to us as a social beverage, its value as a food and a source of nutrients is extremely limited.

Does alcohol affect the absorption or utilization of other nutrients?

Alcohol is a drug, and many drugs have been shown to impair proper nutrition by decreasing absorption of certain nutrients from the intestines, speeding up the excretion of certain nutrients, or disturbing physiological reactions in the body so nutrients cannot be utilized properly.

Alcohol, in some individuals, has been shown to cause inflammation of the stomach, intestines, and pancreas, which would possibly impair proper digestion of food and nutrient absorption. Alcohol and one of its metabolic byproducts have also been known to interfere with vitamin metabolism in the liver. Much of the research in this area has been conducted with heavy drinkers and alcoholics, and significant impairment of vitamin B utilization has been reported, notably vitamin B_1, B_6, B_{12} and folacin. Research with normal healthy individuals has not shown as great a disturbance in vitamin metabolism, but some studies have reported reduced absorption of vitamin B_1 associated with moderate intakes of alcohol. Theoretically, this could impair physical performance of an endurance nature since vitamin B_1 is involved in the aerobic metabolism of carbohydrate. The effect of alcohol upon physical performance is discusssed later.

What happens to alcohol in the body?

Alcohol is rapidly absorbed from the stomach and small intestine, particularly so if little food is present in the digestive tract. It enters the bloodstream and is then distributed to the various body tissues, the concentration in each tissue being dependent upon its water content. There is a constant interchange of water between the blood and the tissues so that alcohol is either being deposited in or removed from the tissues depending upon the concentration in the blood. As the blood circulates through the liver the alcohol begins to be metabolized so that it can be used for energy.

The liver is a remarkable body organ, and one of its major functions is to break down substances foreign to the body, such as drugs. About 95–98 percent of the alcohol ingested is metabolized by the liver, the remaining 2–5 percent is excreted largely unchanged in the urine, breath, or sweat. If alcohol is consumed faster than it can be eliminated, the amount in the blood and body tissues will continue to rise. A blood sample can measure the **blood alcohol level (BAL),** which expresses the alcohol concentration.

The elimination of alcohol proceeds at a relatively constant rate, approximately three-quarters of an ounce per hour. It is oxidized in three stages. First, a key enzyme in the liver, alcohol dehydrogenase, transforms alcohol to acetaldehyde. This first step can only occur so fast and limits the rate at which alcohol can be removed. Second, acetaldehyde is transformed, primarily in the liver, to acetic acid. Finally, acetic acid is subsequently oxidized to carbon dioxide and water.

In this metabolic breakdown, parts of the alcohol may help form other compounds. The following are some of the possible fates of alcohol.

1. Produces fatty acids, which may be released into the blood, used as energy by the liver, or stored as fats in the liver.

2. Produces lactate, which is released into the blood.

3. Produces acetate and ketones, which enter the bloodstream.

Fatty acids, lactate, acetate, and ketones may be used as energy sources. Thus, some have contended that alcohol may be a good source of energy during exercise. The next question explores this issue.

Can alcohol be a significant source of energy during exercise?

Alcohol and physical performance

Although alcohol contains a relatively large number of calories and its metabolic pathways in the body are short, the available evidence suggests that it is not utilized to any significant extent during exercise. First, as you recall, the major sources of energy for exercise are carbohydrates and fats, which are in ample supply in most individuals. Alcohol may help form fats, but there is no evidence that it can substitute for other fat sources in the body. Even if it could, this would be of no benefit since the body has more than enough fat to supply energy during prolonged exercise. Second, the liver is the major body tissue that utilizes the potential Calories found in alcohol. The acetate and other by-products of alcohol metabolism that are released by the liver into the blood may enter the skeletal muscles but appear to be of little importance to exercising muscle. Repeated research studies have found that exercise cannot speed up the elimination of alcohol from the body. Third, even if the energy from alcohol could be used, it would represent an uneconomical source. The amount of oxygen needed to release the Calories from alcohol is greater than for an equivalent amount of carbohydrate and fat. And lastly, the rate at which the liver could metabolize alcohol would limit its use as an energy source during exercise, particularly in an individual working at a high level of intensity. If the liver can metabolize only three-quarters of an ounce of alcohol per hour, this would amount to approximately 160 Calories, or about 15 percent of the energy needs for a competitive runner. In summary, these four factors suggest alcohol is not utilized during exercise, and even if it was it would not offer any advantages over natural supplies of carbohydrate and fat. In fact, it would be a less economical source.

Although alcohol itself does not appear to be used as an energy source during exercise, it may affect various physiological processes important to energy metabolism during exercise.

What are the physiological effects of alcohol that may influence physical performance?

Alcohol affects all cells of the body eliciting psychological or physiological effects, which may, based upon theoretical considerations, either improve or impair physical performance. A key point determining the effect of alcohol is the variation in response of different individuals to a given dose. People differ markedly in their susceptibility to alcohol, especially at low doses whereby it may impair significantly motor performance of one person but not another.

Alcohol is a narcotic, a depressant. It affects the brain. As a depressant, alcohol would not be advocated as a means to improve performance; however, some have contended that the increased feelings of self-confidence and a perceived decrease in sensitivity to pain may offset any depressant effects and possibly benefit performance. Moreover, alcohol in small doses may exert a paradoxical stimulation effect. Parts of the brain that normally inhibit behavior may be depressed by alcohol. Hence, inhibitory controls exerted by the brain are decreased, and a freer expression of behavior may occur. A transitory sensation of excitement may occur, but may eventually be followed by depression effects.

The effects of alcohol on physical performance may be evaluated from two viewpoints—the direct effect on perceptual-motor performance and the effect on various physiological processes important to exercise. **Perceptual-motor activities** involve the perception of a stimulus, integration of this stimulus by the brain and the nervous system, and an appropriate motor response (movement). Physiological processes involve those body systems supporting exercise, such as the cardiovascular system and respiratory system.

Alcohol may adversely affect perceptual-motor activities because it impairs the integrating function of the brain. Reaction time, hand-eye coordination, balance, visual perception, and other perceptual-motor skills deteriorate at low levels of blood alcohol. Simply consider the relationship of alcohol consumption to automobile accidents. Driving a car is a perceptual-motor skill. Individuals involved in activities with a perceptual-motor skill should abstain from alcohol use.

In general, a review of the relevant research has revealed that the acute effects of alcohol in one or two drinks will neither improve nor deteriorate physiological processes associated with maximal exercise. Maximal oxygen uptake, maximal heart rate, and other indicators of maximal performance are unchanged by small doses of alcohol. Strength and local muscular endurance are also not affected.

On the other hand, some recent research has revealed some deleterious effects of alcohol, which may theoretically impair prolonged endurance performance as in long distance running. The following effects of alcohol during exercise have been reported recently:

1. Alcohol may block the formation of glucose by the liver during exercise.

2. Alcohol may decrease the release of glucose from the stomach into the blood.

3. Alcohol may disturb water balance in the muscle cells.

The first two points have caused a decrease in blood glucose during the latter stages of endurance exercise, causing hypoglycemia in some subjects after an hour and a half of exercise. The combination of hypoglycemia and alcohol intake has also been shown to impair temperature regulation in the cold, particularly during recovery. There was also decreased glucose uptake by the legs during the latter stages of exercise, which could contribute to a faster depletion of muscle glycogen. The decrease in muscle cell water may disturb cell enzyme activity and cause fatigue. Although the effect of alcohol on maximal long distance performance has not been studied directly, these other research findings would suggest alcohol consumption is not generally recommended during long distance events.

In summary, although alcohol may elicit subjective sensations in some individuals that may make them believe they may be able to perform better, careful research does not support this viewpoint. As a matter of fact, physical activities characterized by fine neuromuscular control usually deteriorate following alcohol consumption. Although small to moderate doses of alcohol have not been shown to improve or impair tasks involving strength and local muscular endurance, there is some theoretical basis for avoiding alcohol during prolonged endurance activities.

Will consumption of alcohol as a social beverage have any adverse effect upon physical performance?

Only a limited number of studies have investigated this issue, and there is rather general agreement that light social drinking will not impair physical performance on the following day. Tests of reaction time, strength, power, and cardiovascular performance were not adversely affected following the consumption of one drink the night before. On the other hand, heavy drinking may cause problems. Aside from the obvious impairment that may be caused by the symptoms of an alcohol hangover, heavy drinking has been shown to cause such diverse effects as involuntary eye movements and dehydration. The involuntary movements of the eyeball could impair one's ability in critical visual-motor tasks. A state of dehydration, if not corrected prior to endurance performance, could have potentially hazardous consequences, particularly if exercise is performed in a hot environment. This latter topic was discussed in detail in Chapter 14.

At one time alcohol was on the International Olympic Committee (IOC) list of drugs that would ban an athlete from competition if it were detected in their blood. However, due to the fact that many European athletes are accustomed to either wine or beer with their meals, small amounts in the blood of the athletes, with the exception of those in shooting competition, became permissable starting with the Munich Olympics in 1972. Although this is not experimental evidence, it suggests that international class athletes may be expected to perform at top levels even with moderate consumption of alcohol. The drinking practices and running performances of many long distance runners in the United States also suggests that light to moderate social drinking will not adversely affect physical performance, provided it is not done on the day of competition.

Are there any health hazards or benefits associated with alcohol consumption?

Alcohol and your health

This is a rather complex question, and the response is dependent primarily on the amount of alcohol we are talking about. There is some controversy as to whether or not light to moderate alcohol drinking poses a significant health hazard. As a matter of fact, some epidemiological research has shown that moderate consumption of alcohol, about three beers or three glasses of wine per day, was associated with a lesser chance of developing coronary heart disease (CHD). Alcohol is known to relieve emotional tension and has also been associated with increased levels of high density lipoprotein cholesterol (HDL), both of which may help to prevent CHD. On the other hand, other research has shown that three or more drinks per day would increase the risk of developing high blood pressure, another cardiovascular disorder. In addition, alcohol consumption is known to raise the lipid or fat levels in the blood, a risk factor for CHD. However, the current available evidence does not suggest that light to moderate consumption of alcohol (three beers, three glasses of wine, or two highballs) needs to be given up in order to prevent heart disease. Consumed in moderation, along with a balanced diet, alcohol should not pose any health problems to the average individual. However, since alcohol is a significant source of Calories, it should be restricted in weight loss diets.

Heavy alcohol consumption is a different matter as it can produce significant health problems. One of the major body organs affected by alcohol is the liver. Even with a balanced diet high in protein, six drinks a day for less than a month has been shown to cause significant accumulation of fat in the liver. If continued, this could lead to irreversible liver disease, hepatitis, and cirrhosis, the formation of scar tissue. As liver function deteriorates, fat, carbohydrate, and protein metabolism are not regulated properly with possible pathological consequences for other body organs such as the kidney and heart. The health hazards of prolonged excessive alcohol consumption have been well documented, and anyone with such a problem should seek professional help.

In this necessarily brief discussion, only some of the physiological effects of alcohol have been mentioned. As you know, alcohol affects the brain and can have profound effects on thinking processes, motor performance, and emotional behavior. All three of these functions are important for the safe operation of motor vehicles. Excessive alcohol consumption will disturb all three functions and unfortunately is associated with nearly half the number of automobile accidents in our country. This is the major health hazard resulting from the behavioral effects of alcohol.

What is caffeine and where is it found in the diet?

Caffeine is legally classified as a drug. It is a bitter, white compound of organic nature found in several types of plants. Although caffeine may be prepared as an odorless, bitter white powder, it is a natural component of coffee beans, tea leaves, cocoa beans, kola nuts, and other plants. Beverages and other preparations made from these sources contain varying amounts of caffeine. The following represents some typical levels:

Caffeine and physical performance

Cup of perked coffee	125 mg
Cup of instant coffee	70 mg
Cup of tea	70 mg
Glass of cola	65 mg
Glass of diet cola	40 mg
Aspirin tablet	25 mg
Stay-awake tablet	110 mg

A normal therapeutic dose of caffeine may range from 100–300 mg. One to two cups of perked coffee could easily provide this amount.

Caffeine has no food value of any significance to humans. However, it may exert significant effects on the body through its pharmacological properties.

What are the physiological effects of caffeine?

As with alcohol, the physiological effects of caffeine may be dependent upon the individual. A developed tolerance to caffeine may reduce some of the effects, whereas an excessive response may be noted in someone who normally does not consume caffeine. Two cups of coffee, about 250 mg, may make one person more alert, but it may cause a jittery, nervous reaction in another. Individuality of response is an important concept to keep in mind.

Following the ingestion of coffee, tea, or other caffeine-containing beverages the blood levels of caffeine peak within 30–60 minutes. The caffeine is rapidly distributed to the body tissues roughly in proportion to their water content. The physiological effects follow a similar time course, and the effects on any given tissue are dependent upon its caffeine concentration.

The physiological effects of caffeine are many and varied, some of possible significance to the active individual. In general, caffeine is a stimulant. It may exert a direct effect on some tissues or act indirectly through its action on the nervous system. The following are the major physiological effects of caffeine.

Caffeine is a central nervous system stimulant. In doses of 50–200 mg it may cause increased alertness; however, excessive dosages of 300–500 mg may contribute to nervousness and muscular tremor.

Caffeine also stimulates the heart. It will increase the heart rate as well as the force of contraction, thus increasing the amount of blood pumped by the heart. It may cause some irregular heart rate rhythms in some individuals.

It relaxes some of the smooth muscles in the body, particularly those in the blood vessels. This will cause greater circulation to some areas of the body.

Caffeine will stimulate the release of epinephrine (adrenalin) from the adrenal gland. Increased levels of adrenalin in the blood can then stimulate a number of body tissues, including the heart and blood vessels.

In conjunction with the increased levels of adrenalin, caffeine will also increase the amount of free fatty acids (FFA) in the blood, which may be a source of energy for the muscle. Blood glucose levels also rise, but this may be due to decreased uptake of glucose by the tissues rather than by increased glucose release from the liver.

Caffeine may also stimulate an increased secretion of gastric acids. This may give rise to a feeling of an upset stomach.

Finally, caffeine is a **diuretic.** It will stimulate the formation of urine and the removal of water from the body. This dehydration effect may be of concern to the distance runner or cyclist who must perform in the heat.

Can caffeine use improve or impair physical performance?

Some of the physiological effects of caffeine would appear to be beneficial to athletic performance. Stimulation of the nervous system, increased amount of blood from the heart, and the release of adrenalin could, theoretically, improve a variety of physiological processes important during exercise. Indeed, prior to the 1972 Munich Olympics competing athletes were banned from using caffeine by the International Olympic Committee (IOC) because it was thought to increase physical performance. Caffeine was removed from the IOC drug list from 1972–1982, but was recently reinstated as a banned drug for the Los Angeles Olympics. Consumption of 5–6 cups of strong coffee in 1–2 hours would constitute an illegal dose.

Most available research has shown that caffeine will not improve physical performance in events characterized by strength, power, or endurance events lasting less than an hour in duration. Exercise itself is a stimulant, increasing the amount of blood coming from the heart, facilitating blood flow to the active muscles, stimulating the release of epinephrine, and increasing blood levels of FFA and glucose. Hence, in most athletic events these exercise effects appear to override those created by caffeine. There is no additive effect of the caffeine so performance is not improved.

In recent years, however, research has shown that caffeine may be beneficial to individuals involved in long distance events such as marathon running (26.2 miles), which may last well over two hours. In theory, this is what happens. The marathoner relies to a great extent on the muscle and liver glycogen content, which may become depleted during the last six miles or so and hence contribute to fatigue and a reduction in running speed. Caffeine, in conjunction with the increased adrenalin levels, will elevate FFA levels in the blood and increase the utilization of triglycerides stored in the muscle as a source of energy during the run. The increased fat utilization decreases the amount of muscle glycogen used; hence, there is a glycogen sparing effect so the runner has an ample supply of muscle glycogen to help maintain an optimal running speed during the later stages of the race.

Research with caffeine has produced some conflicting results relative to its effects on aerobic endurance performance, but, in general, the following conclusions seem to be supported by the available data. Caffeine will increase the blood FFA at rest, but the increase during exercise does not appear to be any greater than that caused by exercise alone. However, the use of the triglycerides in the muscle appears to increase, and may spare muscle glycogen use. Performance in endurance events lasting less than 30 minutes is not affected by caffeine, but it may improve performance in events of long duration, i.e., greater than 90 minutes. However, the exact mechanism of this improvement has yet to be elucidated. In certain individuals, caffeine may actually impair aerobic endurance. With other types of physical performance, caffeine has not been effective as a means to improve anaerobic capacity while the results relative to psychomotor performance are equivocal. This entire area is in need of additional research.

There may be some possible deleterious effects of caffeine on performance. As a diuretic, caffeine may decrease the body water level prior to competition. As noted in Chapter 14, the opposite effect is usually desired during exercise in the heat. The partial dehydration effect of caffeine may limit the cooling ability of the individual, which may contribute to an excessive body temperature and decreased physical performance capacity. However, a recent study reported no effect of caffeine on temperature regulation in a two hour treadmill run. For those individuals not used to caffeine, it may cause an increase in nervous tension and stomach distress. These sensations may also be detrimental to physical performance.

If you are involved in long distance competition you may desire to experiment with the use of caffeine as an aid to performance. Two cups of brewed coffee is a good dose. If you are not used to caffeine, try it during a practice session rather than during actual competition. Stay-awake tablets may be substituted for coffee. The caffeine should be taken about one hour prior to exercising. Use yourself as an experiment of one subject, repeating the procedure often both with and without caffeine and noting your overall response to the exercise task. Until more evidence is available, your own personal evaluation will provide the best basis for your decision to use caffeine as an aid to your performance.

Are there any health hazards or benefits associated with caffeine?

Caffeine and your health

Since caffeine is known to increase blood levels of FFA some early reports suggested that caffeine may be a risk factor for coronary heart disease as elevated FFA levels may contribute to atherosclerosis or narrowing of the blood vessels in the heart. However, the available research suggests that the moderate intake of caffeine as practiced by most adults is of little importance to the development of CHD. A recently recommended amount was about two cups per day. In a recent thorough review dealing with physiological and psychological effects of caffeine in humans, the general conclusion was that caffeine is a relatively safe drug for the average healthy person. However, large amounts of caffeine may cause some minor problems like sleeplessness. On the other hand, individuals with such health problems as high blood pressure, ulcers, certain cardiovascular diseases, and some nervous disorders should abstain from caffeine. The stimulation effect may aggravate the condition.

Furthermore, recent research has suggested that young children may become addicted to caffeine, demonstrating hyperactivity, irritability, and nervousness. Because of the small size of a child, one twelve-ounce bottle of cola may be the equivalent of three to four cups of coffee to the adult. Thus, excessive consumption of cola-type sodas by young children may lead to a physical dependence. Withdrawal symptoms have been detected in such children, including headaches, upset stomachs, and cold sweats. These possible problems, in combination with the low nutritional quality of cola-type drinks in general, should suggest that those products be limited to rather small amounts in the diets of children.

Are there any other concerns that the physically active individual might have relative to the use of alcohol and caffeine?

Athletes at all levels of competition often wonder if there exists some magical compound that will give them some advantage over their competitors. Both alcohol and caffeine have been used for this purpose. However, research with alcohol has shown it to be ineffective as a means to increase performance capacity, while caffeine may possibly be effective in events that are of very prolonged duration although more research is needed to substantiate this possibility. The key to success in athletic competition is not to be found in special pills or elixers, but rather in the long hours of training essential to develop superior levels of physical fitness and technique for your particular activity. This training should be complemented with a balanced diet plan.

The consumer athlete

16

Within the past decade there has been a phenomenal increase in knowledge relative to all facets of life, the science of nutrition included. Thousands upon thousands of studies have been conducted, revealing facts to help unravel some of the mysteries of human nutrition. Certain individuals may capitalize on these research findings for personal financial gain. For example, isolated nutritional facts may be distorted in order to market a specific nutritional product for the general public. Following a professional advertising campaign, the end result is we end up buying a product that we do not need. This is the essence of quackery.

Quackery is big business. It has been estimated that five to ten billion dollars a year are spent on questionable health practices in the United States. A substantial percentage of this amount has been for unnecessary nutritional products. Authorities in this area have noted the amount of misinformation about nutrition is overwhelming, and it is circulated widely particularly by those who may profit from it. Although we may still think of quacks as sleezy individuals selling patent medicine from a covered wagon, the truth is they are very subtle. Nutrition quacks sound authentic, use modern advertising and marketing techniques, and take advantage of the fact that most people still believe there is something mystical about food.

J. V. Durnin, an international authority in nutrition and exercise, has stated that there is still no sphere of nutrition in which faddism, misconceptions, ignorance, and quackery are more obvious than in athletics. As revealed by interviews with international class athletes at the Montreal Olympics and other surveys, many athletes still believe there is a special diet or special nutritional ingredient essential to their success. One athlete has been reported to take seventy-six tablets of various nutritional compounds—for breakfast. The typical road runner also consumes a wide variety of nutritional compounds specifically advertised to increase endurance performance. Why do these practices exist when the evidence suggests that the nutritional requirements for the individual in physical training depend upon the same fundamental principles that apply to the nonactive person?

The best defense against nutritional quackery is sound knowledge of nutritional principles. Although all facets of consumer awareness about nutritional quackery cannot be covered in this brief chapter, some basic information relative to the nutritional quality of foods, the role of additives, and nutritional quackery specific to the active individual may provide you with some basic knowledge in order to separate fact from fiction and make sound decisions concerning the nutritional products you purchase.

Nutritional value of American foods

Is the nutritional value of our food declining?

The recently developed dietary goals for Americans were discussed in Chapter 1. One of the underlying implications of these goals is that many of our foods are overprocessed. They contain too much refined sugar, extracted oils or white flour, all products of a refinement process. Refined sugar is pure carbohydrate with no nutritional value except Calories. The same can be said for extracted oils, which are pure fat. In the bleaching and processing of wheat to white flour, at least twenty-two known essential nutrients are removed, including the B vitamins, vitamin E, calcium, phosphorus, potassium, and magnesium. In addition, many fruits and vegetables are artificially ripened before they have reached maturity and contain smaller quantities of vitamins and minerals. We also consume many totally synthetic products such as artificial orange juice, nondairy creamers, and imitation ice cream, which do not possess the same nutrient value as their natural counterparts. There appears to be legitimate concern about the declining nutritional value of our food supply. Much of the blame is assigned to the processing of food, but this is not necessarily so.

In the mind of the public, processed foods are being thought of more and more as inferior foods when compared to natural sources, for example, frozen peas versus fresh peas. The major purpose of food processing is to prevent waste through deterioration or spoilage. There are a variety of ways to do this, including heat, dehydration, refrigeration, freezing, and the use of chemicals. Food is processed by companies preparing their products for sale, but food processing also occurs at home in the preparation of a meal. You may wash, cut, cook, and freeze a variety of foods at home. Food processing, both at home and by commercial organizations, will result in the loss of some nutrients. However, a recent respected research report noted that commercial preservation techniques in common use today do not cause major nutrient losses in the foods we eat. Nutrient losses by commerical food processing may be less than foods processed at home. In addition, food companies may enrich or fortify certain products before marketing. Examples include the addition of some B vitamins and iron to grain products, vitamins A and D to milk, vitamin A to margarine, and iodine to table salt. In some cases not all of the nutrients that were removed in processing are returned, but in some products a greater amount is returned or added.

Benjamin Borenstein has noted with some reservations that carbohydrates, lipids, protein, niacin, vitamin K, and minerals are relatively stable during food processing and storage. Vitamins A, D, E, B_2, B_6, B_{12}, pantothenic acid, and folacin are a little less stable, while B_1 and vitamin C may be seriously depleted by commercial and home food processing.

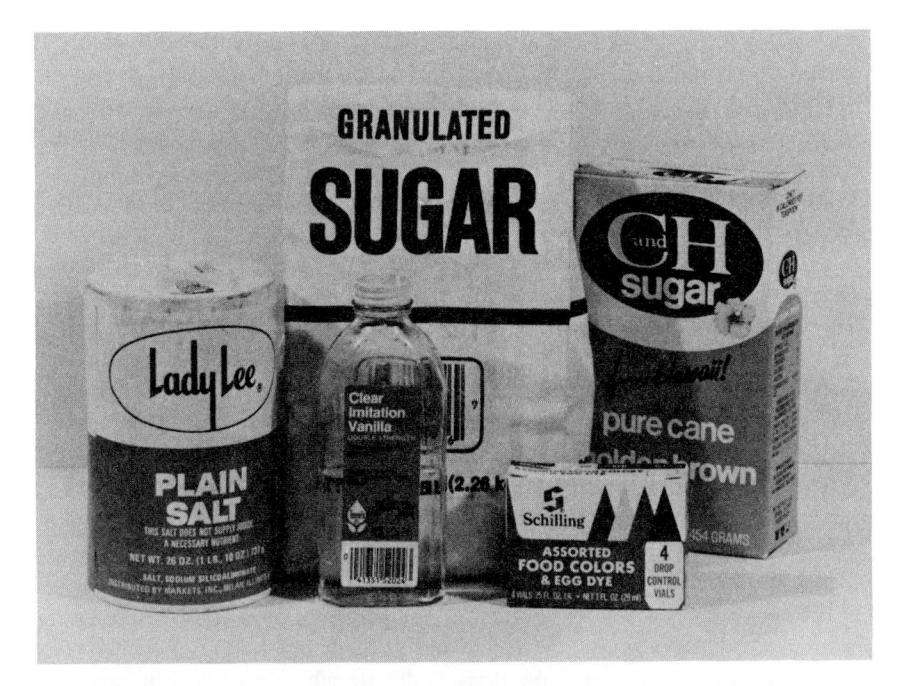

Most food additives are generally recognized as being safe, but excess sugar, fat, and several other chemicals are of dubious value.
(David Corona)

The key point is that food processing will not necessarily produce a nutritionally inferior product. Even if processing does cause a slight decrease in nutritional quality, it will help provide a greater and more varied food supply with adequate amounts of dietary nutrients. The major problem is the excessive use of highly refined products like sugar, oils, unenriched white flour, and those with questionable additives. Wise food selection can help avoid these problems.

What are food additives and should they be avoided?

Do you ever read the list of ingredients on food product labels? If not, check one out in the near future. My guess is you will not know what half the ingredients are or why they are there. A recently purchased pie had the main ingredients of water, sugar, wheat flour, fruit, and margarine, but the following were among the other compounds found in the pie: salt, artificial flavors, artificial colors, agar, locust bean gum, microcrystalline cellulose, sodium propionate, potassium sorbate, polysorbate 60, sorbiton monosterarate, sodium phosphate, carboxymethylcellulose, and calcium carrageenan. The pie was delicious, but were all these additives necessary? Although we will not discuss the role of each of these additives, look at some of the major reasons why they might be there.

The Food and Drug Administration (FDA) classifies **food additives** as any substance added directly to food. Two of the leading additives in the United States are sugar and salt, which may present health problems to certain people. On the other hand, vitamins and minerals are also added to many foods and may help insure adequate intake of those nutrients. There are over forty different reasons why additives are put in the foods we eat, but the four most common are to add flavor, to enhance color, to improve the texture, and to preserve the food. For example, vanilla extract may be added to ice cream to impart a vanilla flavor, vitamin C may be added to fruits and vegetables to prevent discoloration, emulsifiers may be added to help blend oil evenly throughout a product, and sodium propionate may be used to prolong shelf life.

In order to have FDA approval, additives must be **generally recognized as safe (GRAS).** They may be added only to specific foods for specific purposes, and in general must improve the quality of the food without posing any hazards to humans. Only the minimum amount necessary to achieve the desired purpose may be added.

Laboratory tests with animals have shown that certain additives may cause cancer or other health problems. The **Feingold hypothesis** suggests that hyperactivity in some children is due to the consumption of excessive amounts of some additives. Now there is debate whether or not the results of the animal research are of practical significance for humans since the relative doses given to the animals were much greater than humans could consume, and the Feingold hypothesis is controversial. We have seen a government ban or partial ban on several additives during the past decade, including cyclamates, saccharin, and red dye number two.

Although we may realize that absolute safety does not exist in anything we do, including the food we eat, we do have a right to expect that the food we purchase is generally safe for consumption. The government and food manufacturers must take utmost care to insure that food additives do not create any appreciable risks to our health. On the other hand, we as consumers also have a responsibility to select foods necessary for good nutrition. Food product labeling has helped us in this regard, for we can now tell what ingredients we are eating although we may not always know why they are there.

The general consensus appears to be that most additives in our foods are safe. Probably the most hazardous additives to our health are the excessive amounts of refined sugar and oils added to many products, the high caloric content and low nutritive value contributing to excess body weight and possible undernutrition. When you check a food label, the ingredients must be listed in order of concentration in the product with the largest amount of ingredient listed first. If you see sugar and vegetable oils among the first couple of ingredients, you are probably getting a high-Calorie food with little nutrient value, depending what the remaining ingredients are. By avoiding these types of foods, you will be eliminating unnecessary additives to your diet.

Although most additives are considered to be safe, it may be prudent to avoid others that may possibly be harmful. By following these precautions, you will be able to avoid or reduce the most dubious additives found in foods.

1. Eat fresh foods whenever possible, such as fruit, vegetables, fresh meat and poultry, minimally processed bread, and similar products.

2. Read the labels on processed foods and select those products with the least number of additives.

3. Avoid or reduce the consumption of foods that contain the following additives: artificial coloring, dyes, saccharin, sodium nitrate, sodium nitrite, monosodium glutamate, BHT, BHA, sugar, and salt.

Do foods contain enough pesticides to cause concern?

Over two thousand insects, weeds, or plant diseases damage nearly one-third of our nation's farm crop each year. Various herbicides and pesticides are used to counteract these pests, but a number of illnesses and deaths have been attributed to prolonged exposure to these chemicals, including cancer, birth defects, nervous system disorders, genetic mutations, and miscarriages. On the one hand we need to control those pests destructive to our food supply, but on the other hand the health of the public should not be harmed by the chemicals being used. This is the dilemma concerning the use of pesticides and similar chemicals.

Most of the serious diseases from pesticide use have been among farmworkers who may be exposed to high concentrations on a daily basis or in people who live near sprayed areas. However, direct exposure to even small amounts of insect spray as found in many homes has been known to alter brain function, causing irritability, insomnia, and reduced concentration ability. The prudent individual should avoid direct contact with these substances as much as possible, for even thorough washing with soap and water has little effect upon the absorption through the skin of some insect sprays.

Pesticides may also be on the food we eat and in the water we drink. Studies have shown that pesticide levels are increasing in human fat and mother's milk, the latter posing a possible problem to infants who are nursed. The FDA and state government agencies conduct spot surveys to analyze the pesticide content of produce for sale. In general, their results suggest that most produce has no pesticides or negligible amounts within safe limits. However, fish and meat products may contain higher amounts of pesticides as they become more concentrated in these animals when they consume large quantities of plants with pesticide residue. Thus, exposure to certain pesticide sprays plus the amounts in the food and water we consume may lead to the increased amounts found in the human body.

Unfortunately, there is little understanding of how this level of pesticide exposure will affect human health. Based on current knowledge, probably the most prudent behavior we may undertake is to avoid direct skin or breathing exposure to pesticides, wash produce thoroughly, and eat less animal fat. There is some evidence that pesticide-free farming may be effective, but it will take some time before it may be implemented on a large scale so that we may reduce the amount of chemicals we unintentionally consume.

Are natural or organic foods more nutritious?

Almost all the foods we eat are organic and many are in their natural state, especially fresh fruits and vegetables. Those individuals who advertise and sell **natural and organic foods** usually make the following claims about their products:

1. They are grown in soil without artificial fertilizers.

2. No pesticides were used in the growing process.

3. Very little processing has been done.

4. There are no chemical additives.

These points certainly do not detract from the nutrient value of a food, but do they increase the nutrient content above a similar food not grown and processed under similar circumstances?

First, with few exceptions of trace minerals like iodine, zinc, cobalt, and selenium, the composition of the soil has little effect upon the vitamin and mineral content of the plant. Plant development is determined by the genetic aspects of the seed. If the minerals necessary for development of the plant are absent or in low quantity in the soil, the plant will not grow or fewer plants will develop. Vitamin content is also controlled by nature and in order for the plant to develop, it must have its natural amount of vitamins. Otherwise, it would not develop. Natural fertilizer does not provide any significant advantage over artificial fertilizer. Both can provide the necessary substances for plant growth. Second, as noted above, the amount of pesticides on market produce is well within safe limits according to current standards. Moreover, how do you know whether or not an apple or any other plant product was grown free of pesticides or herbicides? In reality, you do not. Third, the major forms of processing used today do not cause major losses of nutrients. The minor amounts lost may be replaced or are of little practical significance. As mentioned earlier, commercial preparation of foods, particularly frozen foods, may more effectively preserve nutrients than home processing. And lastly, most additives to foods today are generally considered to be safe.

In summary, the available evidence does not support the viewpoint that organic and natural foods are more nutritious than their counterparts grown under different conditions. However, they are advertised as being more nutritious and they generally cost more. Hence, the consumer is being exposed to nutritional quackery and economic fraud.

What is the concept of nutrient density?

Due to the increasing use of machines and other laborsaving devices during this past century, the energy requirement of the average individual has decreased significantly. Whereas 3,800 Calories may have been necessary to meet the energy needs of the average worker fifty years ago, 2,800 Calories may now be adequate. The lowered caloric requirement is due to an overall decrease in daily physical activity. However, although the caloric requirement has decreased, the need for adequate amounts of nutrients such as protein, vitamins, and minerals has not. Today one must get a proper balance of nutrients from less food Calories. This may become especially important for those individuals on a diet program to lose weight.

Let's take a look at the concept of *nutrient density*. In essence, a food with high nutrient density possesses a significant amount of a specific nutrient or nutrients per serving or for a certain amount of Calories. Let's look at vitamin C as an example. Two cookies contain 100 Calories and only a trace of vitamin C. On the other hand, a 100-Calorie orange contains over 70 mg of vitamin C, which is more than the daily RDA. The orange has a higher nutrient density of vitamin C. As another example, consider the following nutritional data for three ounces of tuna fish and clams:

Nutrient density

	Calories	*Protein*	*Iron*
Tuna fish:	170	24 g	1.6 mg
Clams:	65	11 g	5.2 mg

The protein density is similar in the two foods, as you get approximately 1 g of protein for 7 Calories of tuna fish (170 ÷ 24) and 1 g of protein for 6 Calories from clams (65 ÷ 11). However, clams contain more than three times the amount of iron per serving, and if you consider the fact that the caloric content of the clams is less than half the value for the tuna fish, the nutrient density of iron in the clams is over eight times greater than in the tuna fish. Both foods are excellent sources of protein for the amount of Calories consumed, and although tuna fish is a fairly good source of iron, clams are a much superior source.

Although the active individual should be knowledgeable about nutrient density, the greater caloric intake due to increased physical activity provides a greater opportunity to obtain adequate amounts of required nutrients. Nevertheless, high nutrient content foods should serve as the basis for food selection. One simple method is to reduce intake of foods high in refined sugar, fat content, and unenriched flour. In addition, by studying the nutritional information provided on the labels of most products you may easily discriminate between high and low nutrient density foods.

A discussion of nutrient density and the Index of Nutritional Quality (INQ) was presented in Chapter 1.

What is nutrition labeling?

With the tremendous increase in manufactured food products over the past twenty to thirty years, it has become increasingly difficult to determine the nutritional quality of the food we eat. For example, how much protein do you get from a frozen potpie? Moreover, food manufacturers have often distorted nutritional facts and made rather extravagant claims for their particular product. The average consumer knows little about the nutrient value of most natural foods, and recent developments have compounded the problem of selecting foods that have high nutrient density. A law was passed in 1973 designed to establish a set of standards so that most Americans could choose what to eat based upon sound nutritional information.

This set of standards resulted in **nutritional labeling,** whereby major nutrients found in a food product are listed on the label. It is not the total solution to the problem of poor food selection existing among many Americans, but combined with an educational program to increase nutritional awareness it may effectively improve the nutritional health of our nation.

The following nutrients must be listed in food labels:

Protein	Niacin
Vitamin A	Vitamin C
Thiamin (B_1)	Calcium
Riboflavin (B_2)	Iron

The following may be listed:

Vitamin D	Pantothenic Acid
Vitamin E	Phosphorus
Vitamin B_6	Iodine
Folacin	Magnesium
Vitamin B_{12}	Zinc

Carbohydrate and fat content are usually listed; the simple refined sugar content, saturated and polyunsaturated fats, and cholesterol may also be listed. Additional information includes Calories, serving size, servings per container, and Calories per serving.

The eight nutrients that must be listed on food labels are known as the key nutrients, or **indicator nutrients.** It is believed that if these eight nutrients are obtained in ample supply in a varied diet, then all of the other essential nutrients also will be supplied. In other words, obtaining 100 percent of the U.S. RDA of the eight indicator nutrients from a wide variety of foods should also provide 100 percent of the other nutrients essential in human nutrition.

In order to be of practical value to the consumer, the nutrient content is listed as a percentage of the United States Recommended Daily Allowance (U.S.RDA). The percentages for most nutrients are based upon the U.S. RDA for the average adult male because he usually has the greatest nutrient requirement. However, the U.S. RDA for iron is based upon the adult female since her need is greater.

Protein is listed twice on the label, once as the amount in grams and second as a percentage of the U.S. RDA. The percentage amount reflects the fact that not all protein quality is the same. For example, 8 g of protein from milk, a complete protein, is listed as 20 percent of the U.S. RDA for protein; however, a similar amount of protein in spaghetti, an incomplete protein, represents only 10 percent of the U.S. RDA.

Also recall that food manufacturers must list ingredients in order of their concentration. A product that lists gravy, turkey, salt, and so forth has more gravy than turkey. What may appear to be a good nutritional buy really is not.

An example of a nutrition label for a quart of skim milk is as follows:

Nutrition Informaton Per Serving

Serving size	One 8-ounce glass
Servings per container	4
Calories	90
Protein	9 g
Carbohydrate	12 g
Fat	0 g

Percentage of U.S. Recommended Daily Allowances (U.S. RDA)

Protein	20	Vitamin D	25
Vitamin A	10	Vitamin B_6	4
Vitamin C	4	Vitamin B_{12}	15
Thiamine	8	Phosphorus	25
Riboflavin	30	Magnesium	10
Niacin	*	Zinc	6
Calcium	30	Pantothenic Acid	6
Iron	*		

*Contains less than 2% of the U.S. RDA of the nutrients

Skim milk would be an excellent source of protein, vitamin A, riboflavin, calcium, vitamin D, vitamin B_{12}, phosphorus, and magnesium; it would be a poor source of vitamin C, niacin, iron, and vitamin B_6. However, the tryptophan in milk could be used to make niacin in the body.

There are a number of other subtle points about nutritional labeling but in general the nutritional information presented may serve as a practical guide for determining nutrient density and choosing foods wisely. For those trying to lose weight, foods with high concentrations of nutrients but low Calorie content may be chosen. High iron content foods may be chosen for women and children. It may serve as a useful guide for those who want or need to restrict saturated fats, cholesterol, or sodium in their diets.

In addition, nutrition labeling can help you to get the most nutrition for your money. Reading labels carefully and comparing brands and prices may reveal significant savings and no loss of nutrient value when a store or generic brand is purchased instead of one that is nationally advertised. Products with large amounts of refined sugars and fats are usually uneconomical as they are high in Calories but low in nutrients. In general, you should look for food products providing the greatest percentages of the U.S. RDA for the major nutrients (protein, vitamins A, B, and C, calcium, and iron), at the lowest price. A low Calorie content may also be desirable for those on a weight reduction diet, but may not be as important to the physically active person.

Do fast-food restaurants provide sound nutrition?

Fast-food chains such as McDonalds, Kentucky Fried Chicken, and Pizza Hut have increased tremendously in our country over the past twenty years, raising the question as to whether or not their products provide sound nutrition. Surveying the menu of a major hamburger chain in relationship to the four food groups, we may find the following items on the lunch menu:

Meat group—Hamburgers, fish sandwich, chicken sandwich
Milk group—Milk, milk shakes, cheese (on burger)
Breads and cereals—Buns
Fruits and vegetables—Orange juice, lettuce and tomato (on sandwiches), assorted fruit pies, French fried potatoes

The hamburgers are 100 percent beef with a moderately low fat content (about 20 percent). The fish and chicken are lower in fat, but usually fried. High quality milk and cheese are served, but the milk shakes may have a high fat and sugar content. The buns are usually enriched, but are not usually whole grain products. The lettuce and tomato serving is relatively small, the fruit pies have a high sugar content, but the orange juice and potatoes may be of high quality although the potatoes may be French fried.

In general, the major fast food chains do provide nutritious products. The fat and sugar content of some foods may be a little high, but the customer may be able to substitute foods with lower fat content. A fish sandwich, an order of French fries, and a glass of milk provides a very nutritious snack and contains a serving from each of the four food groups. Some fast-food chains also provide a salad bar so additional vegetables may be obtained. Food quality control at the major fast-food chains is excellent, the products you buy being grade A quality.

No one is suggesting that you eat only fast-food products, but rather that they may be used sparingly to complement other meals taken in the home or elsewhere. Whole grain products, deep green and yellow vegetables, and low fat meat and milk products should be eaten in other daily meals.

How does food cultism affect the active individual?

Hunger is an innate physiological drive necessary for the preservation of life in all animals. Since eating helps to satisfy this drive it is natural to assume that most individuals would be deeply interested in the composition and quality of their diet. However, such is not generally the case. Although hunger is a basic physiological drive, appetite is responsive to both physiological and psychological factors. For example, snake meat is high quality protein and will satisfy the physiological hunger drive, but psychologically it is not considered too appetizing by most Americans. Since eating is controlled partly by psychological processes, and since the amount of money spent on food products is a substantial proportion of the family budget, is it no wonder that there exists a high prevalence of food cultism and nutritional quackery in our culture today? **Food cultism,** nutritional fads, and quackery go hand in hand.

Nutritional quackery in athletics

Although nutritional faddism persists throughout the general public, there is probably no area of nutrition where faddism, misconceptions, and ignorance are more obvious than in food products marketed for athletes and other active people. Why is this so when the scientific evidence tells us that the nutritional requirements of the individual involved in physical training depend upon the same fundamental principles governing human beings in general?

There are several reasons for food cultism among those involved in some form of athletic competition. First, eating behavior may be patterned after someone who is successful in a given sport. If Olympic champions suggest part of their success was due to brand X vitamin tablets, a vegetarian diet, or the milk of a cow that is in heat, you may be assured these dietary practices will be adopted by aspiring young athletes. Second, many coaches, trainers, and team physicians may suggest that certain foods or food supplements are essential to success. In a recent survey, many athletes reported that they received some of their nutritional information from their coaches, much of which was unfortunately simply a perpetuation of myths and misconceptions. Misinformation also may have been obtained from leading sports magazines that ofttimes present articles on nutrition for the athlete based upon very questionable research.

Probably the most significant factor contributing to food cultism among active individuals is direct advertising. Literally hundreds of products are marketed specifically for the athlete. As just one example a leading runners' magazine recently carried an advertisement that one tablespoon of the advertised product, mixed with your favorite unsweetened fruit juice, would provide improved energy and endurance. It was described as the ultimate food formula for ultimate energy. The major ingredient was dried potassium-rich bananas, and the cost was approximately $12 per pound. Rather expensive bananas, and, incidentally, fresh bananas are also potassium-rich.

Most of these products are economic frauds. The prices are exorbitant in comparison to the same amount of nutrients found in ordinary foods. High protein pills and powders designed for athletes usually cost more than ten times the same amount of protein obtained in milk. Other than economic fraud, these products are an intellectual fraud. There is no scientific evidence to support their claims. Simple basic facts about the physiological functions of the nutrients in these products are distorted, magnified, and advertised in such a way as to make one believe they will increase performance. After all, most people believe you cannot advertise anything but the truth. Unfortunately, in the area of nutrition and physical performance, it is very easy to distort the truth and appeal to the psychological emotions of the athlete.

Active individuals involved in competition, whether at the Olympics or a local hometown 10 km road race, want to do their best. Often they will rely on a variety of different compounds or treatments, usually called ergogenic aids, which are designed to improve physical performance capacity.

What is an ergogenic aid?

Many athletes in training for competition are always searching for the ultimate ingredient to provide that extra winning edge over their opponents. Over the years a number of theoretical ergogenic aids have been utilized in attempts to increase athletic performance capability; the term **ergogenic** is defined as anything that tends to increase work output. A large number of diverse substances or treatments have been utilized in this regard, and the rationale for their use was based on the theory that they would directly benefit the physiological capacity of a particular body system, such as the cardiovascular system, or they would help remove psychological restraints, which might limit physiological capacity.

There are several different classifications of ergogenic aids, grouped according to the general nature of their application. Listed below are several major categories with an example of one theoretical ergogenic aid for each.

Mechanical aids. Heat application may serve as a passive form of warm-up in an attempt to increase blood flow to a body area and possibly increase speed of muscle contraction.

Psychological aids. Hypnosis, through posthypnotic suggestion, may help remove psychological barriers that limit performance capacity.

Physiological aids. Blood doping, or the infusion of blood into the athlete, may increase oxygen transportation capacity and thus increase endurance.

Pharmacological aids. Drugs such as amphetamines have been used in attempts to increase strength and power due to their stimulating effect upon the nervous system.

Nutritional aids. Vitamin E has been taken in attempts to increase endurance capacity, as it has been theorized to improve the utilization of oxygen in the tissues.

Although the theoretical rationale exists for many of these substances, the scientific evidence generally does not support their effectiveness as a means to increase athletic performance. Moreover, although some ergogenic aids like heat applications may pose no health problems, others such as the use of amphetamines and anabolic steroids may have some serious toxic effects. In general, drugs have not been shown to increase performance capacity, and they should be avoided by the active person on this basis as well as the potential medical complications they may create.

Probably the most abused ergogenic aids are those classified as nutritional. As many people, including athletes, believe that certain foods possess magical qualities, it is no wonder that a wide array of nutrients or special food preparations have been used since time immemorial in attempts to run faster, jump higher, or throw farther.

What does research say about the effectiveness of the many nutritional ergogenic aids that are marketed for the athlete or active individual?

It was noted earlier that food has three basic functions in the human body—to build and repair body tissues, to regulate body processes, and to provide energy. These functions are accomplished through an adequate intake of six nutrients—carbohydrate, fat, protein, vitamins, minerals, and water. Previous chapters in this book have examined the role of each of these nutrients as they relate to physical performance, including the possible ergogenic effect of supplementation to a balanced diet.

As a brief review, let us look at each of the six nutrients and their possible effectiveness to increase physical performance capacity. Consult each respective chapter for details. Carbohydrate may benefit performance in prolonged exercise, such as in marathons, ultramarathons, and similar such events. Carbohydrate loading prior to performance and the ingestion of carbohydrate beverages during competition may be helpful. High carbohydrate compounds before most other athletic events are not helpful. Fat supplementation to the diet has no theoretical rationale, as the body possesses significant amounts for energy needs. Expensive protein supplements are not necessary as the balanced American diet is rather high in protein content and meets the needs of both the young developing and mature athlete. The most commonly used vitamin supplements among athletes include the B-complex, C, and E. Research has shown that supplementation with each of these has not increased physical performance. Mineral supplementation, including the major electrolytes found in sport drinks as well as iron, does not improve performance of the individual on a balanced diet. However, iron supplements may be helpful to the female athlete who may be on a low-Calorie diet or who experiences heavy menstrual flow and to male endurance athletes who lose large amounts of sweat in training. Hyperhydration with water before competition may be helpful in long endurance events, particularly when performing in the heat. Taking water during such events is also helpful. Both practices may help prevent the adverse effects of dehydration and high body temperature upon physical performance.

As is evident from the above review, nutrient supplementation will not increase physical performance capacity with the exception of several practices such as carbohydrate loading and hyperhydration, both of which can be done without expensive ergogenic aids. Since any advertised nutritional ergogenic aid contains either one or a combination of the six nutrients, logic suggests that they too will be ineffective. Yet we still see hundreds of different nutritional compounds "scientifically designed" to improve athletic performance, or some single magical nutrient that will work wonders with the athlete. Space limitations do not allow for a lengthy discussion of all nutritional ergogenic aids used, but a few of the more recently used compounds will be evaluated briefly.

Bee pollen or pollen extract has been marketed almost specifically for athletes, primarily runners, as a means to increase performance. However, several sound research studies have shown that bee pollen does not benefit those components in the blood that may contribute to endurance capacity, does not improve recovery between exercise repetitions in a workout so one can train harder, nor does it increase endurance. Another compound that has been reported to cause significant improvements in endurance capacity is the so-called vitamin B_{15}, also known as pangamic acid or dimethylglycine. Recent controlled research with human subjects has revealed that vitamin B_{15} will not improve physical performance. Moreover, a recent review has noted that no specific disease state could be attributed to a deficiency of vitamin B_{15}, thus questioning its classification as a vitamin. Furthermore, a recent report from the American Council on Science and Health noted that B_{15} is a label, not a substance, as sellers of the product have put a variety of different chemical compounds in a bottle and simply labeled it vitamin B_{15}. Dr. Victor Herbert, Director of The Hematology and Nutrition Laboratory at the Veteran's Administration Hospital in New York, stated that these pills may be hazardous because some of the chemicals present have dangerous side effects, including mutagenic compounds suspected of causing cancer.

A number of other nutritional compounds have been popular among athletes throughout the years, including honey, gelatin, lecithin, ginseng, wheat germ oil, and aspartates. Research with each of these compounds has revealed no beneficial effect upon physical performance capacity when utilized as a supplement to the normal balanced diet. However, some recent research with alkaline salts, such as sodium bicarbonate, has revealed a possible beneficial effect upon anaerobic exercise performance, such as running a half-mile, but needs further documentation.

In summary, the general consensus is that a balanced diet is all that is necessary to provide the nutrients necessary for maximal performance potential. If you have trained properly, obtained adequate rest, and eaten the appropriate foods, commercial nutritional supplements designed for athletes or the active individual will not provide any additional benefits.

17 Special considerations for active people

The major thrust of this book has been toward the nutritional needs of the physically active individual; and whether discussing such topics as human energy sources and systems, exercise in the heat, or each of the six specific nutrients, an attempt was made to suggest dietary modifications if and when necessary. For example, the technique of glycogen loading and hyperhydration were discussed in the carbohydrate and water chapters, respectively, and the myth of protein supplementation was discredited in Chapters 4 and 11.

The purpose of this chapter is to synthesize some of this nutritional information and relate it to some of the special dietary considerations and health concerns of the physically active person. The topic of additional nutritional demands for athletes is one of the most abused issues in athletic nutrition; it will be discussed in light of the available research reviewed for this book. The nutritional needs of the active female, as well as the active younger and older individual, are also discussed.

What to eat before competition is of interest to almost all physically active persons, so some general guidelines are presented to help you avoid some unnecessary problems during competitive events.

Certain individuals, such as diabetics, must be cautious about the interaction of diet and exercise, as do individuals with a family history of coronary heart disease and high blood pressure. The role of diet and/or exercise in these and other health-related problems is covered, including the techniques of extreme weight loss in certain sports.

Finally, the viewpoints of several international authorities in athletic nutrition are presented, which are reinforced by the general viewpoint of this book.

Does the stress of exercise impose any additional nutritional demands on the body?

If you read some of the articles about nutrition for athletes in popular sports magazines or pay any attention to athletic food supplements advertised therein, you would probably get the impression that athletes have special nutrition requirements above those of the nonathlete. Vitamin and mineral supplements are often highly recommended. However, if you have progressed through this text to this point, you are probably aware that such is not the case.

Exercise and nutritional requirements

Nutrition for the active person may be viewed from two aspects, one stressing the acute effects while the other focuses on the chronic, or training, effects of habitual exercise. An **acute exercise bout** will utilize specific body energy sources and systems, depending upon the intensity and duration of the exercise. Briefly, the high-energy phosphates are utilized during short, high-intensity exercise, muscle glycogen is used in intense exercise lasting about one to three minutes, and the oxidation of glycogen and fats becomes increasingly important in endurance activities greater than five minutes. High levels of muscle glycogen would be important to an individual performing a long duration exercise bout. Reviewing Chapter 8 will help reinforce these concepts. The energy changes in each one of these systems may require certain vitamins and minerals for optimal efficiency. If exercise is performed repeatedly, such as on a daily basis, the body will begin to make adjustments in these energy systems so that they become more efficient. This is the so-called **chronic training effect,** and many of the body adjustments incorporate certain specific nutrients. For example, one of the chronic effects of long distance running is an increased hemoglobin content in the blood and increased myoglobin and cytochromes in the muscle cells; all three compounds need iron in order to be formed. Hence, increased muscle glycogen, or carbohydrate, stores would benefit performance in an acute exercise bout such as a marathon run, and the daily diet would need to contain adequate amounts of iron in order to make effective body adjustments due to the chronic effects of training.

If an individual is well nourished, an acute bout of exercise will not impose any special demands for any of the six nutrients, with several possible exceptions. Body energy stores of carbohydrate and fat are adequate to satisfy the energy demands of most activities lasting less than one hour. Protein is not generally considered a significant energy source during exercise, although recent research has indicated it may contribute about 10 percent of the energy demand when a person has low muscle glycogen stores. The vitamin and mineral content of the body will be sufficient to help regulate the increased levels of metabolic activity, and body water supply will be adequate under normal environmental conditions. The general exceptions are exercise bouts of long duration and exercise in warm or hot weather. Endurance-type exercise at a moderately high level may benefit from carbohydrate loading and/or carbohydrate intake during the exercise; those methods were discussed in Chapter 2. Drinking water before and during exercise in the heat may also benefit performance, as it may help to reduce the heat stress to the body. A discussion was presented in Chapters 7 and 14.

During a training period, the amount of calorie intake needed to maintain body weight may increase considerably, being an additional 1,000 Calories or more per day in certain activities. If these additional calories are selected wisely from among the Basic Four Food Groups, then you should obtain an adequate amount of all nutrients essential for the formation of new body tissues and proper functioning of the energy systems that increase during exercise. A balanced intake of carbohydrate, fat, protein, vitamins, minerals, and water is all that is necessary. The guidelines presented in Chapter 1 will help insure adequate nutrition.

In activities where excess body weight may serve to handicap performance, a loss of some body fat may be helpful. Guidelines for safe losses of body fat for sports competition were presented in Chapters 12 and 13, but in those cases where a very low-Calorie diet is used in conjunction with an exercise program to achieve a desirable competitive weight, nutrient supplementation with vitamins and minerals may be recommended. More is said about weight control in wrestlers later in this chapter.

Does the active female have any special nutritional requirements?

From birth until puberty there is little or no difference in the nutritional requirements of boys and girls. However, between the ages of approximately eleven to fourteen, endocrine changes during the onset of puberty produce significant differences in body size and composition. Throughout adolescence and adulthood, males are taller and weigh more. From a nutritional standpoint, the smaller body size and greater percentage of body fat of the female are the major differences between the sexes. Thus, the average female has a lower basal metabolic rate and expends less energy during physical activity than the average male. Consequently, her need for calories is less.

Along with a decreased need for Calories, the smaller body size and lower metabolic rate place lesser demands for some of the nutrients. Females in general need slightly lower amounts of protein, vitamins A and E, thiamin, niacin, riboflavin, and vitamin B_6. The decreased amount of these nutrients corresponds to the decreased caloric intake, so the nutritional density of the food remains constant. Although the RDA for vitamin D, vitamin C, folacin, vitamin B_{12}, calcium, phosphorus, and zinc is the same for males and females, females probably need slightly lesser amounts of these nutrients due to their smaller body size. Since the average caloric requirement for the adult female is about 700 Calories less than the adult male, she needs to have a greater nutrient density in the food she eats in order to get the RDA of these nutrients. A balanced intake of foods throughout the Basic Four Food Groups will ensure adequate amounts of these nutrients. Moreover, the physically active woman may expend more Calories per day, permitting a greater caloric intake with no gain in body weight and a greater opportunity to obtain these nutrients.

Women should keep in mind that the U.S. RDA, which is used in nutritional labeling, is based upon the RDA of the adult male, with the exception of iron. Hence, if a certain product will supply 25 percent of the RDA for a male, it may supply about 30 percent for the average female.

Iron is the only nutrient that females require in greater amounts than males, the RDA being 18 mg per day for females and only 10 for males. Since the U.S. RDA used in nutritional labeling uses the adult female requirement for iron as the RDA, a food with 10 percent of the RDA for iron will contain almost 20 percent of the male RDA. The importance of iron in physical performance was discussed in chapter 6, and since women must get their RDA of iron with fewer amount of calories, they should select foods high in iron content and may possibly benefit from iron supplementation if body iron stores are low.

One possible problem for the physically active female is the development of amenorrhea, which has been reported recently in several surveys of endurance athletes. There appears to be no identifiable cause at present, but certain nutritional factors such as a rapid loss of body weight, a low percentage of body fat, and a decreased intake of protein and fat have been associated with its development. A disturbed endocrine balance as a result of amenorrhea may also contribute to the development of osteoporosis. Physically active women should also stress the intake of calcium in the diet, skim milk and low-fat yogurt being excellent sources.

Many women who are physically active continue with their conditioning program throughout the greater part of pregnancy and during the lactation period. Nutritional requirements increase considerably during this time when the woman must eat nutrients for two. The American College of Obstetricians and Gynecologists issued a position statement that recommends, in general, the following points for pregnant women:

1. Increase protein consumption, preferably from animal foods.

2. Increase caloric consumption about 15 percent, or about 300 Calories per day more than the nonpregnant female.

3. Weight gain should not be restricted unduly; a gain of 10–12 kg, or 22–27 lbs, is acceptable.

4. Increase intake of the essential nutrients including all vitamins and minerals.

5. Take an iron supplement of about 30–60 mg per day. Since the need for nutrients may increase considerably during pregnancy and lactation, the female must become increasingly conscious about the food she eats. Foods with high nutrient density must be the basis for the diet. Physicians may recommend vitamin and mineral supplements. The active female will have a greater opportunity to get a proper balance of nutrients due to her greater caloric intake.

Aside from their main purpose, oral contraceptive pills alter the metabolism of almost all the nutrients in the body. Research has shown that the pill may cause subnormal levels of some water soluble vitamins, such as B_1, B_2, B_6, B_{12}, folacin, and C. As some of these vitamins are involved in the energy processes in the body, there may be some

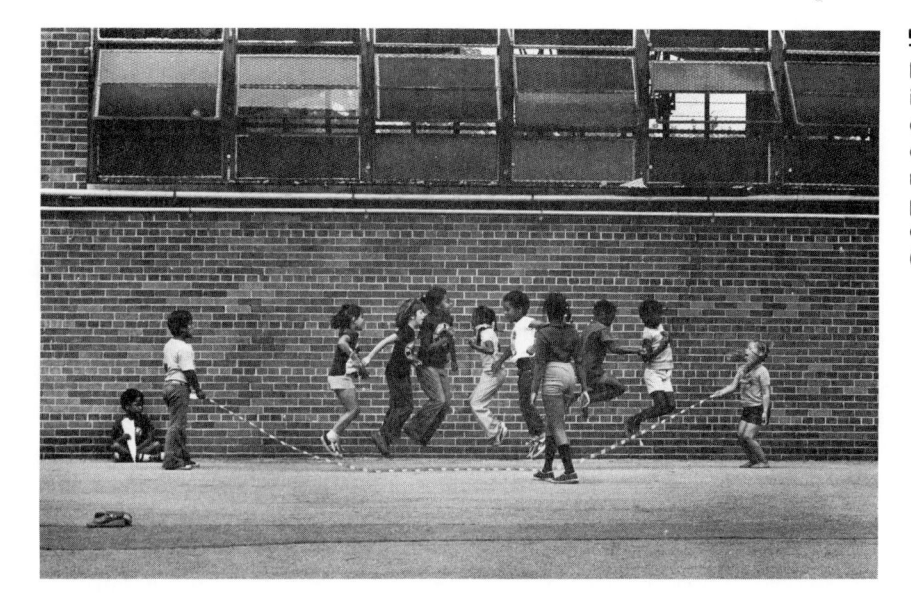

Regular exercise is important in the growth and development of young children and is probably the most important factor in the prevention of childhood obesity.
(Jean-Claude Lejeune)

implications for the active female who is taking oral contraceptive tablets. However, little research has been conducted to see what effects, if any, the pill can exert on physical performance. Moreover, there is very little evidence to support the theory that females using the pill need increased amounts of these nutrients if they are getting the RDA. On the other hand, vitamin supplements may be recommended if the diet is poor. Again, the active female, as contrasted to one who is inactive, will be better assured of receiving these nutrients as she can consume more Calories due to her increased energy expenditure through exercise.

Are there any special nutrient requirements at different ages?

During the growth and development years of childhood, the need for major nutrients such as protein, calcium, phosphorus, and iron, as well as many of the other nutrients, is relatively high due to the rapid increase in muscle, bone, and other body tissues. For example, a young child of age six needs 40 mg/kg body weight of calcium, whereas an adult only needs about 11 mg/kg. Similar relationships hold true for the other nutrients. The child also needs more Calories per unit body weight than the adult; in our example above, corresponding values would be 85 Calories/kg body weight for the child, and only about 40 Calories/kg for the adult. This higher Calorie-to-body weight ratio for the child helps to insure adequate nutrient intake, but foods rich in protein, calcium, phosphorus, and iron should be selected from among the Basic Four Food Groups.

Although children make some of the decisions relative to the food they eat, the parent is primarily responsible for providing sound nutrition. Presently there is a high rate of childhood obesity in the United States. Also, some studies with children have revealed high blood cholesterol and triglyceride levels, which are risk factors for coronary heart disease. Since dietary habits may be formed early in life, it is important for parents to educate their children about sound nutritional principles and provide examples in the home. Adherence to the recently published dietary goals of the United States, as discussed in Chapter 1, would be a good general guideline. These guidelines for children have been generally approved by the American Academy of Pediatrics and the American Heart Associations.

The major nutritional problem during childhood is an excess of Calories resulting in obesity. Research has shown that obese children normally become obese adults. Although the development of obesity may have a variety of causes, excess consumption of food and physical inactivity appear to be the most important causes in childhood. Since prevention of obesity may usually be more successful than treatment, children should be encouraged to become involved in physical activities and to eat foods of high nutrient density in the home.

Following the onset of puberty, adolescents go through a growth spurt where major nutrient needs remain relatively high. In particular, calcium, potassium, and iron are needed for proper bone and blood development, and slightly increased amounts of protein are needed to sustain muscle development. A balanced intake of the four food groups stressing dairy products high in calcium and phosphorus as well as foods rich in iron will provide the RDA of all nutrients necessary for growth and development during this time of life.

During adolescence boys and girls may become more conscious about weight conrol. In general girls may want to lose excess fat whereas boys may want to increase their muscle mass. Whatever the case for either sex, the principles discussed in Chapter 11 for gaining weight and in Chapters 12 and 13 for losing weight may be helpful. Parental involvement appears to be very important in the comprehensive weight control program for children.

Throughout adulthood and into the senior years nutrient needs may be obtained from a balanced diet. However, as the basal metabolic rate decreases with age, and in general as people become less active physically, caloric consumption should decrease if a set body weight is to be maintained. But, the RDA of most nutrients does not decrease, with the exception of several of the B vitamins; thus, the older person should select foods with a high nutrient density as discussed in Chapter 16, particularly high calcium foods for elderly females.

Coronary heart disease is the major cause of death in the United States today, and although its development may begin in childhood, it generally strikes during adulthood, especially in the advanced years. A modified diet as discussed in Chapter 3 and an aerobics exercise program as explained in Chapter 13 may help reduce some of the risk factors associated with this disease.

Individuals may be active at all ages. There are soccer and basketball leagues for children as young as five or six, and a five-year-old has completed a 26.2-mile marathon. Adolescents are active in high school and college sports, and the fitness boom in the United States has involved millions of adults in daily physical exercise and athletic competition. Specific Masters and Senior competition exists for those individuals in the middle and advanced years. In essence, the nutritional principles in this book hold true for the physically active person at all ages. Beyond a good balanced diet for a given age, little can be done nutritionally to increase physical performance, with those exceptions noted earlier in this chapter.

As an additional point, exercise in itself may be an effective therapeutic measure for elderly individuals, particularly females, who may be prone to osteoporosis. Osteoporosis is a softening of the bones due to loss of calcium. Recent research at the University of Wisconsin has revealed that a proper exercise program may prevent the development of osteoporosis in elderly women. Exercise was just as effective as calcium supplements for preventing loss of bone calcium.

When and what should you eat prior to competition?

It is a well-established fact that the ingestion of food prior to competition will not benefit physical performance, yet the pregame meal, so to speak, is one of the major topics of discussion among athletes. A number of special meals have been utilized throughout the years because of their alleged benefits upon physical performance, and special products have been marketed as pre-event nutritional supplements. Although research has not substantiated the value of any one particular pregame meal, there are some general guidelines that have been developed from practical experience over the years.

Pre-event nutrition should not be construed to mean the meal immediately before the game. Sound nutrition must be obtained throughout the training season and during the days prior to competition. For example, the marathon runner will benefit little from what is eaten the day of the run, but may obtain significant nutritional help by a carbohydrate-loading technique several days prior. However, most individuals do think of the pregame meal as the last meal prior to competition.

There are several major purposes of the pregame meal that may be achieved through proper timing and composition. In general, the pregame meal should:

1. Allow for the stomach to be empty at the start of competition.

2. Help avoid a sensation of hunger.

3. Not adversely affect body energy supplies.

Eating for physical performance

4. Help minimize gastrointestinal distress.

5. Provide for an adequate amount of body water.

In general, a solid meal should be eaten about three to four hours prior to competition. This should allow ample time for digestion to occur so that the stomach is relatively empty, and yet hunger sensations are minimized. However, pre-event emotional tension or anxiety may delay digestive time, as will a meal with a high fat or protein content. Hence, the composition of the meal is critical. It should be high in carbohydrate and low in fat and protein, providing an easily digestible meal.

Large amounts of concentrated carbohydrate foods such as sugar and honey should not be ingested within an hour of most types of competition. Research has shown that a rapid rise in blood glucose will elicit an insulin response that will quickly remove the glucose from the blood, possibly creating a reactive hypoglycemia, or low blood sugar, which may produce symptoms of weakness and fatigue. Also, the insulin may block the utilization of free fatty acids by the muscles so that the muscle glycogen stores will be utilized at a faster rate. This may be of critical importance in endurance competition lasting over an hour. Moreover, high sugar compounds may create a reverse osmotic effect, possibly increasing the fluid content of the stomach, which may cause a feeling of distress, cramps, or nausea. Large amounts of concentrated sugar products are not recommended prior to competition. However, as noted in Chapter 2, the use of glucose polymers may be helpful to endurance athletes. Consult that chapter for details.

The composition of the pregame meal should not contribute to any gastrointestinal distress, such as flatulance, increased acidity in the stomach, heartburn, or increased bulk that may stimulate the need for a bowel movement during competition. In general, foods to be avoided include gas formers like beans, spicy foods that may elicit heartburn, and bulk foods like bran products. Through experience, you should learn what foods disagree with you during performance, and of course, you should avoid these prior to competition.

Adequate fluid intake should be assured prior to an event, particularly so if it will be of long duration or conducted under hot environmental conditions. Diuretics, such as caffeine and alcohol, that increase the excretion of body water should be avoided. Large amounts of protein increase the water output of the kidneys, and thus should be avoided. Fluids may be taken up to fifteen to thirty minutes prior to competition, and will help to insure adequate hydration.

A wide variety of foods may be selected for the pregame meal. It should consist of foods that are high in complex carbohydrates with moderate to low amounts of protein. Examples of such foods have been presented in previous chapters and may also be found in Appendix C, particularly those in the bread list.

The foods should be agreeable to you. You should eat what you like within the guidelines presented above.

Two examples of pregame meals, each containing about 500–600 Calories, are as follows:

Glass of skim milk	Glass of orange juice
Toasted cheese sandwich	2 poached eggs
Several cookies	2 pieces of toast with jelly
Banana	Sliced peaches with skim milk

One important last point. Meals other than the precompetition meal eaten on the same day should not be skipped. They should adhere to the basic principles set forth in Chapter 1.

Are liquid pregame meals more advantageous than solid meals?

Liquid meals may have some advantages over solid meals for pregame nutrition. The available liquid meals are well balanced in nutrition value, have a high carbohydrate content, have no bulk, are easily digested and assimilated, and may be more practical and economical than a solid pregame meal.

There are a number of different liquid meal products available commercially, including Nutrament®, Sustagen®, SustaCal®, Ensure®, and Ensure-Plus®. The composition of each may vary somewhat, and checking the label will reveal the exact content of the various nutrients. The energy content of two popular brands are as follows:

	Sustagen	*Nutrament*
Calories	390	375
Carbohydrate (g)	66.5	50.3
Fat (g)	3.5	8.9
Protein (g)	23.5	23.5

Vitamins and minerals may be added in varying amounts.

Since the liquid meal may be assimilated more readily than a solid meal, it may be taken closer to competition, say two to three hours before. Research has shown that there is no difference between a liquid meal and a solid meal relative to subsequent hunger, nausea, diarrhea, or weight changes prior to competition.

From a practical standpoint, liquid meals may save time and money. The time and expense of stopping for a solid meal prior to an event may be avoided by the proper use of liquid meals. Although they are rather economically priced in comparison to a solid meal, they may be prepared even more economically at home. The following formula will provide one quart of a tasty liquid meal:

1/2 cup water
1/2 cup of nonfat dry milk
1/4 cup of sugar
3 cups of skim milk
1 teaspoon of flavoring (cherry, vanilla, or chocolate extract)

Finally, although liquid meals may have some advantages, they do not produce an ergogenic effect. They will not affect physical performance any differently than a well-planned, solid pregame meal. Moreover, they should be used primarily as a substitute during pre-event nutrition and should not be used on a long-term basis to replace the balanced diet concept.

What should you eat after competition or a hard training session?

In general, a balanced diet is all that is necessary to meet your nutrient needs and restore your nutritional status to normal following competition or daily, hard physical training. Carbohydrate and fat are the main nutrients used during exercise and can be replaced easily from foods among the four food groups. The increased caloric intake that is needed to replace your energy expenditure will also help provide you with the additional small amounts of protein, vitamins, and minerals, which may be necessary for effective recovery. Thirst will normally help replace water losses on a day-to-day basis.

Those individuals involved in daily physical activity of a prolonged nature, such as long distance running and swimming or prolonged tennis bouts, should stress complex carbohydrate foods in their daily diet. This will help to replenish muscle glycogen, which is necessary for continued daily workouts at high intensity. Complex carbohydrates are also rich in the vitamins and minerals necessary for their metabolism in the body.

For those persons who must compete several times daily and eat between competitions, such as in tennis tournaments or swim meets, the principles relative to pregame meals may be relevant. These principles have been discussed previously in this chapter.

Is breakfast important to the physically active person?

A balanced breakfast may provide a significant amount of calories and other nutrients in the daily diet of the physically active person. A breakfast of skim milk, poached eggs, toast, and orange juice will help provide a substantial part of the RDA for protein, calcium, vitamin C, and other nutrients. A balanced breakfast with an average amount of protein also will help to prevent the onset of midmorning hunger. The protein will help maintain blood glucose levels normal throughout the morning, whereas a breakfast of refined carbohydrates, like doughnuts, may trigger an insulin response and produce hypoglycemia in the middle of the morning. The resultant hunger is typically satisfied by eating other refined carbohydrates, which will satisfy the hunger urge only until about lunch time. The high nutrient density of the balanced breakfast is preferable to one based on refined carbohydrate products.

Several studies have been conducted relative to the effect of breakfast upon physical performance. In general, the results of these studies suggest that omitting breakfast will cause a decrease in maximal work capacity, particularly so if the individual normally eats breakfast. Skipping breakfast would be comparable to a small fast, as the individual might not eat for twelve to fourteen hours. This could conceivably produce hypoglycemia, low blood sugar levels, and result in a decrease in physical performance.

The available evidence does not prove conclusively that physical performance will be adversely affected by missing breakfast. Although individual preferences should be taken into account, a balanced breakfast could provide a good source of some major nutrients to the individual who is involved in a physical conditioning program.

Can exercise supplement dietary modifications in the prevention and treatment of certain health problems?

Diet, exercise, and your health

There are a number of different diseases and health problems treated, in part, by dietary modification. Exercise is also used as a treatment modality for certain health conditions and may serve as a beneficial supplement to dietary control. The beneficial effects of exercise are usually indirect, that is, exercise may improve upon some factor, which may contribute to the development of the disease. For example, exercise can reduce blood lipids, high levels of which are suspected of contributing to atherosclerosis and coronary heart disease. In other cases exercise exerts direct effects, such as its role in burning excess Calories in cases of obesity. Although exercise is not to be considered a panacea for all health problems, and although some of its beneficial effects are theoretical in nature, the available scientific evidence suggests it may be an effective adjunct in the prevention and treatment of several major health problems.

Dietary modifications in the prevention and treatment of coronary heart disease (CHD) may involve reduced intake of saturated fats, cholesterol, and refined carbohydrate foods. Caloric restriction in order to lose excess body weight is also recommended. Exercise can assist the dietary effects in this regard, as it can help to lower blood lipid levels and also burn excess Calories. Exercise may also increase the proportion of HDL cholesterol, which may exert a protective effect against coronary heart disease. In addition, exercise can exert some direct effects on the heart by increasing its efficiency; as the heart becomes trained through a proper exercise regimen, it works less both at rest and during submaximal exercise. A cardiac risk index is found in Appendix G, which may be useful in evaluating your predisposition to CHD.

Hypertension, or high blood pressure, is usually treated by a dietary program similar to the one for coronary heart disease. A low sodium diet is advocated. Exercise has been shown to reduce the blood pressure in hypertensive individuals, but will have no effect on those who have normal blood pressure. Much of the blood pressure lowering effect may be attributed to losses in body weight incurred through exercise and diet.

The role of exercise in the treatment of obesity and excess body fat was covered in Chapter 13. Exercise may be a very effective means to remove excess fat Calories.

Diabetics usually have a medically supervised diet that avoids concentrated sugars, and is also balanced in Calories to help maintain normal body weight as overweight or obesity may aggravate the condition. The major physiological problem with the diabetic is the lack of insulin or insulin receptors which normally facilitate the transfer of glucose from the blood into the tissues, particularly the liver and muscle. High blood glucose levels may occur and produce some serious health problems. Although the interaction of exercise, blood glucose and insulin on the diabetic is complex, the general overall effect of exercise tends to be beneficial. Weight loss through exercise is helpful to some diabetics. Exercise can have an insulin effect and help reduce blood glucose levels. If the diabetic who exercises also takes insulin, there may be a compounding effect and hypoglycemia, or low blood sugar, may occur. When exercising, the diabetic should be aware of this possibility and carry something sweet to eat in case hypoglycemia occurs.

Dr. David Costill has noted that in order for diabetics to exhibit nearly normal metabolism during running, they must have some active insulin available to facilitate glucose uptake by the muscle. He suggests that 25–50 percent of the daily dose should be injected two and one half to three hours prior to the daily run. A light carbohydrate meal should be consumed about two hours prior to the run. Costill also notes that the only major threat to the diabetic runner under these conditions is hypoglycemia. Exercising diabetics should work closely with their physicians.

Although chemical studies have not shown any proven value of the usual dietary restrictions in the treatment of ulcers, diet therapy is still part of the medical treatment of this condition. The dietary modifications are designed to inhibit acid output or neutralize it in the stomach. The usual medical advice is to avoid gastric irritating foods, such as caffeine and alcohol, and consume more products like milk. Exercise per se has not been shown to prevent ulcers or to serve as a useful treatment. However, it is theorized that exercise can serve to reduce psychic stress and tension, which may be involved as contributing factors to the onset of ulcers.

Individuals with any of the above health problems are undoubtedly under medical care. Dietary modifications and an exercise program should be individually prescribed by your physician who will explain the reasons for and the possible precautions and benefits for such a prescription. Although exercise may be an effective therapeutic treatment and preventative medicine, it should be designed individually since there may be some exceptions to its advisability.

Are there any health hazards associated with rapid weight loss for sports competition such as wrestling?

In sports where athletes compete in weight classes, such as wrestling and boxing, most competitors and their coaches believe that it is best to attain the lowest weight possible in order to increase chances of success. Athletes training for such competition usually reduce their weight gradually during the preseason so they are close to their competitive weight. Then, several days prior to competition they may undergo a period of starvation, dehydration, and hard exercise to lose those extra pounds to make their weight. As noted in Chapter 12, these techniques may cause significant losses of both body fluids and lean tissue mass such as muscle. Although these techniques have been shown to cause decreases in strength and endurance in some studies, others have shown no changes in these performance measures. Moreover, even if the athlete thinks he will lose some strength, he still believes he will be relatively stronger at the lower weight class.

Aside from performance measures, these weight loss techniques have been associated with several acute health problems. Studies with starvation and dehydration in humans have suggested these techniques may contribute to kidney problems, liver damage, inflammation of the pancreas, and ulceration in the gastrointestinal tract. These conditions, however, are believed to be temporary and return to normal following several days of balanced food and fluid intake.

The potential health problems arise when a youngster sets an unrealistically low body weight goal for himself and utilizes starvation, dehydration, diuretics, and appetite suppressant drugs to accomplish his goal. Anyone who has been involved in wrestling has known individuals such as these and in most cases no apparent harm is immediately done. Unfortunately, we do not know the long-range effects, if any. What is the effect of these practices on the developing adolescent? What are the long-term effects on the liver and other organs of alternating starvation and refeeding? These and other related questions are unanswered by current scientific data.

Nevertheless, based upon the data that is available, organizations such as the American Medical Association and the American College of Sports Medicine have made some general recommendations to help alleviate potential problems:

1. Body composition should be assessed, and anyone below 5–7 percent body fat would need a physician's permission to compete.

2. Weight loss should be done gradually. A balanced diet between 1,200–2,400 C is necessary to provide minimum amounts of necessary nutrients.

3. Dehydration techniques such as saunas, steam baths, and diuretics should be prohibited.

4. Wrestlers should weigh-in immediately prior to performance. This would discourage rapid dehydration and weight gain techniques used between weigh-in and match time.

5. More wrestlers should be allowed in the intermediate weight classes since there are more boys at these weight levels.

There are a number of difficulties in establishing effective weight control methods for young wrestlers. Many coaches and wrestlers still remain unconvinced that current weight control practices pose any immediate or future health hazard. The available scientific data is very limited, and this general area is in dire need of long-term research to either substantiate or reject some of the contentions being made. In the meantime, the coach and team physician should exercise their best professional judgement to protect the health of the athlete.

What do most authorities say about nutrition for the athlete?

Nutrition for athletes

As a summarization, it would appear to be appropriate to see what experts in the field of nutrition and physical performance suggest relative to the diet of the athlete. J. V. Durnin, a renowned British scientist, emphasized the point that the nutritional requirements for the athlete in training depend upon the same basic principles that govern human beings in general. Ernst Simonson, an eminent authority in the area of exercise physiology, had studied the concept of fatigue throughout his career and concluded that no type of diet supplement will improve any type of physical performance for someone who is already on a balanced diet. J. Williams, an authority in sports medicine stated that no specific diet will change a moderately endowed athlete into a champion, but a balanced diet is necessary to guarantee maximal performance. Roger Banister, a prominent physician and the first man to run a four-minute mile, indicated that athletes do not need special foods or extra vitamin supplements as long as they eat a well-balanced diet. Jean Mayer, an international authority, has echoed these general statements.

Although there may be some benefits to the athlete from such nutritional practices as carbohydrate loading, hyperhydration, and several others noted in this book, the recommendation of the Food and Nutrition Board of the National Research Council represents the best general advice. The NRC noted that even though athletic activity increases energy expenditure, the increased needs for any essential nutrients should be met by the larger quantities of foods consumed, provided they are chosen wisely.

Appendixes

Appendix A

1980 Recommended dietary allowances

Food and Nutrition Board, National Academy of Sciences-National Research Council Recommended Daily Dietary Allowance[a]
Revised 1980

	Age (years)	Weight (kg)	Weight (lbs)	Height (cm)	Height (in)	Protein (g)	Vitamin A (μg R.E.)[b]	Vitamin D (μg)[c]	Vitamin E (mg α T.E.)[d]	Vitamin C (mg)	Thiamin (mg)
Infants	0.0–0.5	6	13	60	24	kg×2.2	420	10	3	35	0.3
	0.5–1.0	9	20	71	28	kg×2.0	400	10	4	35	0.5
Children	1–3	13	29	90	35	23	400	10	5	45	0.7
	4–6	20	44	112	44	30	500	10	6	45	0.9
	7–10	28	62	132	52	34	700	10	7	45	1.2
Males	11–14	45	99	157	62	45	1,000	10	8	50	1.4
	15–18	66	145	176	69	56	1,000	10	10	60	1.4
	19–22	70	154	177	70	56	1,000	7.5	10	60	1.5
	23–50	70	154	178	70	56	1,000	5	10	60	1.4
	51+	70	154	178	70	56	1,000	5	10	60	1.2
Females	11–14	46	101	157	62	46	800	10	8	50	1.1
	15–18	55	120	163	64	46	800	10	8	60	1.1
	19–22	55	120	163	64	44	800	7.5	8	60	1.1
	23–50	55	120	163	64	44	800	5	8	60	1.0
	51+	55	120	163	64	44	800	5	8	60	1.0
Pregnant						+30	+200	+5	+2	+20	+0.4
Lactating						+20	+400	+5	+3	+40	+0.5

[a]The allowances are intended to provide for individual variations among most normal persons as they live in the United States under usual environmental stresses. Diets should be based on a variety of common foods in order to provide other nutrients for which human requirements have been less well defined.
[b]Retinol equivalents. 1 Retinol equivalent = 1 μg retinol or 6 μg carotene.
[c]As cholecaliciferol. 10 μg cholecaliciferol = 400 I.U. vitamin D.
[d]α tocopheral equivalents. 1 mg d-α-tocopheral = 1αT.E.
[e]1 NE (niacin equivalent) is equal to 1 mg of niacin or 60 mg of dietary tryptophan.
[f]The folacin allowances refer to dietary sources as determined by *Lactobacillus casei* assay after treatment with enzymes ("conjugases") to make polyglutamyl forms of the vitamin available to the test organism.
[g]The RDA for vitamin B_{12} in infants is based on average concentration of the vitamin in human milk. The allowances after weaning are based on energy intake (as recommended by the American Academy of Pediatrics) and consideration of other factors such as intestinal absorption.
[h]The increased requirement during pregnancy cannot be met by the iron content of habitual American diets nor by the existing iron stores of many women; therefore the use of 30–60 mg of supplement iron is recommended. Iron needs during lactation are not substantially different from those of non-pregnant women, but continued supplementation of the mother for 2–3 months after parturition is advisable in order to replenish stores depleted by pregnancy.

Water-soluble Vitamins					Minerals						
Riboflavin (mg)	Niacin (mg N.E.)[e]	Vitamin B₆ (mg)	Folacin[f] (μg)	Vitamin B₁₂ (μg)	Calcium (mg)	Phosphorus (mg)	Magnesium (mg)	Iron (mg)	Zinc (mg)	Iodine (μg)
0.4	6	0.3	30	0.5[g]	360	240	50	10	3	40
0.6	8	0.6	45	1.5	540	360	70	15	5	50
0.8	9	0.9	100	2.0	800	800	150	15	10	70
1.0	11	1.3	200	2.5	800	800	200	10	10	90
1.4	16	1.6	300	3.0	800	800	250	10	10	120
1.6	18	1.8	400	3.0	1,200	1,200	350	18	15	150
1.7	18	2.0	400	3.0	1,200	1,200	400	18	15	150
1.7	19	2.2	400	3.0	800	800	350	10	15	150
1.6	18	2.2	400	3.0	800	800	350	10	15	150
1.4	16	2.2	400	3.0	800	800	350	10	15	150
1.3	15	1.8	400	3.0	1,200	1,200	300	18	15	150
1.3	14	2.0	400	3.0	1,200	1,200	300	18	15	150
1.3	14	2.0	400	3.0	800	800	300	18	15	150
1.2	13	2.0	400	3.0	800	800	300	18	15	150
1.2	13	2.0	400	3.0	800	800	300	10	15	150
+0.3	+2	+0.6	+400	+1.0	+400	+400	+150	[h]	+5	+25
+0.5	+5	+0.5	+100	+1.0	+400	+400	+150	[h]	+10	+50

1980 RDAs—Mean Heights and Weights and Recommended Energy Intake

Category	Age (years)	Weight (kg)	Weight (lb)	Height (cm)	Height (in)	Energy Needs (with range) (Calories)	(MJ)
Infants	0.0–0.5	6	13	60	24	kg × 115 (95–145)	kg × .48
	0.5–1.0	9	20	71	28	kg × 105 (80–135)	kg × .44
Children	1–3	13	29	90	35	1,300 (900–1,800)	5.5
	4–6	20	44	112	44	1,700 (1,300–2,300)	7.1
	7–10	28	62	132	52	2,400 (1,650–3,300)	10.1
Males	11–14	45	99	157	62	2,700 (2,000–3,700)	11.3
	15–18	66	145	176	69	2,800 (2,100–3,900)	11.8
	19–22	70	154	177	70	2,900 (2,500–3,300)	12.2
	23–50	70	154	178	70	2,700 (2,300–3,100)	11.3
	51–75	70	154	178	70	2,400 (2,000–2,800)	10.1
	76+	70	154	178	70	2,050 (1,650–2,450)	8.6
Females	11–14	46	101	157	62	2,200 (1,500–3,000)	9.2
	15–18	55	120	163	64	2,100 (1,200–3,000)	8.8
	19–22	55	120	163	64	2,100 (1,700–2,500)	8.8
	23–50	55	120	163	64	2,000 (1,600–2,400)	8.4
	51–75	55	120	163	64	1,800 (1,400–2,200)	7.6
	76+	55	120	163	64	1,600 (1,200–2,000)	6.7
Pregnancy						+300	
Lactation						+500	

1980 RDAs—Estimated Safe and Adequate Daily Dietary Intakes of Additional Selected Vitamins and Minerals[a]

Subjects	Age (years)	Vitamin K (μg)	Biotin (μg)	Pantothenic Acid (mg)	Copper (mg)	Manganese (mg)	Fluoride (mg)	Chromium (mg)
Infants	0–0.5	12	35	2	0.5–0.7	0.5–0.7	0.1–0.5	0.01–0.04
	0.5–1	10–20	50	3	0.7–1.0	0.7–1.0	0.2–1.0	0.02–0.06
Children and Adolescents	1–3	15–30	65	3	1.0–1.5	1.0–1.5	0.5–1.5	0.02–0.08
	4–6	20–40	85	3–4	1.5–2.0	1.5–2.0	1.0–2.5	0.03–0.12
	7–10	30–60	120	4–5	2.0–2.5	2.0–3.0	1.5–2.5	0.05–0.2
	11	50–100	100–200	4–7	2.0–3.0	2.5–5.0	1.5–2.5	0.05–0.2
Adults		70–140	100–200	4–7	2.0–3.0	2.5–5.0	1.5–4.0	0.05–0.2

[a]Because there is less information on which to base allowances, these figures are not given in the main table of the RDA and are provided here in the form of ranges of recommended intakes.
[b]Since the toxic levels for many trace elements may be only several times usual intakes, the upper levels for the trace elements given in this table should not be habitually exceeded.

From: Recommended Dietary Allowances, Revised 1980. Food and Nutrition Board National Academy of Sciences-National Research Council, Washington, D.C.

The data in this table (facing page, top) has been assembled from the observed median heights and weights of children, together with desirable weights for adults for the mean heights of men (70 inches) and women (64 inches), between the ages to 18 and 34 years as surveyed in the U.S. population
(HEW/NCHS data).

The energy allowances for the young adults are for men and women doing light work. The allowances for the two older age groups represent mean energy needs over these age spans, allowing for a 2 percent decrease in basal (resting) metabolic rate per decade and a reduction in activity of 200 Calories/years and 400 Calories for women over 75. The customary range of daily energy output is shown for adults in parentheses, and is based on a variation in energy needs of ± 400 Calories at any one age, emphasizing the wide range of energy intakes appropriate for any group of people.

Energy allowances for children through age 18 are based on median energy intakes of children these ages followed in longitudinal growth studies. The values in parentheses are 10th and 90th percentiles of energy intake, to indicate the range of energy consumption among children of these ages.

		Electrolytes		
Selenium (mg)	Molybdenum (mg)	Sodium (mg)	Potassium (mg)	Chloride (mg)
0.01–0.04	0.03–0.06	115–350	350–925	275–700
0.02–0.06	0.04–0.08	250–750	425–1275	400–1200
0.02–0.08	0.05–0.1	325–975	550–1,650	500–1,500
0.03–0.12	0.06–0.15	450–1,350	775–2,325	700–2,100
0.05–0.2	0.10–0.3	600–1,800	1,000–3,000	925–2,775
0.05–0.2	0.15–0.5	900–2,700	1,525–4,575	1,400–4,200
0.05–0.2	0.15–0.5	1,100–3,300	1,875–5,625	1,700–5,100

Food exchange list

Appendix B

Exchange lists represent groups of foods, in specific measured amounts, that contain approximately the same amount of energy, carbohydrate, fat, and protein. Thus, foods within a particular exchange list may be substituted for one another.

Meals should be planned so as to contain a selection from each of the exchange groups. A balanced selection should be used to total your daily caloric intake. The exchange list is patterned after the Basic Four Food Groups and the principles discussed in Chapters 1 and 12 are relevant for sound nutritional practices and dieting. The Exchange Lists for Meal Planning were prepared by a number of organizations, primarily the American Dietetic Association and the American Diabetes Association in cooperation with the National Institute of Arthritis, Metabolism, and Digestive Diseases and the National Heart and Lung Institute; National Institutes of Health, Public Health Service; and the United States Department of Health, Education, and Welfare.

(1) The Milk List

A *Milk Exchange* is a serving of food which is equivalent to one cup of skim milk in its energy nutrient content. One milk exchange contains substantial amounts of carbohydrate and protein and about 80 Calories.

(12 grams carbohydrate, 8 grams protein)

Nonfat Fortified Milk

1 cup	skim or nonfat milk
1 cup	buttermilk made from skim milk
1 cup	yogurt made from skim milk (plain, unflavored)
1/3 cup	powdered, nonfat dry milk, before adding liquid
1/2 cup	canned evaporated skim milk, before adding liquid

Low-fat Fortified Milk

1 cup	1% fat fortified milk (add 1/2 fat exchange)*
1 cup	2% fat fortified milk (add 1 fat exchange)*
1 cup	yogurt made from 2% fortified milk (plain, unflavored) (add 1 fat exchange*)

Whole Milk (add 2 fat exchanges*)

1 cup	whole milk
1 cup	buttermilk made from whole milk
1 cup	yogurt made from whole milk (plain, unflavored)
1/2 cup	canned, evaporated whole milk, before adding liquid

*These foods contain more fat than skim milk. When calculating fat values, add fat exchanges as indicated. (1 fat exchange = 5 grams fat.)

(2) The Vegetable List

A VEGETABLE EXCHANGE is a serving of any vegetable that contains a moderate amount of carbohydrate, a small but significant amount of protein, and about 25 Calories.

(5 grams carbohydrate, 2 grams protein)

1/2 cup asparagus
1/2 cup bean sprouts
1/2 cup beets
1/2 cup broccoli
1/2 cup Brussels sprouts
1/2 cup cabbage
1/2 cup carrots
1/2 cup cauliflower
1/2 cup celery
1/2 cup cucumbers
1/2 cup eggplant
1/2 cup green pepper

Greens:

1/2 cup beet greens
1/2 cup chards
1/2 cup collard greens
1/2 cup dandelion greens
1/2 cup kale

Greens continued:

1/2 cup mustard greens
1/2 cup spinach
1/2 cup turnip greens
1/2 cup mushrooms
1/2 cup okra
1/2 cup onions
1/2 cup rhubarb
1/2 cup rutabaga
1/2 cup sauerkraut
1/2 cup string beans, green or yellow
1/2 cup summer squash
1/2 cup tomatoes
1/2 cup tomato juice
1/2 cup turnips
1/2 cup vegetable juice cocktail
1/2 cup zucchini

The following vegetables may be assumed to have negligible carbohydrate, protein, and Calories:

chicory
Chinese cabbage
endive
escarole

lettuce
parsley
radishes
watercress

Starchy vegetables are found on the Bread Exchange List.

(3) The Fruit List

A FRUIT EXCHANGE is a serving of fruit which contains about 10 grams of carbohydrate and 40 Calories. The protein and fat content of fruit is negligible.

(10 grams carbohydrate)

1 small	apple	1/8 medium	honeydew melon
1/3 cup	apple juice	1/2 small	mango
1/2 cup	applesauce (unsweetened)	1 small	nectarine
2 medium	apricots, fresh	1 small	orange
4 halves	apricots, dried	1/2 cup	orange juice
1/2 small	banana	3/4 cup	papaya
1/2 cup	blackberries	1 medium	peach
1/2 cup	blueberries	1 small	pear
1/4 small	cantaloupe melon	1 medium	persimmon
10 large	cherries	1/2 cup	pineapple
1/3 cup	cider	1/3 cup	pineapple juice
2	dates	2 medium	plums
1	fig, fresh	2 medium	prunes
1	fig, dried	1/4 cup	prune juice
1 half	grapefruit	1/2 cup	raspberries
1/2 cup	grapefruit juice	2 tbsp	raisins
12	grapes	3/4 cup	strawberries
1/4 cup	grape juice	1 medium	tangerine
		1 cup	watermelon

Cranberries may be assumed to have negligible carbohydrate and Calories if used without sugar.

Appendix B

(4) The Bread List (Includes Bread, Cereals, and Starchy Vegetables)

A BREAD EXCHANGE is a serving of bread, cereal, or starchy vegetable which contains appreciable carbohydrate and a small but significant amount of protein, totaling about 70 Calories.

(15 grams carbohydrate, 2 grams protein)

Bread

1 slice	white (including French and Italian)
1 slice	whole wheat
1 slice	rye or pumpernickel
1 slice	raisin
1 half	small bagel
1 half	small English muffin
1	plain roll, bread
1 half	frankfurter roll
1 half	hamburger bun
3 tbsp	dried bread crumbs
1 6-inch	tortilla

Cereal

1/2 cup	bran flakes
3/4 cup	other ready-to-eat cereal, unsweetened
1 cup	puffed cereal (unfrosted)
1/2 cup	cereal (cooked)
1/2 cup	grits (cooked)
1/2 cup	rice or barley (cooked)
1/2 cup	pasta (cooked): spaghetti, noodles, or macaroni
3 cups	popcorn (popped, no fat added)
2 tbsp	cornmeal (dry)
2 1/2 tbsp	flour
1/4 cup	wheat germ

Crackers

3	arrowroot
2	graham, 2 1/2" square
1 half	matzoth, 4" × 6"
20	oyster
25	pretzels, 3 1/8" long × 1/8" diameter
3	rye wafers, 2" × 3 1/2"
6	saltines
4	soda, 2 1/2" square

Dried Beans, Peas, and Lentils

1/2 cup	beans, peas, lentils (dried and cooked)
1/4 cup	baked beans, no pork (canned)

Starchy Vegetables

1/3 cup	corn
1 small	corn on cob
1/2 cup	lima beans
2/3 cup	parsnips
1/2 cup	peas, green (canned or frozen)
1 small	potato, white
1/2 cup	potato (mashed)
3/4 cup	pumpkin
1/2 cup	squash: winter, acorn, or butternut
1/4 cup	yam or sweet potato

Prepared Foods*

1 biscuit, 2" diameter (add 1 fat exchange)
1 corn bread, 2" × 2" × 1" (add 1 fat exchange)
1 corn muffin, 2" diameter (add 1 fat exchange)
5 crackers, round butter type (add 1 fat exchange)
1 muffin, plain, small (add 1 fat exchange)
8 potatoes, French fried, length 2" by 3 1/2" (add 1 fat exchange)
15 potato chips or corn chips (add 2 fat exchanges)
1 pancake, 5" × 1/2" (add 1 fat exchange)
1 waffle, 5" × 1/2" (add 1 fat exchange)

*These foods contain more fat than bread. When calculating fat values, add fat exchanges as indicated. (1 fat exchange = 5 grams fat.)

(5) The Meat List

A MEAT EXCHANGE is a serving of protein-rich food which contains negligible carbohydrate, but a significant amount of protein and fat, roughly equivalent to the amounts in one ounce of lean meat; contains about 55 Calories.

(7 grams protein, 3 grams fat)

Low-Fat Meat

1 ounce beef:	baby beef (very lean), chipped beef, chuck, flank steak, tenderloin, plateribs, plate skirt steak, round (bottom, top), all cuts rump, spare ribs, tripe
1 ounce lamb:	leg, rib, sirloin, loin (roast and chops), shank, shoulder
1 ounce pork:	leg (whole rump, center shank), ham, smoked (center slices)
1 ounce veal:	leg, loin, rib, shank, shoulder, cutlets
1 ounce poultry:	meat-without-skin of chicken, turkey, cornish hen, guinea hen, pheasant
1 ounce fish:	any fresh or frozen
1/4 cup fish:	canned salmon, tuna, mackerel, crab, and lobster
5 (or 1 ounce):	clams, oysters, scallops, shrimp
3	sardines, drained
1 ounce cheese:	containing less than 5% butterfat
1/4 cup	cottage cheese, dry and 2% butterfat
1/2 cup	dried beans and peas (add 1 bread exchange*)

Medium-Fat Meat (Add 1/2 Fat Exchange*)

1 ounce beef:	ground (15% fat), corned beef (canned), rib eye, round (ground commercial)
1 ounce pork:	loin (all cuts tenderloin), shoulder arm (picnic), shoulder blade, Boston butt, Canadian bacon, boiled ham
1 ounce	liver, heart, kidney, and sweetbreads (these are high in cholesterol)
1/4 cup	cottage cheese, creamed
1 ounce cheese:	mozzarella, ricotta, farmer's cheese, Neufchatel
3 tbsp	Parmesan cheese
1	egg (high in cholesterol)

High-Fat Meat (Add 1 Fat Exchange*)

1 ounce beef:	brisket, corned beef (brisket), ground beef (more than 20% fat), hamburger (commercial), chuck (ground commercial), roasts (rib), steaks (club and rib)
1 ounce lamb:	breast
1 ounce pork:	spare ribs, loin (back ribs), pork (ground), country style ham, deviled ham
1 ounce veal:	breast
1 ounce poultry:	capon, duck (domestic), goose
1 ounce chese:	cheddar types
1 slice	cold cuts, 4 1/2" $\times$ 1/8" slice
1 small	frankfurter

Peanut Butter

2 tbsp	peanut butter (add 2 1/2 fat exchanges*)

*These foods contain more carbohydrate or fat than lean meat. When calculating carbohydrate or fat values, add bread or fat exchanges as indicated.

(6) The Fat List

A FAT EXCHANGE is a serving of any food which contains negligible carbohydrate and protein, but appreciable fat, totaling about 45 Calories.

(5 grams fat)

Polyunsaturated Fat

1 tsp margarine, soft, tub, or stick*

1 eighth avocado (4″ in diameter)†

1 tsp oil, corn, cottonseed, safflower, soy, sunflower

1 tsp oil, olive†

1 tsp oil, peanut†

5 small olives†

10 whole almonds†

2 large whole pecans†

20 whole peanuts, Spanish†

10 whole peanuts, Virginia†

6 small walnuts

6 small nuts, other†

Saturated Fat

1 tsp margarine, regular stick	1 tbsp cream cheese
1 tsp butter	1 tbsp French dressing‡
1 tsp bacon fat	1 tbsp Italian dressing‡
1 strip bacon, crisp	1 tsp lard
2 tbsp cream, light	1 tsp mayonnaise‡
2 tbsp cream, sour	2 tsp salad dressing, mayonnaise type‡
1 tbsp cream, heavy	3/4 inch salt pork cube

Unlimited Foods

These are *free foods*, which contain negligible carbohydrate, protein, and fat, and therefore negligible Calories.

Diet Calorie-free beverage	Paprika	Chili powder
Coffee	Garlic	Onion salt or powder
Tea	Celery salt	Horseradish
Bouillon without fat	Parsley	Vinegar
Unsweetened gelatin	Nutmeg	Mint
Unsweetened pickles	Lemon	Cinnamon
Salt and pepper	Mustard	Lime
Red pepper		

*Made with corn, cottonseed, safflower, soy, or sunflower oil only.
†Fat content is primarily monounsaturated.
‡If made with corn, cottonseed, safflower, soy, or sunflower oil, can be assumed to contain polyunsaturated fat.

Appendix C

Caloric expenditure per minute for various physical activities

Body Weight													
KG		45	48	50	52	55	57	59	61	64	66	68	70
Pounds		100	105	110	115	120	125	130	135	140	145	150	155

Sedentary Activities

lying quietly		.99	1.0	1.1	1.1	1.2	1.3	1.3	1.4	1.4	1.5	1.5	1.5
sitting and writing, card playing, etc.		1.2	1.3	1.4	1.5	1.5	1.6	1.7	1.7	1.8	1.8	1.9	2.0
standing with light work, cleaning, etc.		2.7	2.9	3.0	3.1	3.3	3.4	3.5	3.7	3.8	3.9	4.1	4.2

Physical Activities

archery		3.1	3.3	3.5	3.6	3.8	4.0	4.1	4.3	4.5	4.6	4.8	4.9
badminton													
recreational singles		3.6	3.8	4.0	4.2	4.4	4.6	4.7	4.9	5.1	5.3	5.4	5.6
social doubles		2.7	2.9	3.0	3.1	3.3	3.4	3.5	3.7	3.8	3.9	4.1	4.2
competitive		5.9	6.1	6.4	6.7	7.0	7.3	7.6	7.9	8.2	8.5	8.8	9.1
baseball													
player		3.1	3.3	3.4	3.6	3.8	4.0	4.1	4.3	4.4	4.5	4.7	4.8
pitcher		3.9	4.1	4.3	4.5	4.7	4.9	5.1	5.3	5.5	5.7	5.9	6.0
basketball													
half court		3.0	3.1	3.3	3.5	3.6	3.8	3.9	4.1	4.2	4.4	4.5	4.7
recreational		4.9	5.2	5.5	5.7	6.0	6.2	6.5	6.7	7.0	7.2	7.5	7.7
vigorous competition		6.5	6.8	7.2	7.5	7.8	8.2	8.5	8.8	9.2	9.5	9.9	10.2
bicycling, level													
(mph)	(min/mile)												
5	12:00	1.9	2.0	2.1	2.2	2.3	2.4	2.5	2.6	2.7	2.8	2.9	3.0
6	10:00	2.7	2.8	3.0	3.1	3.2	3.4	3.5	3.6	3.8	3.9	4.0	4.2
8	7:30	3.4	3.6	3.8	4.0	4.1	4.3	4.5	4.7	4.8	5.0	5.2	5.4
10	6:00	4.2	4.4	4.6	4.8	5.1	5.3	5.5	5.7	5.9	6.1	6.4	6.6
11	5:28	5.0	5.2	5.5	5.7	6.0	6.2	6.5	6.7	7.0	7.2	7.5	7.8
12	5:00	5.7	6.0	6.3	6.6	6.9	7.2	7.5	7.8	8.1	8.4	8.7	9.0
13	4:37	6.8	7.1	7.5	7.8	8.2	8.5	8.8	9.2	9.5	9.9	10.2	10.6

73	75	77	80	82	84	86	89	91	93	95	98	100
160	165	170	175	180	185	190	195	200	205	210	215	220
1.6	1.6	1.7	1.7	1.8	1.8	1.9	1.9	2.0	2.0	2.1	2.1	2.2
2.0	2.1	2.2	2.2	2.3	2.4	2.4	2.5	2.5	2.6	2.7	2.7	2.8
4.4	4.5	4.6	4.8	4.9	5.0	5.2	5.3	5.4	5.6	5.7	5.9	6.0
5.1	5.3	5.4	5.6	5.7	5.9	6.0	6.2	6.4	6.5	6.7	6.9	7.0
5.8	6.0	6.2	6.4	6.6	6.7	6.9	7.1	7.3	7.4	7.6	7.8	8.0
4.4	4.5	4.6	4.8	4.9	5.0	5.2	5.3	5.4	5.6	5.7	5.9	6.0
9.4	9.7	10.0	10.3	10.6	10.9	11.2	11.5	11.8	12.1	12.4	12.7	13.0
5.0	5.2	5.3	5.5	5.6	5.8	5.9	6.1	6.3	6.4	6.6	6.8	6.9
6.3	6.5	6.7	6.9	7.1	7.3	7.4	7.7	7.9	8.0	8.2	8.5	8.6
4.8	5.0	5.1	5.3	5.4	5.6	5.7	5.9	6.0	6.2	6.4	6.5	6.7
8.0	8.2	8.5	8.7	9.0	9.2	9.5	9.7	10.0	10.2	10.5	10.7	11.0
10.5	10.9	11.2	11.5	11.9	12.2	12.5	12.9	13.2	13.5	13.8	14.2	14.5
3.1	3.2	3.3	3.4	3.5	3.6	3.7	3.8	3.9	4.0	4.1	4.2	4.3
4.3	4.4	4.6	4.7	4.9	5.0	5.1	5.3	5.4	5.5	5.7	5.8	6.0
5.5	5.7	5.9	6.1	6.3	6.4	6.6	6.8	6.9	7.1	7.3	7.5	7.7
6.8	7.0	7.2	7.4	7.6	7.9	8.1	8.3	8.5	8.7	8.9	9.1	9.4
8.0	8.3	8.5	8.8	9.0	9.3	9.5	9.8	10.0	10.3	10.6	10.8	11.1
9.3	9.5	9.8	10.1	10.4	10.7	11.0	11.3	11.6	11.9	12.2	12.5	12.8
10.9	11.3	11.6	12.0	12.3	12.6	13.0	13.3	13.7	14.0	14.4	14.7	15.0

Body Weight

KG	45	48	50	52	55	57	59	61	64	66	68	70
Pounds	100	105	110	115	120	125	130	135	140	145	150	155
bowling	2.7	2.8	3.0	3.1	3.3	3.4	3.5	3.7	3.8	3.9	4.1	4.2
calisthenics												
light type	3.4	3.6	3.8	4.0	4.1	4.3	4.5	4.7	4.8	5.0	5.2	5.4
timed vigorous	9.7	10.1	10.6	11.1	11.6	12.1	12.6	13.1	13.6	14.1	14.6	15.1
canoeing												
(mph) (min/mile)												
2.5 24	1.9	2.0	2.1	2.2	2.3	2.4	2.5	2.6	2.7	2.8	2.9	3.0
4.0 15	4.4	4.6	4.9	5.1	5.3	5.5	5.8	6.0	6.2	6.4	6.7	6.9
5.0 12	5.7	6.0	6.3	6.6	6.9	7.2	7.5	7.8	8.1	8.4	8.7	9.0
dancing												
moderately (waltz)	3.1	3.3	3.5	3.6	3.8	4.0	4.1	4.3	4.5	4.6	4.8	4.9
active (square, disco)	4.5	4.7	5.0	5.2	5.4	5.6	5.9	6.1	6.3	6.6	6.8	7.0
aerobic (vigorously)	6.0	6.3	6.7	7.0	7.3	7.6	7.9	8.2	8.5	8.8	9.1	9.4
fencing												
moderately	3.3	3.5	3.6	3.8	4.0	4.1	4.3	4.5	4.6	4.8	5.0	5.2
vigorously	6.6	7.0	7.3	7.7	8.0	8.3	8.7	9.0	9.4	9.7	10.0	10.4
field hockey	5.0	6.3	6.7	7.0	7.3	7.6	7.9	8.2	8.5	8.8	9.1	9.4
football												
moderate	3.3	3.5	3.6	3.8	4.0	4.1	4.3	4.5	4.6	4.8	5.0	5.2
touch, vigorous	5.5	5.8	6.1	6.4	6.6	6.9	7.2	7.5	7.8	8.0	8.3	8.6
golf												
2-some (carry clubs)	3.6	3.8	4.0	4.2	4.4	4.6	4.7	4.9	5.1	5.3	5.4	5.6
4-some (carry clubs)	2.7	2.9	3.0	3.1	3.3	3.4	3.5	3.7	3.8	3.9	4.1	4.2
power-cart	1.9	2.0	2.1	2.2	2.3	2.4	2.5	2.6	2.7	2.8	2.9	3.0
handball												
moderate	6.5	6.8	7.2	7.5	7.8	8.2	8.5	8.8	9.2	9.5	9.9	10.2
competitive	7.7	8.0	8.4	8.8	9.2	9.6	10.0	10.4	10.8	11.1	11.5	11.9
hiking, pack (3 mph)	4.5	4.7	5.0	5.2	5.4	5.6	5.9	6.1	6.3	6.6	6.8	7.0
hocky, ice	6.6	7.0	7.3	7.7	8.0	8.3	8.7	9.0	9.4	9.7	10.0	10.4

73	75	77	80	82	84	86	89	91	93	95	98	100
160	165	170	175	180	185	190	195	200	205	210	215	220
4.4	4.5	4.6	4.8	4.9	5.0	5.2	5.3	5.5	5.6	5.7	5.9	6.0
5.5	5.7	5.9	6.1	6.3	6.4	6.6	6.8	7.0	7.1	7.3	7.5	7.7
15.6	16.1	16.6	17.1	17.6	18.1	18.6	19.1	19.6	20.0	20.5	21.0	21.5
3.1	3.2	3.3	3.4	3.5	3.6	3.7	3.8	3.9	4.0	4.1	4.2	4.3
7.1	7.4	7.6	7.8	8.0	8.2	8.5	8.7	8.9	9.1	9.4	9.6	9.8
9.3	9.5	9.8	10.1	10.4	10.7	11.0	11.3	11.6	11.9	12.2	12.5	12.8
5.1	5.3	5.4	5.6	5.7	5.9	6.0	6.2	6.4	6.5	6.7	6.9	7.0
7.3	7.5	7.7	7.9	8.2	8.4	8.6	8.9	9.1	9.3	9.5	9.8	10.0
9.7	10.0	10.3	10.6	10.9	11.2	11.5	11.8	12.1	12.4	12.7	13.0	13.3
5.3	5.5	5.7	5.8	6.0	6.2	6.3	6.5	6.7	6.8	7.0	7.1	7.3
10.7	11.0	11.4	11.7	12.1	12.4	12.7	13.1	13.4	13.8	14.1	14.4	14.8
9.7	10.0	10.3	10.6	10.9	11.2	11.5	11.8	12.1	12.4	12.7	13.0	13.3
5.3	5.5	5.7	5.8	6.0	6.2	6.3	6.5	6.7	6.8	7.0	7.1	7.3
8.9	9.2	9.4	9.7	10.0	10.3	10.6	10.8	11.1	11.4	11.7	12.0	12.2
5.8	6.0	6.2	6.4	6.6	6.7	6.9	7.1	7.3	7.4	7.6	7.8	8.0
4.4	4.5	4.6	4.8	4.9	5.0	5.2	5.3	5.4	5.6	5.7	5.9	6.0
3.1	3.2	3.3	3.4	3.5	3.6	3.7	3.8	3.9	4.0	4.1	4.2	4.3
10.5	10.9	11.2	11.5	11.9	12.2	12.5	12.9	13.2	13.5	13.8	14.2	14.5
12.3	12.7	13.1	13.5	13.9	14.3	14.7	15.0	15.4	15.8	16.2	16.6	17.0
7.3	7.5	7.7	7.9	8.2	8.4	8.6	8.9	9.1	9.3	9.5	9.8	10.0
10.7	11.0	11.4	11.7	12.1	12.4	12.7	13.1	13.4	13.8	14.1	14.4	14.8

Body Weight

KG	45	48	50	52	55	57	59	61	64	66	68	70
Pounds	100	105	110	115	120	125	130	135	140	145	150	155
horseback riding												
walk		1.9	2.0	2.1	2.2	2.3	2.4	2.5	2.6	2.7	2.8	2.9	3.0
sitting to trot		2.7	2.9	3.0	3.1	3.3	3.4	3.5	3.7	3.8	3.9	4.1	4.2
posting to trot		4.2	4.4	4.6	4.8	5.1	5.3	5.5	5.7	5.9	6.1	6.4	6.6
gallop		5.7	6.0	6.3	6.6	6.9	7.2	7.5	7.8	8.1	8.4	8.7	9.0
horseshoes	2.5	2.6	2.8	2.9	3.0	3.1	3.3	3.4	3.5	3.7	3.8	3.9
jogging (see running)												
judo	8.5	8.9	9.3	9.8	10.2	10.6	11.0	11.5	11.9	12.3	12.8	13.2
karate	8.5	8.9	9.3	9.8	10.2	10.6	11.0	11.5	11.9	12.3	12.8	13.2
mountain climbing	6.5	6.8	7.2	7.5	7.8	8.2	8.5	8.8	9.2	9.5	9.8	10.2
paddle ball	5.7	6.0	6.3	6.6	6.9	7.2	7.5	7.8	8.1	8.4	8.7	9.0
pool (billiards)	1.5	1.6	1.6	1.7	1.8	1.9	1.9	2.0	2.1	2.2	2.2	2.3
racketball	6.5	6.8	7.1	7.5	7.8	8.1	8.4	8.8	9.1	9.4	9.8	10.1
roller skating (9 mph)	4.2	4.4	4.6	4.8	5.1	5.3	5.5	5.7	5.9	6.1	6.4	6.6
running (steady state)												
(mph)	(min/mile)											
5.0	12:00	6.0	6.3	6.6	7.0	7.3	7.6	7.9	8.2	8.5	8.8	9.1	9.4
5.5	10:55	6.7	7.0	7.3	7.7	8.0	8.4	8.7	9.0	9.4	9.7	10.0	10.4
6.0	10:00	7.2	7.6	8.0	8.4	8.7	9.1	9.5	9.8	10.2	10.6	10.9	11.3
7.0	8:35	8.5	8.9	9.3	9.0	10.2	10.6	11.0	11.5	11.9	12.3	12.8	13.2
8.0	7:30	9.7	10.2	10.7	11.2	11.6	12.1	12.6	13.1	13.6	14.1	14.6	15.1
9.0	6:40	10.8	11.3	11.9	12.4	12.9	13.5	14.0	14.6	15.1	15.7	16.2	16.8
10.0	6:00	12.1	12.7	13.3	13.9	14.5	15.1	15.7	16.4	17.0	17.6	18.2	18.8
11.0	5:28	13.3	14.0	14.6	15.3	16.0	16.7	17.3	18.0	18.7	19.4	20.0	20.7
12.0	5:00	14.5	15.2	16.0	16.7	17.4	18.2	18.9	19.7	20.4	21.1	21.9	22.6
sailing, small boat	2.7	2.9	3.0	3.1	3.3	3.4	3.5	3.7	3.8	3.9	4.1	4.2
skating, ice (9 mph)	4.2	4.4	4.6	4.8	5.1	5.2	5.5	5.7	5.9	6.1	6.4	6.6
skiing, cross country												
(mph)	(min/mile)											
2.5	24:00	5.0	5.2	5.5	5.7	6.0	6.2	6.5	6.7	7.0	7.2	7.5	7.8
4.0	15:00	6.5	6.8	7.2	7.5	7.8	8.2	8.5	8.8	9.2	9.5	9.9	10.2
5.0	12:00	7.7	8.0	8.4	8.8	9.2	9.6	10.0	10.4	10.8	11.1	11.5	11.9

73	75	77	80	82	84	86	89	91	93	95	98	100
160	165	170	175	180	185	190	195	200	205	210	215	220
3.1	3.2	3.3	3.4	3.5	3.6	3.7	3.8	3.9	4.0	4.1	4.2	4.3
4.4	4.5	4.6	4.8	4.9	5.0	5.2	5.3	5.4	5.6	5.7	5.9	6.0
6.8	7.0	7.2	7.4	7.6	7.9	8.1	8.3	8.5	8.7	8.9	9.1	9.4
9.3	9.5	9.8	10.1	10.4	10.7	11.0	11.3	11.6	11.9	12.2	12.5	12.8
4.0	4.2	4.3	4.4	4.5	4.7	4.8	4.9	5.2	5.2	5.3	5.4	5.6
13.6	14.1	14.5	14.9	15.4	15.8	16.2	16.6	17.1	17.5	17.9	18.4	18.8
13.6	14.1	14.5	14.9	15.4	15.8	16.2	16.6	17.1	17.5	17.9	18.4	18.8
10.5	10.8	11.2	11.5	11.8	12.1	12.5	12.8	13.1	13.5	13.8	14.1	14.5
9.3	9.5	9.8	10.1	10.4	10.7	11.0	11.2	11.6	11.9	12.2	12.5	12.8
2.4	2.5	2.6	2.6	2.7	2.8	2.9	2.9	3.0	3.1	3.2	3.2	3.3
10.4	10.7	11.1	11.4	11.7	12.0	12.4	12.7	13.0	13.4	13.7	14.0	14.4
6.8	7.0	7.2	7.4	7.6	7.9	8.1	8.3	8.5	8.7	8.9	9.1	9.4
9.7	10.0	10.3	10.6	10.9	11.2	11.6	11.9	12.2	12.5	12.8	13.1	13.4
10.7	11.1	11.4	11.7	12.1	12.4	12.8	13.1	13.4	13.8	14.1	14.5	14.8
11.7	12.0	12.4	12.8	13.1	13.5	13.8	14.3	14.6	15.0	15.4	15.7	16.1
13.6	14.1	14.5	14.9	15.4	15.8	16.2	16.6	17.1	17.5	17.9	18.4	18.8
15.6	16.1	16.6	17.1	17.6	18.1	18.5	19.0	18.5	20.0	20.5	21.0	21.5
17.3	17.9	18.4	19.0	19.5	20.1	20.6	21.2	21.7	22.2	22.8	23.3	23.9
19.4	20.0	20.7	21.3	21.9	22.5	23.1	23.7	24.2	24.8	25.4	26.0	26.7
21.4	22.1	22.7	23.4	24.1	24.8	25.4	26.1	26.8	27.5	28.1	28.8	29.5
23.3	24.1	24.8	25.6	26.3	27.0	27.8	28.5	29.2	30.0	30.7	31.5	32.2
4.4	4.5	4.6	4.8	4.9	5.0	5.2	5.3	5.4	5.6	5.7	5.9	6.0
6.8	7.0	7.2	7.4	7.6	7.9	8.1	8.3	8.5	8.7	8.9	9.1	9.4
8.0	8.3	8.5	8.8	9.0	9.3	9.5	9.8	10.0	10.3	10.6	10.8	11.1
10.5	10.9	11.2	11.5	11.9	12.2	12.5	12.9	13.2	13.5	13.8	14.2	14.5
12.3	12.7	13.1	13.5	13.9	14.3	13.7	15.0	15.4	15.8	16.2	16.6	17.0

Body Weight												
KG		45	48	50	52	55	57	59	61	64	66	68	70
Pounds		100	105	110	115	120	125	130	135	140	145	150	155
skiing, downhill	6.5	6.8	7.2	7.5	7.8	8.2	8.5	8.8	9.2	9.5	9.9	10.2
soccer	5.9	6.2	6.6	6.9	7.2	7.5	7.8	8.1	8.4	8.7	9.0	9.3
squash												
normal	6.7	7.0	7.3	7.7	8.0	8.4	8.7	9.1	9.5	9.8	10.1	10.5
competition	7.7	8.0	8.4	8.8	9.2	9.6	10.0	10.4	10.8	11.1	11.5	11.9
swimming (yards/min)												
backstroke												
25	2.5	2.6	2.8	2.9	3.0	3.1	3.3	3.4	3.5	3.7	3.8	3.9
30	3.5	3.7	3.9	4.1	4.2	4.4	4.6	4.8	4.9	5.1	5.3	5.5
35	4.5	4.7	5.0	5.2	5.4	5.6	5.9	6.1	6.3	6.6	6.8	7.0
40	5.5	5.8	6.1	6.4	6.6	6.9	7.2	7.5	7.8	8.0	8.3	8.6
breaststroke												
20	3.1	3.3	3.5	3.6	3.8	4.0	4.1	4.3	4.5	4.6	4.8	4.9
30	4.7	5.0	5.2	5.4	5.7	5.9	6.2	6.4	6.7	6.9	7.1	7.4
40	6.3	6.7	7.0	7.3	7.6	8.0	8.3	8.6	8.9	9.3	9.6	9.9
front crawl												
20	3.1	3.3	3.5	3.6	3.8	4.0	4.1	4.3	4.5	4.6	4.8	4.9
25	4.0	4.2	4.4	4.6	4.8	5.0	5.2	5.4	5.6	5.8	6.0	6.2
35	4.8	5.1	5.4	5.6	5.9	6.1	6.4	6.6	6.8	7.0	7.3	7.5
45	5.7	6.0	6.3	6.6	6.9	7.2	7.5	7.8	8.1	8.4	8.7	9.0
50	7.0	7.4	7.7	8.1	8.5	8.8	9.2	9.5	9.9	10.3	10.6	11.0
table tennis	3.4	3.6	3.8	4.0	4.1	4.3	4.5	4.7	4.8	5.0	5.2	5.4
tennis												
singles, recreational	5.0	5.2	5.5	5.7	6.0	6.2	6.5	6.7	7.0	7.2	7.5	7.8
doubles, recreational	3.4	3.6	3.8	4.0	4.1	4.3	4.5	4.7	4.8	5.0	5.2	5.4
competition	6.4	6.7	7.1	7.4	7.7	8.1	8.4	8.7	9.1	9.4	9.8	10.1
volleyball												
moderate, recreational	2.9	3.0	3.2	3.3	3.5	3.6	3.8	3.9	4.1	4.2	4.4	4.5
vigorous, competition	6.5	6.8	7.1	7.5	7.8	8.1	8.4	8.8	9.1	9.4	9.8	10.1

73	75	77	80	82	84	86	89	91	93	95	98	100
160	165	170	175	180	185	190	195	200	205	210	215	220
10.5	10.9	11.2	11.5	11.9	12.2	12.5	12.9	13.2	13.5	13.8	14.2	14.5
9.6	9.9	10.2	10.5	10.8	11.1	11.4	11.7	12.0	12.3	12.6	12.9	13.2
10.8	11.2	11.5	11.8	12.2	12.5	12.9	13.2	13.5	13.9	14.2	14.6	14.9
12.3	12.7	13.1	13.5	13.9	14.3	14.7	15.0	15.4	15.8	16.2	16.6	17.0
4.0	4.2	4.3	4.4	4.5	4.7	4.8	4.9	5.1	5.2	5.3	5.4	5.6
5.6	5.8	6.0	6.2	6.4	6.5	6.7	6.9	7.1	7.2	7.4	7.6	7.8
7.3	7.5	7.7	7.9	8.2	8.4	8.6	8.9	9.1	9.3	9.5	9.8	10.0
8.9	9.2	9.4	9.7	10.0	10.3	10.6	10.8	11.1	11.4	11.7	12.0	12.2
5.1	5.3	5.4	5.6	5.7	5.9	6.0	6.2	6.4	6.5	6.7	6.9	7.0
7.6	7.9	8.1	8.3	8.6	8.8	9.1	9.3	9.5	9.8	10.0	10.3	10.5
10.2	10.5	10.9	11.2	11.5	11.9	12.2	12.5	12.8	13.1	13.5	13.8	14.1
5.1	5.3	5.4	5.6	5.7	5.9	6.0	6.2	6.4	6.5	6.7	6.9	7.0
6.4	6.6	6.8	7.0	7.2	7.4	7.6	7.8	8.0	8.2	8.4	8.6	8.8
7.8	8.0	8.3	8.5	8.8	9.0	9.2	9.4	9.7	9.9	10.2	10.4	10.7
9.3	9.5	9.8	10.1	10.4	10.7	11.0	11.3	11.6	11.9	12.2	12.5	12.8
11.3	11.7	12.0	12.4	12.8	13.1	13.5	13.8	14.2	14.5	14.9	15.2	15.6
5.5	5.7	5.9	6.1	6.3	6.4	6.6	6.8	7.0	7.1	7.3	7.5	7.7
8.0	8.3	8.5	8.8	9.0	9.3	9.5	9.8	10.0	10.3	10.6	10.8	11.1
5.5	5.7	5.9	6.1	6.3	6.4	6.6	6.8	7.0	7.1	7.3	7.5	7.7
10.4	10.8	11.1	11.4	11.8	12.1	12.4	12.8	13.1	13.4	13.7	14.1	14.4
4.7	4.8	5.0	5.1	5.3	5.4	5.6	5.7	5.9	6.0	6.1	6.3	6.4
10.4	10.7	11.1	11.4	11.7	12.0	12.4	12.7	13.0	13.4	13.7	14.0	14.4

Appendix C

Body Weight													
KG		45	48	50	52	55	57	59	61	64	66	68	70
Pounds		100	105	110	115	120	125	130	135	140	145	150	155
walking													
(mph)	(Min/mile)												
1.0	60:00	1.5	1.6	1.7	1.8	1.8	1.9	2.0	2.1	2.2	2.2	2.3	2.4
2.0	30:00	2.1	2.2	2.3	2.4	2.5	2.6	2.8	2.9	3.0	3.1	3.2	3.3
2.3	26:00	2.3	2.4	2.5	2.7	2.8	2.9	3.0	3.1	3.2	3.4	3.5	3.6
3.0	20.00	2.7	2.9	3.0	3.1	3.3	3.4	3.5	3.7	3.8	3.9	4.1	4.2
3.2	18:45	3.1	3.3	3.4	3.6	3.8	4.0	4.1	4.3	4.4	4.5	4.7	4.8
3.5	17:10	3.3	3.5	3.7	3.9	4.0	4.2	4.4	4.6	4.7	4.9	5.1	5.3
4.0	15:00	4.2	4.4	4.6	4.8	5.1	5.3	5.5	5.7	5.9	6.1	6.4	6.6
4.5	13:20	4.7	5.0	5.2	5.4	5.7	5.9	6.2	6.4	6.7	6.9	7.1	7.4
5.0	12:00	5.4	5.7	6.0	6.3	6.5	6.8	7.1	7.4	7.7	7.9	8.2	8.4
5.4	11:10	6.2	6.6	6.9	7.2	7.5	7.9	8.2	8.5	8.8	9.2	9.5	9.8
5.8	10:20	7.7	8.0	8.4	8.8	9.2	9.6	10.0	10.4	10.8	11.1	11.5	11.9
water skiing		5.0	5.2	5.5	5.7	6.0	6.2	6.5	6.7	7.0	7.2	7.5	7.8
weight training		5.2	5.4	5.7	6.0	6.2	6.5	6.8	7.0	7.3	7.6	7.8	8.1
wrestling		8.5	8.9	9.3	9.8	10.2	10.6	11.0	11.5	11.9	12.3	12.8	13.2

73	75	77	80	82	84	86	89	91	93	95	98	100
160	165	170	175	180	185	190	195	200	205	210	215	220
2.4	2.5	2.6	2.7	2.8	2.9	2.9	3.0	3.1	3.2	3.2	3.3	3.4
3.4	3.5	3.6	3.7	3.9	4.0	4.1	4.2	4.3	4.4	4.5	4.6	4.7
3.7	3.8	4.0	4.1	4.2	4.3	4.4	4.5	4.7	4.8	4.9	5.0	5.1
4.4	4.5	4.6	4.8	4.9	5.0	5.2	5.3	5.4	5.6	5.7	5.9	6.0
5.0	5.2	5.3	5.5	5.6	5.8	5.9	6.1	6.3	6.4	6.6	6.8	6.9
5.4	5.6	5.8	6.0	6.2	6.3	6.5	6.7	6.9	7.0	7.2	7.4	7.6
6.8	7.0	7.2	7.4	7.6	7.9	8.1	8.3	8.5	8.7	8.9	9.1	9.4
7.6	7.9	8.1	8.3	8.6	8.8	9.1	9.3	9.5	9.8	10.0	10.3	10.5
8.7	9.0	9.2	9.5	9.8	10.1	10.4	10.6	10.9	11.2	11.5	11.8	12.0
10.1	10.4	10.8	11.1	11.4	11.8	12.1	12.4	12.7	13.0	13.4	13.7	14.0
12.3	12.7	13.1	13.5	13.9	14.3	14.7	15.0	15.4	15.8	16.2	16.6	17.0
8.0	8.3	8.5	8.8	9.0	9.3	9.5	9.8	10.0	10.3	10.6	10.8	11.1
8.3	8.6	8.9	9.1	9.4	9.7	9.9	10.2	10.5	10.7	11.0	11.2	11.5
13.6	14.1	14.5	14.9	15.4	15.8	16.2	16.6	17.1	17.5	17.9	18.4	18.8

Appendix C

Appendix D

Units of measurement: English system—metric system equivalents

The Metric System and Equivalents

To measure ingredients, a standardized system has been established that is interpreted on an international basis. However, in our country we also employ another set of measure and weight. In the field of dietetics, both systems are employed. The following tables give the quantities of the measures besides stating equivalents. With this information it is possible to calculate in either system of measure and weight.

Household Measures (Approximations)

For easy computing purposes, the cubic centimeter (cc.) is considered equivalent to 1 gram:

    1 cc. = 1 gram = 1 milliliter (ml)

For easy computing purposes, one ounce equals 30 grams or 30 cubic centimeters.

1 quart	=	960 grams
1 pint	=	480 grams
1 cup	=	240 grams
1/2 cup	=	120 grams
1 glass (8 ounces)	=	240 grams
1/2 glass (4 ounces)	=	120 grams
1 orange juice glass	=	100 to 120 grams
1 tablespoon	=	15 grams
1 teaspoon	=	5 grams

Level Measures and Weights

1 teaspoon	=	5 cc. / 5 grams
3 teaspoons	=	1 tablespoon / 15 cc. / 15 grams
2 tablespoons	=	30 cc. / 30 grams / 1 ounce (fluid)
4 tablespoons	=	1/4 cup / 60 cc. / 60 grams
8 tablespoons	=	1/2 cup / 120 cc. / 120 grams
16 tablespoons	=	1 cup / 240 grams / 240 ml. (fluid) / 8 ounces (fluid) / 1/2 pound
2 cups	=	1 pint / 480 grams / 480 ml. (fluid) / 16 ounces (fluid) / 1 pound
4 cups	=	2 pints / 1 quart / 1,000 or 960 cc. / 1,000 or 960 ml. (fluid) / 1 kilogram / 2.2 pounds
4 quarts	=	1 gallon

Units of Weight

		Ounce	Pound	Gram	Kilogram
1 ounce	=	1.0	0.06	28.4	0.028
1 pound	=	16.0	1.0	454	0.454
1 gram	=	0.035	.002	1.0	0.001
1 kilogram	=	35.3	2.2	1,000	1.0

Units of Volume

	Ounce	Pint	Quart	Milliliter	Liter
1 ounce	1.0	0.062	0.031	29.57	0.029
1 pint	16.0	1.0	0.5	473	.473
1 quart	32.0	2.0	1.0	946	.946
1 milliliter	0.034	0.002	0.001	1.0	0.001
1 liter	33.8	2.112	1.056	1,000	1.0

Units of Length

	Millimeter	Centimeter	Inch	Foot	Yard	Meter
1 millimeter	1.0	0.1	0.0394	0.0033	0.0011	0.001
1 centimeter	10.0	1.0	0.394	0.033	0.011	0.01
1 inch	25.4	2.54	1.0	0.083	0.028	0.025
1 foot	304.8	30.48	12.0	1.0	0.333	0.305
1 yard	914.4	91.44	36.0	3.0	1.0	0.914
1 meter	1,000	100	39.37	3.28	1.094	1.0

Appendix E — Desirable body weights for boys and girls

Boys
(Weight Is Expressed in Pounds)

Ht. Ins.	5 Yrs.	6 Yrs.	7 Yrs.	8 Yrs.	9 Yrs.	10 Yrs.	11 Yrs.	12 Yrs.	13 Yrs.	14 Yrs.	15 Yrs.	16 Yrs.	17 Yrs.	18 Yrs.	19 Yrs.	Ht. Ins.
38	34	34														38
39	35	35														39
40	36	36														40
41	38	38	38													41
42	39	39	39	39												42
43	41	41	41	41												43
44	44	44	44	44												44
45	46	46	46	46	46											45
46	47	48	48	48	48											46
47	49	50	50	50	50	50										47
48		52	53	53	53	53										48
49		55	55	55	55	55	55									49
50		57	58	58	58	58	58	58								50
51			61	61	61	61	61	61								51
52			63	64	64	64	64	64	64							52
53			66	67	67	67	67	68	68							53
54				70	70	70	70	71	71	72						54
55				72	72	73	73	74	74	74						55
56				75	76	77	77	77	78	78	80					56
57					79	80	81	81	82	83	83					57
58					83	84	84	85	85	86	87					58
59						87	88	89	89	90	90	90				59
60						91	92	92	93	94	95	96				60
61							95	96	97	99	100	103	106			61
62							100	101	102	103	104	107	111	116		62
63							105	106	107	108	110	113	118	123	127	63
64								109	111	113	115	117	121	126	130	64
65								114	117	118	120	122	127	131	134	65
66									119	122	125	128	132	136	139	66
67									124	128	130	134	136	139	142	67
68										134	134	137	141	143	147	68
69										137	139	143	146	149	152	69
70										143	144	145	148	151	155	70
71										148	150	151	152	154	159	71
72											153	155	156	158	163	72
73											157	160	162	164	167	73
74											160	164	168	170	171	74

The following percentages of net weight have been added for clothing (shoes and sweaters not included): 35 to 64 pounds: 3.5 percent; 64 pounds and over: 2.0 per cent.

Girls
(Weight Is Expressed in Pounds)

Ht. Ins.	5 Yrs.	6 Yrs.	7 Yrs.	8 Yrs.	9 Yrs.	10 Yrs.	11 Yrs.	12 Yrs.	13 Yrs.	14 Yrs.	15 Yrs.	16 Yrs.	17 Yrs.	18 Yrs.	Ht. Ins.
38	33	33													38
39	34	34													39
40	36	36	36												40
41	37	37	37												41
42	39	39	39												42
43	41	41	41	41											43
44	42	42	42	42											44
45	45	45	45	45	45										45
46	47	47	47	48	48										46
47	49	50	50	50	50	50									47
48		52	52	52	52	53									48
49		54	54	55	55	56	56								49
50		56	56	57	58	59	61	62							50
51			59	60	61	61	63	65							51
52			63	64	64	64	65	67							52
53			66	67	67	68	68	69	71						53
54				69	70	70	71	71	73						54
55				72	74	74	74	75	77	78					55
56					76	78	78	79	81	83					56
57					80	82	82	82	84	88	92				57
58						84	86	86	88	93	96	101			58
59						87	90	90	92	96	100	103	104		59
60						91	95	95	97	101	105	108	109	111	60
61							99	100	101	105	108	112	113	116	61
62							104	105	106	109	113	115	117	118	62
63								110	110	112	116	117	119	120	63
64								114	115	117	119	120	122	123	64
65								118	120	121	122	123	125	126	65
66									124	124	125	128	129	130	66
67									128	130	131	133	133	135	67
68									131	133	135	136	138	138	68
69										135	137	138	140	142	69
70										136	138	140	142	144	70
71										138	140	142	144	145	71

The following percentages of net weight have been added for clothing (shoes and sweaters not included): 35 to 65 pounds: 3.0 percent; 66 to 82 pounds: 2.5 percent; 83 pounds and over: 2 percent.

Appendix E 275

Appendix F

Calories in fast-food restaurant products

Specialty Food Items

Food Item and Description	kcal
Arthur Treacher's Fish and Chips	
2 pieces of fish, 4 oz of chips	275
Baskin-Robbins Ice Cream	
one scoop (2 1/2 oz) with sugar cone	
Chocolate Fudge	229
French Vanilla	217
Rocky Road	204
Butter Pecan	195
Jamoca Almond Fudge	190
Chocolate Mint	189
Jamoca	182
Fresh Strawberry	168
Fresh Peach	165
Mango Sherbet	132
Banana Daiquiri Ice	129
Burger King	
The "Whopper"	606
The "Whaler"	744
French fries (2 3/4 oz)	214
Large shake	332
Hamburger	252
Cheeseburger	305
Hot dog	291
Chocolate shake	317
Vanilla shake	322
Strawberry shake	315
Taco Bell	
Taco	159
Tostada	188
Frijoles	178

Food Item and Description	kcal
Enchirito	418
Burrito	319
"Bell Burger"	243
White Castle	
Hamburger	157
French fries	219
Cheeseburger	198
Fish sandwich	200
Milk shake	213
Onion rings	341
Cinnamon roll	305
Cherry roll	334
Arby's	
Junior roast beef sandwich	240
Regular roast beef sandwich	429
Turkey sandwich without dressing	337
Turkey sandwich with dressing	402
Ham 'n Cheese	458
Super roast beef sandwich	705
Carvel Ice Cream	
Standard 3-oz. cup of:	
Vanilla	148
Chocolate	147
Sherbet	105
"Thinny Thin": chocolate, coffee, or vanilla	56
Colonel Sanders Kentucky Fried Chicken	
15-piece bucket	3300
Drumstick	220
3-piece special	660
"Dinner," with 3 pieces of chicken, cole slaw, mashed potatoes, gravy, roll	980

Food Item and Description	kcal
Diary Queen Ice Cream	
Banana split	547
"Super Brazier"	907
Chicken snack	342
Dunkin Donuts	
Hole-in-the-middle "cake" donuts	
Plain cake	240
Plain honey-dipped	260
Plain with white icing	265
Plain with chocolate icing	235
Chocolate cake	240
Chocolate honey-dipped	250
"Yeast raised," with jelly, custard, or cream fillings:	
Honey-dipped	225
Sugar	205
(add 45 Calories for filling)	
Hardee's	
Huskee Delux	525
Huskee Junior	475
Fish sandwich	275
Hot dog	265
Apple turnover	290
French fries (2 oz.)	155
Milk shake (8 oz.)	320

Food Item and Description	kcal
Howard Johnson's	
Small cone	
Sherbet (any flavor)	136
Vanilla	186
Chocolate	195
Medium cone	
Vanilla	247
Chocolate	261
Large cone	
Vanilla	370
Chocolate	390
McDonald's	
Egg McMuffin	312
Hamburger	249
Cheeseburger	309
Quarter Pounder	414
Quarter Pounder with cheese	521
Big Mac	557
Filet-O-Fish	406
French fries	215
Apple pie	265

From *Nutrition, Weight Control, and Exercise* by Frank I. Katch and William D. MacArdle. Copyright © 1977 by Houghton Mifflin Company. Used by permission.

Appendix G

A cardiac risk index

1. *Age*	10 to 20	21 to 30	31 to 40	41 to 50	51 to 60	61 to 70 and over
	1	2	3	4	6	8
2. *Heredity*	No known history of heart disease	1 relative with cardiovascular disease over 60	2 relatives with cardiovascular disease over 60	1 relative with cardiovascular disease under 60	2 relatives with cardiovascular disease under 60	3 relatives with cardiovascular disease under 60
	1	2	3	4	6	8
3. *Weight*	More than 5 lbs. below standard weight	Standard weight	5–20 lbs. overweight	21–35 lbs. overweight	36–50 lbs. overweight	51–65 lbs. overweight
	0	1	2	3	5	7
4. *Tobacco Smoking*	Nonuser	Cigar and/or pipe	10 cigarettes or less a day	20 cigarettes a day	30 cigarettes a day	40 cigarettes a day or more
	0	1	2	3	5	8
5. *Exercise*	Intensive occupational and recreational exertion	Moderate occupational and recreational exertion	Sedentary work and intense recreational exertion	Sedentary occupational and moderate recreational exertion	Sedentary work and light recreational exertion	Complete lack of all exercise
	1	2	3	5	6	8
6. *Cholesterol or % fat in diet*	Cholesteral below 180 mg. Diet contains no animal or solid fats	Cholesterol 181–205 mg. Diet contains 10% animal or solid fats	Cholesterol 206–230 mg. Diet contains 20% animal or solid fats	Cholesterol 231–255 mg. Diet contains 30% animal or solid fats	Cholesterol 256–280 mg. Diet contains 40% animal or solid fats	Cholesterol 281–330 mg. Diet contains 50% animal or solid fats
	1	2	3	4	5	7
7. *Blood Pressure*	100 upper reading	120 upper reading	140 upper reading	160 upper reading	180 upper reading	200 or over upper reading
	1	2	3	4	6	8
8. *Sex*	Female	Female over 45	Male	Bald Male	Bald short male	Bald short stocky male
	1	2	3	4	6	7

Total Score: _____

Reprinted with permission of Dr. John Boyer, San Diego State University. San Diego, California.

To score your cardiac risk index, total the point values from the small boxes as they relate to you for each of the eight factors listed.

Cardiovascular Disease Risk Index Scoring Table

Group I	6 to 11 = very low risk
Group II	12 to 17 = low risk
Group III	18 to 25 = average risk
Group IV	26 to 32 = high risk
Group V	33 to 42 = dangerous risk
Group VI	42 to 60 = extremely dangerous risk

Appendix H

A polyunsaturated fat, low cholesterol diet plan

Polyunsaturated Fat, Low Cholesterol*

Allowed	Omitted
Beverage Coffee, tea; carbonated beverage; cereal beverage	

Meat
Meat, fish, or fowl without visible fat or skin; cottage cheese; egg white; peanut butter
Two egg yolks per week; **one** of the following may be used in place of **one** egg yolk:
  Cheese   2 ounces
  Cold cuts   2 ounces
  Frankfurters   2 (8–9/lb)
  Organ meats   2 ounces
  Shellfish   2 ounces
	Fried

Fat Listed in order of preference for increasing ratio of polyunsaturated to saturated fat: Vegetable oils: safflower, corn, soybean, sesame, cottonseed Margarine: liquid safflower oil margarine, liquid corn oil margarine Nuts: walnuts, pecans, almonds Salad dressings: mayonnaise; other salad dressings except "Omitted"	Butter; hydrogenated fats, coconut, olive, or peanut oils; avocado; bacon; cream, non-dairy cream substitutes; cream cheese; salad dressings with cream or cheese; nuts not "Allowed"; olives
Milk Skim milk, buttermilk	Whole milk, chocolate milk
Bread Bread, quick breads, rolls, crackers except "Omitted"; cereals Potato and potato substitutes except "Omitted"	Any with butter, cream, hydrogenated fat, egg yolk, whole milk; butter or cheese crackers; commercially prepared baked goods Potato chips; buttered popcorn
Vegetable Any	
Fruit* Any	

*No free-sugar diet: omit foods with sugar added.

From Committee on Dietetics of the Mayo Clinic. *Mayo Clinic Diet Manual.* Philadelphia: W. B. Saunders Company, 1971. Reprinted with permission from the W. B. Saunders Company.

Polyunsaturated Fat, Low Cholesterol*

Allowed	Omitted
Soup Fat-free broth, bouillon, or soups made of foods "Allowed"	Commercial; cream soup
Dessert* Gelatin; sherbet; any cake, cookies, pastry, or pudding prepared from "Allowed" foods	Any with butter, chocolate, coconut, cream, egg yolk, nuts not "Allowed," whole milk; commercially prepared mixes
Sweets* Any except "Omitted"	Chocolate and cream candies
Miscellaneous Salt, spices, herbs; condiments; cocoa; pickles; vinegar	Gravy, cream sauce; chocolate

		Polyunsaturated Fat, Low Cholesterol	Polyunsaturated Fat, No Free Sugar, Low Cholesterol
Breakfast	Fruit	1 serving	1 serving*
	Cereal	1 serving	1 serving
	Toast	1 slice	2 slices
	Fat	2 teaspoons	2 teaspoons
	Skim milk	1 cup	1 cup
	Sugar, jelly	2 tablespoons	...
	Beverage	1 cup	1 cup
Noon Meal	Meat	3 ounces	3 ounces
	Potato	1 serving	1 serving
	Vegetable	1 serving	1 serving
	Salad	1 serving	1 serving
	Bread	1 slice	2 slices
	Fat	5 teaspoons	5 teaspoons
	Fruit	1 serving	2 servings*
	Skim milk	1 cup	1 cup
	Sugar, jelly	1 tablespoon	...
	Beverage	1 cup	1 cup
Evening Meal	Meat	3 ounces	3 ounces
	Potato	1 serving	1 serving
	Vegetable	1 serving	1 serving
	Salad	1 serving	1 serving
	Bread	1 slice	2 slices
	Fat	5 teaspoons	5 teaspoons
	Dessert	1 serving	2 servings*
	Skim milk	1 cup	1 cup
	Sugar, jelly	1 tablespoon	...
	Beverage	1 cup	1 cup

*Unsweetened fruit.

Appendix I

Diet plans: 1,000–3,000 Calories

1,000 Calories: carbohydrate 120 Gm; protein 65 Gm; fat 30 Gm
(approximately)

Daily Menu Guide

The foods allowed in your diet should be selected from the seven exchange lists on this page. Menus should be planned on the basis of the menu guide given below. Foods in the same list are interchangeable, because, in the quantities specified, they provide approximately the same amounts of carbohydrate, protein, and fat. For example, when your menu calls for one bread exchange, any item in List 4 may be used in the amount stated. If two bread exchanges are allowed, double the specified amount or use a single exchange of *two* foods in List 4. See pages A-69–A-73 for exchange lists 1–7. Note that this numbering system is different than Appendix B, and applies to all the diet plans in this Appendix.

Breakfast

1 fruit exchange (List 3)
1 bread exchange (List 4)
1 meat exchange (List 5)
1/2 milk (skim) exchange (List 7)
Coffee or tea (any amount)

Lunch

2 meat exchanges (List 5)
2 bread exchanges (List 4)
Vegetable(s) as desired (List 1)
1 fruit exchange (List 3)
1/2 milk (skim) exchange (List 7)
1/2 fat exchange (List 6)
Coffee or tea (any amount)

Dinner

2 meat exchanges (List 5)
1 bread exchange (List 4)
Vegetable(s) as desired (List 1)
2 vegetable exchanges (List 2)
1 fruit exchange (List 3)
1 milk (skim) exchange (List 7)
1/2 fat exchange (List 6)
Coffee or tea (any amount)

1,200 Calories: carbohydrate 150 Gm; protein 60 Gm; fat 40 Gm
(approximately)

Daily Menu Guide

The foods allowed in your diet should be selected from the seven exchange lists on this page. Menus should be planned on the basis of the menu guide given below. Foods in the same list are interchangeable, because, in the quantities specified, they provide approximately the same amounts of carbohydrate, protein, and fat. For example, when your menu calls for one bread exchange, any item in List 4 may be used in the amount stated. If two bread exchanges are allowed, double the specified amount or use a single exchange of *two* foods in List 4.

Breakfast

1 fruit exchange (List 3)
1 bread exchange (List 4)
1 meat exchange (List 5)
1 milk (skim) exchange (List 7)
Coffee or tea (any amount)

Reprinted with permission from Lilly and Company. Modified to approximate recommended dietary goals for Americans (55–60% carbohydrate; 25–30% fat; 12–15% protein). Note that the milk and meat exchanges are different in caloric values than those in Appendix B.

Lunch

2 meat exchanges (List 5)
2 bread exchanges (List 4)
Vegetable(s) as desired (List 1)
2 fruit exchanges (List 3)
1 milk (skim) exchange (List 7)
2 fat exchanges (List 6)
Coffee or tea (any amount)

Dinner

2 meat exchanges (List 5)
2 bread exchanges (List 4)
Vegetable(s) as desired (List 1)
2 vegetable exchanges (List 2)
1 fruit exchange (List 3)
1 fat exchange (List 6)
Coffee or tea (any amount)

1,500 Calories: carbohydrate 195 Gm; protein 80 Gm; fat 45 Gm (approximately)

Daily Menu Guide

The foods allowed in your diet should be selected from the seven exchange lists on this page. Menus should be planned on the basis of the menu guide given below. Foods in the same list are interchangeable, because, in the quantities specified, they provide approximately the same amounts of carbohydrate, protein, and fat. For example, when your menu calls for one bread exchange, any item in List 4 may be used in the amount stated. If two bread exchanges are allowed, double the specified amount or use a single exchange of *two* foods in List 4.

Breakfast

1 fruit exchange (List 3)
2 bread exchanges (List 4)
1 meat exchange (List 5)
1 milk (skim) exchange (List 7)
2 fat exchanges (List 6)
Coffee or tea (any amount)

Lunch

2 meat exchanges (List 5)
2 bread exchanges (List 4)
Vegetable(s) as desired (List 1)
2 fruit exchanges (List 3)
1 milk (skim) exchange (List 7)
1 fat exchange (List 6)
Coffee or tea (any amount)

Dinner

2 meat exchanges (List 5)
2 bread exchanges (List 4)
Vegetable(s) as desired (List 1)
2 vegetable exchanges (List 2)
2 fruit exchanges (List 3)
1 milk (skim) exchange (List 7)
1 fat exchange (List 6)
Coffee or tea (any amount)

2,000 Calories: carbohydrate 250 Gm; protein 105 Gm; fat 65 Gm
(approximately)

Daily Menu Guide

The foods allowed in your diet should be selected from the seven exchange lists on this page. Menus should be planned on the basis of the menu guide given below. Foods in the same list are interchangeable, because, in the quantities specified, they provide approximately the same amounts of carbohydrate, protein, and fat. For example, when your menu calls for one bread exchange, any item in List 4 may be used in the amount stated. If two bread exchanges are allowed, double the specified amount or use a single exchange of *two* foods in List 4.

Breakfast

2 fruit exchanges (List 3)
3 bread exchanges (List 4)
2 meat exchanges (List 5)
1 milk (skim) exchange (List 7)
2 fat exchanges (List 6)
Coffee or tea (any amount)

Lunch

3 meat exchanges (List 5)
2 bread exchanges (List 4)
Vegetable(s) as desired (List 1)
2 vegetable exchanges (List 2)
2 fruit exchanges (List 3)
1 milk (skim) exchange (List 7)
2 fat exchanges (List 6)
Coffee or tea (any amount)

Dinner

3 meat exchanges (List 5)
3 bread exchanges (List 4)
Vegetable(s) as desired (List 1)
2 vegetable exchanges (List 2)
2 fruit exchanges (List 3)
1 milk (skim) exchange (List 7)
2 fat exchanges (List 6)
Coffee or tea (any amount)

2,200 Calories: carbohydrate 280 Gm; protein 110 Gm; fat 70 Gm
(approximately)

Daily Menu Guide

The foods allowed in your diet should be selected from the seven exchange lists on this page. Menus should be planned on the basis of the menu guide given below. Foods in the same list are interchangeable, because, in the quantities specified, they provide approximately the same amounts of carbohydrate, protein, and fat. For example, when your menu calls for one bread exchange, any item in List 4 may be used in the amount stated. If two bread exchanges are allowed, double the specified amount or use a single exchange of *two* foods in List 4.

Breakfast

2 fruit exchanges (List 3)
3 1/2 bread exchanges (List 4)
2 meat exchanges (List 5)
1 milk (skim) exchange (List 7)
2 fat exchanges (List 6)
Coffee or tea (any amount)

Lunch

3 meat exchanges (List 5)
4 bread exchanges (List 4)
Vegetable(s) as desired (List 1)
2 fruit exchanges (List 3)
1 milk (skim) exchange (List 7)
2 fat exchanges (List 6)
Coffee or tea (any amount)

Dinner

3 meat exchanges (List 5)
4 bread exchanges (List 4)
Vegetable(s) as desired (List 1)
2 vegetable exchanges (List 2)
2 fruit exchanges (List 3)
1 milk (skim) exchange (List 7)
2 fat exchanges (List 6)
Coffee or tea (any amount)

2,500 Calories: carbohydrate 310 Gm; protein 120 Gm; fat 80 Gm
(approximately)

Daily Menu Guide

The foods allowed in your diet should be selected from the seven exchange lists on this page. Menus should be planned on the basis of the menu guide given below. Foods in the same list are interchangeable, because, in the quantities specified, they provide approximately the same amounts of carbohydrate, protein, and fat. For example, when your menu calls for one bread exchange, any item in List 4 may be used in the amount stated. If two bread exchanges are allowed, double the specified amount or use a single exchange of *two* foods in List 4.

Breakfast

2 fruit exchanges (List 3)
4 bread exchanges (List 4)
3 meat exchanges (List 5)
1 milk (skim) exchange (List 7)
2 fat exchanges (List 6)
Coffee or tea (any amount)

Lunch

3 meat exchanges (List 5)
4 bread exchanges (List 4)
Vegetable(s) as desired (List 1)
1 vegetable exchange (List 2)
2 fruit exchanges (List 3)
1 milk (skim) exchange (List 7)
2 fat exchanges (List 6)
Coffee or tea (any amount)

Dinner

3 meat exchanges (List 5)
5 bread exchanges (List 4)
Vegetable(s) as desired (List 1)
2 vegetable exchanges (List 2)
2 fruit exchanges (List 3)
1 milk (skim) exchange (List 7)
3 fat exchanges (List 6)
Coffee or tea (any amount)

Bedtime Feeding

(Only when directed by physician)

1/2 milk exchange (1/2 cup milk)
1/2 bread exchange (2 crackers)
} will add approximately 120 Calories to daily diet

3,000 Calories: carbohydrate 375 Gm; protein 150 Gm; fat 95 Gm
(approximately)

Daily Menu Guide

The foods allowed in your diet should be selected from the seven exchange lists on this page. Menus should be planned on the basis of the menu guide given below. Foods in the same list are interchangeable, because, in the quantities specified, they provide approximately the same amounts of carbohydrate, protein, and fat. For example, when your menu calls for one bread exchange, any item in List 4 may be used in the amount stated. If two bread exchanges are allowed, double the specified amount or use a single exchange of *two* foods in List 4.

Breakfast

2 fruit exchanges (List 3)
4 bread exchanges (List 4)
3 meat exchanges (List 5)
1 milk (skim) exchange (List 7)
2 fat exchanges (List 6)
Coffee or tea (any amount)

Lunch

3 meat exchanges (List 5)
4 bread exchanges (List 4)
Vegetable(s) as desired (List 1)
2 fruit exchanges (List 3)
1 milk (skim) exchange (List 7)
2 fat exchanges (List 6)
Coffee or tea (any amount)

Midafternoon Feeding

1 meat exchange (List 5)
1 bread exchange (List 4)
1 milk (skim) exchange (List 7)

Dinner

3 meat exchanges (List 5)
5 bread exchanges (List 4)
Vegetable(s) as desired (List 1)
2 vegetable exchanges (List 2)
2 fruit exchanges (List 3)
1 milk (skim) exchange (List 7)
2 fat exchanges (List 6)
Coffee or tea (any amount)

Bedtime Feeding

2 bread exchanges (List 4)
2 meat exchanges (List 5)
1 milk (skim) exchange (List 7)

List 1: Allowed As Desired (Need Not Be Measured)

Seasonings: Cinnamon, celery salt, garlic, garlic salt,* lemon, mustard, mint, nutmeg, parsley, pepper, saccharin* and other sugarless sweeteners, spices, vanilla, and vinegar.

Other Foods: Coffee or tea (without sugar or cream), fat-free broth, bouillon, unflavored gelatin, rennet tablets, sour or dill pickles,* cranberries (without sugar), rhubarb (without sugar).

Vegetables: Group A—insignificant carbohydrate or calories. You may eat as much as desired of raw vegetable. If cooked vegetable is eaten, limit amount to 1 cup.

Asparagus	Lettuce
Broccoli	Mushrooms
Brussels sprouts	Okra
Cabbage	Peppers, green or red
Cauliflower	Radishes
Celery	Sauerkraut
Chicory	String beans
Cucumbers	Summer squash
Eggplant	Tomatoes
Escarole	Watercress
Greens: beet, chard, collard, dandelion, kale, mustard, spinach, turnip	

---

*Consumption of salt, high salt foods and saccharin-containing products should be restricted.

List 2: Vegetable Exchanges

Each portion supplies approximately 7 Gm. of carbohydrate and 2 Gm. of protein, or 36 Calories.

Vegetables: Group B—One serving equals 1/2 cup, or 100 Gm.

Beets	Pumpkin
Carrots	Rutabagas
Onions	Squash, winter
Peas, green	Turnips

Appendix I

List 3: Fruit Exchanges (Fresh, Dried, or Canned without Sugar)

Each portion supplies approximately 10 Gm. of carbohydrate, or 40 Calories.

	Household Measurement	Weight of Portion
Apple	1 small (2″ diam.)	80 Gm.
Applesauce	1/2 cup	100 Gm.
Apricots, fresh	2 med	100 Gm.
Apricots, dried	4 halves	20 Gm.
Banana	1/2 small	50 Gm.
Berries	1 cup	150 Gm.
Blueberries	2/3 cup	100 Gm.
Cantaloupe	1/4 (6″ diam.)	200 Gm.
Cherries	10 large	75 Gm.
Dates	2	15 Gm.
Figs, fresh	2 large	50 Gm.
Figs, dried	1 small	15 Gm.
Grapefruit	1/2 small	125 Gm.
Grapefruit juice	1/2 cup	100 Gm.
Grapes	12	75 Gm.
Grape juice	1/4 cup	60 Gm.
Honeydew melon	1/8 (7″)	150 Gm.
Mango	1/2 small	70 Gm.
Orange	1 small	100 Gm.
Orange juice	1/2 cup	100 Gm.
Papaya	1/3 med	100 Gm.
Peach	1 med	100 Gm.
Pear	1 small	100 Gm.
Pineapple	1/2 cup	80 Gm.
Pineapple juice	1/3 cup	80 Gm.
Plums	2 med	100 Gm.
Prunes, dried	2	25 Gm.
Raisins	2 tbsp	15 Gm.
Tangerine	1 large	100 Gm.
Watermelon	1 cup	175 Gm.

List 4: Bread Exchanges

Each portion supplies approximately 15 Gm. of carbohydrate and 2 Gm. of protein, or 68 Calories.

	Household Measurement	Weight of Portion
Bread	1 slice	25 Gm.
Biscuit, roll	1 (2" diam.)	35 Gm.
Muffin	1 (2" diam.)	35 Gm.
Cornbread	1 1/2" cube	35 Gm.
Flour	2 1/2 tbsp	20 Gm.
Cereal, cooked	1/2 cup	100 Gm.
Cereal, dry (flakes or puffed)	3/4 cup	20 Gm.
Rice, or grits, cooked	1/2 cup	100 Gm.
Spaghetti, noodles, etc.	1/2 cup	100 Gm.
Crackers, graham	2	20 Gm.
Crackers, oyster	20 (1/2 cup)	20 Gm.
Crackers, saltine	5	20 Gm.
Crackers, soda	3	20 Gm.
Crackers, round	6–8	20 Gm.
Vegetables		
Beans (Lima, navy, etc.), dry, cooked	1/2 cup	90 Gm.
Peas (split peas, etc.), dry, cooked	1/2 cup	90 Gm.
Baked beans, no pork	1/4 cup	50 Gm.
Corn	1/3 cup	80 Gm.
Parsnips	2/3 cup	125 Gm.
Potato, white, baked or boiled	1 (2" diam.)	100 Gm.
Potatoes, white mashed	1/2 cup	100 Gm.
Potatoes, sweet, or yams	1/4 cup	50 Gm.

List 5: Meat Exchanges*

Each portion supplies approximately 7 Gm. of protein and 5 Gm. of fat, or 73 Calories. (30 Gm. equal 1 oz.)

	Household Measurement	Weight of Portion
Meat and poultry (beef, lamb, pork, liver, chicken, etc.) (med. fat)	1 slice (3″ × 2″ × 1/8″)	30 Gm.
Cold cuts	1 slice (4 1/2″ sq., 1/8″ thick)	45 Gm.
Frankfurter	1 (8–9 per lb.)	50 Gm.
Codfish, mackerel, etc.	1 slice (2″ × 2″ × 1″)	30 Gm.
Salmon, tuna, crab	1/4 cup	30 Gm.
Oysters, shrimp, clams	5 small	45 Gm.
Sardines	3 med	30 Gm.
Cheese, cheddar, American	1 slice (3 1/2″ × 1 1/2″ × 1/4″)	30 Gm.
Cheese, cottage	1/4 cup	45 Gm.
Egg	1	50 Gm.
Peanut butter	2 tbsp	30 Gm.

Limit peanut butter to one exchange per day unless allowance is made for carbohydrate in the diet plan.

List 6: Fat Exchanges

Each portion supplies approximately 5 Gm. of fat, or 45 Calories.

	Household Measurement	Weight of Portion
Butter or margarine	1 tsp.	5 Gm.
Bacon, crisp	1 slice	10 Gm.
Cream, light	2 tbsp	30 Gm.
Cream, heavy	1 tbsp	15 Gm.
Cream cheese	1 tbsp	15 Gm.
French dressing	1 tbsp	15 Gm.
Mayonnaise	1 tsp	5 Gm.
Oil or cooking fat	1 tsp	5 Gm.
Nuts	6 small	10 Gm.
Olives	5 small	50 Gm.
Avocado	1/8 (4″ diam.)	25 Gm.

*Meat exchange in Appendix B contains only 3 Gm. of fat and 55 Calories.

List 7: Milk Exchanges*

Each portion supplies approximately 12 Gm. of carbohydrate, 8 Gm. of protein, and 10 Gm. of fat, or 170 Calories.

	Household Measurement	Weight of Portion
Milk, whole	1 cup	240 Gm.
Milk, evaporated	1/2 cup	120 Gm.
*Milk, powdered	1/4 cup	35 Gm.
*Buttermilk	1 cup	240 Gm.

*Add 2 fat exchanges if milk is fat-free. Skim milk has only 80 Calories.

Appendix J — Generalized equations for predicting body fat

Women*

$BD = 1.0994921 - 0.0009929 (X_1) + 0.0000023 (X_1)^2 - 0.0001392 (X_2)$

BD = Body density
X_1 = Sum of triceps, thigh and suprailium skinfolds
X_2 = Age

Men**

$BD = 1.10938 - 0.0008267 (X_1) + .0000016 (X_1)^2 - 0.0002574 (X_2)$

BD = Body density
X_1 = Sum of chest, abdomen and thigh skinfolds
X_2 = Age

To calculate percent body fat, plug into Siri's equation $\left(\dfrac{4.95}{BD} - 4.5\right) \times 100$

---

*From Jackson, A.; Pollock, M.; and Ward, A. 1980. Generalized equations for predicting body density of women. *Medicine and Science in Sports and Exercise,* 12: 175–182.

**Jackson, A., and Pollock, M. 1978. Generalized equations for predicting body density of men. *British Journal of Nutrition* 40: 497–504.

Glossary

acclimitization The ability of the body to undergo physiological adaptations so that the stress of a given environment, such as high environmental temperature, is less severe.

acetaldehyde An intermediate breakdown product of alcohol.

acetic acid A naturally occurring saturated fatty acid; a precursor for the Krebs cycle when converted into acetyl CoA.

acetyl CoA The major fuel for the oxidative processes in the body, being derived from the breakdown of glucose and fatty acids.

acid-base balance A relative balance of acid and base products in the body so that an optimal pH is maintained in the tissues, particularly the blood.

acute exercise bout A single bout of exercise that will produce various physiological reactions dependent upon the nature of the exercise; a single workout.

additives Substances added to food to improve color, texture, stability, or similar such purposes.

adenosinetriphosphate *See* ATP.

ADH The antidiuretic hormone secreted by the pituitary gland; its major action is to conserve body water by decreasing urine formation.

adrenalin A hormone secreted by the adrenal medulla gland; it is a stimulant and prepares the body for "fight or flight."

aerobic Relating to energy processes that occur in the presence of oxygen.

aerobic walking Rapid walking designed to elevate the HR so that a training effect would occur; more strenuous than ordinary leisure walking.

alanine A nonessential amino acid.

alcohol A colorless liquid with depressant effects; ethyl alcohol or ethanol is the alcohol designed for human consumption.

alcohol dehydrogenase An enzyme in the liver that initiates the breakdown of alcohol to acetaldehyde.

aldosterone The main electrolyte-regulating hormone secreted by the adrenal cortex; primarily controls sodium and potassium balance.

alpha-tocopherol The most biologically active alcohol in vitamin E.

amenorrhea Cessation of blood flow in the menstrual cycle.

amino acids The chief structural material of protein, consisting of an amino group (NH_2) and an acid group (COOH) plus other components.

amino group The nitrogen containing component of amino acids (NH_2).

aminostatic theory A theory suggesting that hunger is controlled by the presence or absence of amino acids in the blood acting upon a receptor in the hypothalamus.

ammonia A metabolic byproduct of the oxidation of glutamine; it may be transformed into urea for excretion from the body.

anabolic steroids Drugs designed to mimic the actions of testosterone to build muscle tissue (anabolism) while minimizing the androgenic effects (masculinization).

anabolism Constructive metabolism, the process whereby simple body compounds are formed into more complex ones.

anaerobic Relating to energy processes that occur in the absence of oxygen.

anaerobic threshold The point during exercise when lactic acid begins to accumulate rapidly in the blood, indicative of a greater reliance on anaerobic production of energy.

anemia In general, below normal levels of circulating RBC's and hemoglobin; there are many different types of anemia.

anion A negatively charged ion, or electrolyte.

anorexia nervosa A serious nervous condition, particularly among teenage girls, marked by a loss of appetite and leading to various degrees of emaciation.

antibodies Protein substances developed in the body in reaction to the presence of a foreign substance, called an antigen; natural antibodies are also present in the blood. They are protective in nature.

antidiuretic hormone *See* ADH.

appetite A pleasant desire for food for the purpose of enjoyment that is developed through previous experience; controlled in humans by an appetite center, or appestat, in the hypothalamus.

arginine An essential amino acid.

arteriosclerosis Hardening of the arteries; *also see* atherosclerosis.

ascorbic acid Vitamin C.

atherosclerosis A specific form of arteriosclerosis characterized by the formation of plaques on the inner layers of the arterial wall.

ATP Adenosinetriphosphate, a high-energy phosphate compound found in the body; one of the major forms of energy available for immediate use in the body.

ATP–PC system The energy system for fast, powerful muscle contractions; uses ATP as the immediate energy source, the spent ATP being quickly regenerated by breakdown of the PC. ATP and PC are high energy phosphates in the muscle cell.

BAL Blood alcohol level; the concentration of alcohol in the blood.

basal metabolic rate *See* BMR.

Basic Four Food Groups Grouping of foods into four categories that can be used as a means to educate individuals how to obtain essential nutrients. The four groups are meat, milk, bread-cereals, and fruit-vegetable.

bee pollen A nutritional product containing minute amounts of protein and some vitamins that has been advertised to be possibly ergogenic for some athletes.

behavioral patterns Relative to weight control methods, behavioral patterns, or the way one acts, may be modified to help achieve weight loss.

bile A fluid secreted by the liver into the intestine that aids in the breakdown process of fats.

biotin A component of the B complex.

blood alcohol level *See* BAL.

blood glucose Blood sugar; the means by which carbohydrate is carried in the blood; normal range is 70–120 mg/ml.

BMR The basal metabolic rate; measurement of energy expenditure in the body under resting, post-absorptive conditions, indicative of the energy needed to maintain life under these basal conditions.

caffeine A stimulant drug found in many food products such as coffee, tea, and cola drinks; stimulates the central nervous system.

calciferol A synthetic vitamin D, vitamin D_2.

calcium A silver-white metallic element essential to human nutrition.

caloric concept of weight control The concept that calories are the basis of weight control. Excess calories will add body weight while caloric deficiencies will contribute to weight loss.

caloric deficit A negative caloric balance whereby more calories are expended than consumed; a weight loss will occur.

Calorie A Calorie is a measure of heat energy. A small calorie represents the amount of heat needed to raise one gram of water one degree Celsius. A large Calorie (kilocalorie, KC, or C) is 1,000 small calories.

calorimeter A device used to measure the caloric value of a given food, or heat production of animals or man.

carbohydrate A group of compounds containing carbon, hydrogen and oxygen. Glucose, glycogen, sugar, starches, fiber, cellulose, and the various saccharides are all carbohydrates.

carbohydrate loading A dietary method utilized by endurance-type athletes to help increase the carbohydrate (glycogen) levels in their muscles and liver.

catabolism Destructive metabolism whereby complex chemical compounds in the body are degraded to simpler ones.

cation A positively charged ion or electrolyte.

cellulose The fibrous carbohydrate that provides the structural backbone for plants; plant fiber.

Celsius A thermometer scale that has a freezing point of 0° and a boiling point at 100°; often known as the centigrade scale.

cerebrospinal fluid The fluid found in the brain and spinal cord.

CHD Coronary Heart Disease; a degenerative disease of the heart caused primarily by arteriosclerosis or atherosclerosis of the coronary vessels of the heart.

chloride A compound of chlorine present in a salt form carrying a negative charge; Cl^-, an anion.

cholecalciferol The product of irradiation of 7-dehydrocholesterol found in the skin.

cholesterol A fatlike pearly substance, an alcohol, found in all animal fats and oils; a main constituent of some body tissues and body compounds.

choline A substance associated with the B complex that is widely distributed in both plant and animal tissues; involved in carbohydrate, fat and protein metabolism.

chromium A whitish metal essential to human nutrition; it is involved in carbohydrate metabolism via its role with insulin.

chronic training effect Repeated bouts of exercise will elicit physiological changes in the body that will help make the body more efficient during exercise.

chylomicron A particle of emulsified fat found in the blood following the digestion and assimilation of fat.

cirrhosis A degenerative disease of the liver, one cause being excessive consumption of alcohol.

cobalamin The cobalt-containing complex common to all members of the vitamin B_{12} group; often used to designate cyanocobalamin.

cobalt A gray, hard metal which is a component of vitamin B_{12}.

coenzyme An activator of an enzyme; many vitamins are coenzymes.

complex carbohydrates A term used to describe foods high in starch such as bread, cereals, fruits, and vegetables as contrasted to simple carbohydrates such as table sugar.

conduction In relation to body temperature, the transfer of heat from one substance to another by direct contact.

convection In relation to body temperature, the transfer of heat by way of currents in either the air or water.

cool down A phase after an exercise bout where the individual gradually tapers the level of activity, for example by jogging slowly after a fast run.

copper A reddish metallic element essential to human nutrition; it functions with iron in the formation of hemoglobin and the cytochromes.

core temperature The temperature of the deep tissues of the body, usually measured orally or rectally; also see shell temperature.

coronary heart disease *See* CHD.

coronary risk factors Behaviors (smoking) or body properties (cholesterol levels) that may predispose an individual to coronary heart disease.

cyanocobalamin Vitamin B_{12}.

cysteine A breakdown product of cystine. It is also a sulfur-containing amino acid.

cystine A sulfur-containing amino acid.

cytochromes Any one of a class of pigment compounds that plays an important role in cellular oxidative processes.

deamination Removal of an amine group, or nitrogen, from an amino acid.

dehydration A reduction of the body water to below the normal of hydration; water output exceeds water intake.

depressant Drugs or agents that will depress or lower the level of bodily functions, particularly central nervous system functioning.

diabetes mellitus A disorder of carbohydrate metabolism due to inadequate production of insulin; results in high blood glucose levels and loss of sugar in the urine.

diarrhea Frequent passage of a watery fecal discharge due to a gastrointestinal disturbance.

dietary fiber Fiber in plant foods that cannot be hydrolyzed by the digestive enzymes.

disaccharides Any one of a class of sugars that yields two monosaccharides on hydrolysis; sucrose is the most common.

diuretics A class of agents that stimulate the formation of urine; used as a means to reduce body fluids.

DNA Deoxyribonucleic acid; a complex protein found in chromosomes that is the carrier of genetic information and the basis of heredity.

duration concept One of the major concepts of aerobics exercise; duration refers to the amount of time spent exercising during each bout.

electrolytes A solution that contains ions and can conduct electricity; often the ions of salts such as sodium and chloride are called electrolytes; *also see* ions.

electron transport system A highly structured array of chemical compounds in the cell that transport electrons and harness energy for later use in the process.

element Relative to chemistry, a substance that cannot be subdivided into substances different from itself; many elements are essential to human life.

EMR Exercise metabolic rate; an increased metabolic rate due to the need for increased energy production during exercise; the BMR may be increased more than twenty-fold.

energy The ability to do work; energy exists in various forms, notably mechanical, heat, and chemical in the human body.

English system A measurement system based upon the foot, pound, quart, and other nonmetric units; *also see* metric system.

enzyme A complex protein in the body that serves as a catalyst, facilitating reactions between various substances without being changed itself.

epithelial cells The layer of cells that covers the outside and inside surfaces of the body, including the skin and the lining of the gastrointestinal system.

ergogenic Work-enhancing; agents which are utilized in attempts to increase athletic or physical performance capacity.

ergogenic effect The physiological or psychological effect that an ergogenic substance is designed to produce.

essential amino acids Those amino acids that must be obtained in the diet and cannot be synthesized in the body.

essential fat Fat in the body that is an essential part of the tissues, such as cell membrane structure, nerve coverings, and the brain; *also see* storage fat.

essential fatty acids Those unsaturated fatty acids that may not be synthesized in the body and must be obtained in the diet; linoleic, linolenic, arachidonic.

essential nutrients Those nutrients found to be essential to human life and optimal functioning.

ethanol Alcohol; ethyl alcohol.

ethyl alcohol Alcohol; ethanol.

evaporation The conversion of a liquid to a vapor that consumes energy; evaporation of sweat cools the body by using body heat as the energy source.

exercise frequency In an aerobic exercise program, the number of times per week that an individual exercises.

exercise intensity The tempo, speed, or resistance of an exercise. Intensity can be increased by working faster, doing more work in a given amount of time.

exercise metabolic rate *See* EMR.

exercise sequence Relative to a weight training workout, the lifting sequence is designed so that different muscle groups are utilized sequentially in order to be fresh for each exercise.

exercise stimulus The means whereby one elicits a physiological response; running, for example, can be the stimulus to increase the heart rate and other physiological functions.

extracellular water Body water that is located outside the cells; often subdivided into the intravascular water and the intercellular, or interstitial, water.

faddism Relative to nutrition, the utilization of dietary fads based upon theoretical principles that may or may not be valid; usually used in a negative sense, as in quackery.

fasting Starvation; abstinence from eating that may be partial or complete.

fast twitch fibers Muscle fibers characterized by high contractile speed.

fatigue A generalized or specific feeling of tiredness that may have a multitude of causes; may be mental or physical.

fats Triglycerides; a combination, or ester, of three fatty acids and glycerol.

fatty acids Any one of a number of aliphatic acids containing only carbon, oxygen, and hydrogen; they may be saturated or unsaturated.

feeding center A collection of nerve cells in the hypothalamus that are involved in the control of feeding reflexes.

Feingold hypothesis The hypothesis that certain food additives contribute to hyperactivity and socioemotional problems in children.

FFA Free fatty acids; formed by the hydrolysis of triglycerides.

fiber In general, the indigestible carbohydrate in plants that forms the structural network; *also see* cellulose.

first law of thermodynamics The law that energy cannot be created nor destroyed; energy can be converted from one form to another.

flatulence Gas or air in the gastrointestinal tract, particularly the intestines.

fluoride A salt of hydrofluoric acid; a compound of fluorine that may be helpful in the prevention of dental decay.

folacin Folic acid.

folic acid A water soluble vitamin that appears to be essential in preventing certain types of anemia.

food additives *See* additives.

food cultism Treating a particular food as if it possesses special properties, such as prevention or treatment of disease or improvement of athletic performance, usually without scientific justification.

foot-pound A unit of work whereby the weight of one pound is moved through a distance of one foot.

free fatty acids *See* FFA.

fructose A monosaccharide known also as levulose or fruit sugar; found in all sweet fruits.

fruitarian A type of vegetarian who subsists solely on fruits and fruit products.

glucogenic amino acids Amino acids that may undergo deamination and be converted into glucose through the process of gluconeogenesis.

gluconeogenesis The formation of carbohydrates from molecules that are not themselves carbohydrate, such as amino acids and the glycerol from fat.

glucose A monosaccharide; a thick, sweet, syrupy liquid.

glucose–electrolyte replacement solutions A solution containing varying proportions of water, glucose, sodium, potassium, chloride, and other electrolytes designed to replace sweat losses.

glucose polymer A combination of several glucose molecules into a more complex carbohydrate.

glucostatic theory The theory that hunger and satiety are controlled by the glucose level in the blood; the receptors that respond to the blood glucose level are in the hypothalamus.

glycerol Glycerin, a clear syrupy liquid; combines with fatty acids to form triglycerides.

glycogen A polysaccharide that is the chief storage form of carbohydrate in animals; it is stored primarily in the liver and muscles.

glycogen sparing effect The theory that certain dietary techniques, such as the utilization of caffeine, may facilitate the oxidation of fatty acids for energy and thus spare the utilization of glycogen.

glycolysis The degradation of sugars into smaller compounds; the main quantitative anaerobic energy process in the muscle tissue.

gout The deposit of uric acid byproducts in and about the joints contributing to inflammation and pain; usually occurs in the knee or foot.

gram calorie A small calorie; *see* calorie.

GRAS Generally recognized as safe; a classification for food additives indicating that they most likely are not harmful for human consumption.

HDL cholesterol High density lipoprotein cholesterol; one mechanism whereby cholesterol is transported in the blood. High HDL levels are somewhat protective against CHD.

heat balance equation Heat balance is dependent upon the interrelationships of metabolic heat production and loss or gain of heat by radiation, convection, conduction, and evaporation.

heat cramps Painful muscular cramps or tetanus following prolonged exercise in the heat without water or salt replacement.

heat exhaustion Weakness or dizziness from overexertion in a hot environment.

heat stroke Elevated body temperature of 106°F or greater caused by exposure to excessive heat gains or production and diminished heat loss.

heat syncope Fainting caused by excessive heat exposure.

hemoglobin The protein-iron pigment in the red blood cells that transports oxygen.

hepatitis An inflammatory condition of the liver.

herbicide A chemical agent designed to kill weeds and other undesired plants.

high blood pressure *See* hypertension.

high density lipoprotein A protein-lipid complex in the blood that facilitates the transport of triglycerides, cholesterol, and phospholipids. *See* HDL cholesterol.

histidine An essential amino acid for children.

homeostasis A term used to describe a condition of normalcy in the internal body environment.

hormones A chemical substance produced by specific body cells, secreted into the blood and then acting on some specific target tissues.

HR max The normal maximal heart rate of an individual during exercise.

hunger A basic physiological desire to eat that is normally caused by a lack of food; may be accompanied by stomach contractions.

hydrogenated fats Fats to which hydrogen has been added, usually causing them to be saturated.

hydrolysis A mechanism for splitting substances into smaller compounds by the addition of water; enzyme action.

hypercholesteremia Elevated blood cholesterol levels.

hyperglycemia Elevated blood glucose levels.

hyperhydration The practice of increasing the body water stores by fluid consumption prior to an athletic event; a state of increased water content in the body.

hyperlipidemia Elevated blood lipid levels.

hypertension A condition with various causes whereby the blood pressure is higher than normal.

hypertonic Relative to osmotic pressure, a solution that has a greater concentration of solute or salts, hence higher osmotic pressure, in comparison to another solution.

hypertriglyceridemia Elevated blood levels of triglycerides.

hypervitaminosis A pathological condition due to an excessive vitamin intake, particularly the fat-soluble vitamins A and D.

hypoglycemia A low blood sugar level.

hypohydration Dehydration; a state of decreased water content in the body.

hypothalamus A part of the brain involved in the control of involuntary activity in the body; contains many centers for neural control such as temperature, hunger, appetite, and thirst.

hypotonic Having an osmotic pressure lower than that of the solution to which it is compared.

index of nutritional quality *See* INQ.

indicator nutrients These eight nutrients, if provided in adequate supply through a varied diet, should provide adequate amounts of the other essential nutrients. The eight are protein, vitamin A, thiamin, riboflavin, niacin, vitamin C, calcium, and iron.

initial fitness level The physical fitness level of an individual prior to the onset of a physical conditioning program.

inositol A member of the B-complex although its role in human nutrition has not been established.

INQ Index of nutritional quality; a mathematical means of determining the quality of any given food relative to its content of a specific nutrient.

insensible perspiration Perspiration on the skin not detectable by ordinary senses.

insulin A hormone secreted by the pancreas involved in carbohydrate metabolism.

insulin response Blood insulin levels rise following the ingestion of sugar and the resultant hyperglycemia; the insulin causes the sugar to be taken up by the muscles and liver, possibly creating a reactive hypoglycemia.

intercellular water Body water found between the cells; also known as interstitial water.

International Unit *See* IU.

International Unit System *See* SI.

interstitial water *See* intercellular water.

intracellular water Body water that is found within the cells.

intravascular water Body water found in the vascular system, or blood vessels.

iodine A nonmetallic element that is necessary for the proper development and functioning of the thyroid gland.

ions A particle with an electrical charge; anions are negative and cations are positive.

iron A metallic element essential for the development of several chemical compounds in the body, notably hemoglobin.

iron deficiency anemia Anemia caused by an inadequate intake or absorption of iron, resulting in impaired hemoglobin formation.

isoleucine An essential amino acid.

isotonic Pertaining to a state of equal tension or activity; *i.e.,* equal osmotic pressures between two solutions.

IU International Unit; a method of expressing the quantity of some substance, such as vitamins, which is an internationally developed and accepted standard.

jogging A term used to designate slow running; although the distinction between running and jogging is relative to the individual involved, a common value used for jogging is a nine-minute mile or slower.

joule A measure of work in the metric system; a newton of force applied through a distance of one meter.

KC Kilocalorie or KCAL; *see* Calorie.

ketogenic amino acids Amino acids that may be deaminated, converted into ketones, and eventually into fat.

ketones An organic compound containing a carbonyl group; ketone acids in the body, such as acetone, are the end products of fat metabolism.

key nutrient concept The concept that if certain key nutrients are adequately supplied by the diet, the other essential nutrients will also be present in adequate amounts.

KGM Kilogram-meter; a measure of work in the metric system whereby one kilogram of weight is moved through a distance of one meter; however, the joule is the recommended unit to express work.

kidney stones Compounds in the pelvis of the kidney formed from various salts such as carbonates, oxalates, and phosphates.

kilocalorie A large Calorie; *see* Calorie.

kilogram A unit of mass in the metric system; in ordinary terms 1 kilogram is the equivalent of 2.2 pounds.

kilogram-meter *See* KGM.

kilojoule One thousand joule; one kilojoule (KJ) is approximately 0.25 kilocalorie.

Krebs cycle The main oxidative reaction sequence in the body that generates ATP; also known as the citric acid or tricarboxylic acid cycle.

lactic acid The anaerobic end product of glycolysis; it has been implicated as a causative factor in the etiology of fatigue.

lactic acid system The energy system that produces ATP anaerobically by the breakdown of glycogen to lactic acid; used primarily in events of maximal effort for one to two minutes.

lactose A white crystalline disaccharide that yields glucose and galactose upon hydrolysis; also known as milk sugar.

lactovegetarian A vegetarian who includes milk products in the diet as a form of high quality protein.

LDL cholesterol Low density lipoprotein cholesterol; a mechanism whereby cholesterol is transported in the blood. High blood levels are associated with increased incidence of CHD.

lean body mass The body weight minus the body fat, composed primarily of muscle, bone, and other nonfat tissue.

lecithin A fatty substance of a class known as phospholipids; said to have the therapeutic properties of phosphorus.

legume The fruit or pod of vegetables including soybeans, kidney beans, lima beans, garden peas, black-eyed peas, and lentils; high in protein.

leucine An essential amino acid.

lipase An enzyme that catabolizes fats into fatty acids and glycerol.

lipoic acid A coenzyme that functions in oxidative decarboxylation, or removal of carbon dioxide from a compound.

lipoprotein A combination of lipid and protein, possessing the general properties of proteins. Practically all the lipids of the plasma are present in this form.

lipostatic theory The theory that hunger and satiety are controlled by the lipid level in the blood.

liquid meals Food in a liquid form designed to provide a balanced intake of essential nutrients.

liquid protein diets Protein in a liquid form; a common form consists of predigested protein into simple amino acids.

liver glycogen The major storage form of carbohydrate in the liver.

long haul concept Relative to weight control, the idea that weight loss via exercise should be gradual and one should not expect to lose large amounts of weight in a short period of time.

low density lipoprotein A protein-lipid complex in the blood that facilitates the transport of triglycerides, cholesterol, and phospholipids. *Also see* LDL cholesterol.

lysine An essential amino acid.

magnesium A white metallic mineral element essential in human nutrition.

major minerals Those minerals essential to human nutrition with an RDA in excess of 100 mg/day: calcium, magnesium, phosphorus, sodium, potassium, chloride.

maltose A white crystalline disaccharide that upon hydrolysis yields two molecules of glucose.

manganese A metallic element essential in human nutrition.

maximal heart rate *See* HR max.

maximal heart rate reserve The difference between the maximal HR and resting HR. A percentage of this reserve, usually 60–90 percent, is added to the resting HR to get the target HR for aerobics training programs.

maximal oxygen uptake *See* VO_2 max.

megadose An excessive amount of a substance in comparison to a normal dose of RDA; usually used with vitamin megadoses.

metabolic aftereffects The theory that the aftereffects of exercise will cause the metabolic rate to be elevated for a period of time, thus expending calories and contributing to weight loss.

metabolic rate The energy expended in order to maintain all physical and chemical changes occurring in the body.

metabolic water The water that is a byproduct of the oxidation of carbohydrate, fat, and protein in the body.

metabolism The sum total of all physical and chemical processes occurring in the body.

methionine An essential amino acid.

metric system A method of measurement based upon units of ten.

METS A measurement unit of energy expenditure; one MET equals approximately 3.5 ml O_2/kg body weight/minute.

microgram One millionth of a gram.

milligram One thousandth of a gram.

mineral An inorganic element occurring in nature.

mitochondria Structures within the cells that serve as the location for the aerobic production of ATP.

molybdenum A hard, heavy, silvery-white metallic element.

monosaccharides Simple sugars (glucose, fructose, and galactose) that cannot be broken down by hydrolysis.

muscle glycogen The form in which carbohydrate is stored in the muscle.

myoglobin An iron-containing compound, similar to hemoglobin, found in the muscle tissues; it binds oxygen in the muscle cells.

narcotic Any agent that produces insensibility to pain.

natural, organic foods Foods that are stated to be grown without the use of man-made chemicals such as pesticides and artificial fertilizers.

Nautilus A brand of exercise equipment designed for strength training programs; uses a principle to help provide optimal resistance throughout the full range of motion.

negative caloric balance A condition whereby the caloric output exceeds the caloric intake, thus contributing to a weight loss.

net protein utilization *See* NPU.

newton A unit of force that will accelerate one kilogram of mass one meter per second per second.

niacin Nicotinamide; nicotinic acid; part of the B complex and an important part of several coenzymes involved in aerobic energy processes in the cells.

niacin equivalent A unit of measure of niacin activity in a food related to both the amount of niacin present and that obtainable from tryptophan; about 60 mg tryptophan can be converted to 1 mg niacin.

nickel A silvery-white metallic element.

nicotinamide An amide of nicotinic acid; niacin.

nicotinic acid Niacin.

nitrogen A colorless, tasteless, odorless gas comprising about 80 percent of the atmospheric gas; an essential component of protein that is formed in plants during their developmental process.

nonessential amino acids Amino acids that may be formed in the body and thus need not be obtained in the diet; *also see* essential amino acids.

normohydration The state of normal hydration, or normal body water levels as compared to dehydration and hyperhydration.

NPU Net protein utilization; a technique utilized to assess protein quality.

nutrient density A concept related to the degree of concentration of nutrients in a given food; *also see* the related concept INQ.

nutritional labeling A listing of selected key nutrients and calories on the label of commercially prepared food products.

obesity An excessive accumulation of body fat; usually reserved for those individuals who are 20–30 percent or greater above the average weight for their size.

oral contraceptives Birth control pills utilized to prevent conception.

osmoreceptors Receptors in the body that react to changes in the osmotic pressure of the blood.

osmotic pressure A pressure that produces a diffusion between solutions which have different concentrations.

osteoporosis Increased porosity or softening of the bone.

overload principle The major concept of physical training whereby one imposes a stress greater than that normally imposed upon a particular body system.

overweight Body weight greater than that which is considered normal; *also see* obesity.

ovolactovegetarian A vegetarian who also consumes eggs and milk products as a source of high quality animal protein.

ovovegetarian A vegetarian who includes eggs in the diet to help obtain adequate amounts of protein.

oxalates Salts of oxalic acid found in certain foods, such as spinach, that retards the absorption of some minerals like calcium.

oxygen consumption The total amount of oxygen utilized in the body for the production of energy; it is directly related to the metabolic rate.

oxygen system The energy system that produces ATP via the oxidation of various foodstuffs, primarily fats and carbohydrates.

PABA Para-aminobenzoic acid; a member of the B complex vitamins.

pantothenic acid A vitamin of the B complex.

para-aminobenzoic acid *See* PABA.

PC Phosphocreatine; a high energy phosphate compound found in the body cells; part of the ATP-PC energy system.

pellagra A deficiency disease caused by inadequate amounts of niacin in the diet.

peptides Small compounds formed by the union of two or more amino acids; known also as dipeptides, tripeptides, etc., depending upon the number of amino acids combined.

perceptual-motor activities Physical activities characterized by the perception of a given stimulus and culminating in an appropriate motor, or movement, response.

periactin A drug used to conteract some allergic reactions such as skin irritation.

pesticides Poisons utilized to destroy pests of various types, including plants and animals.

pH The symbol utilized to express the level of acidity of a solution; a low pH represents high acidity.

phenylalanine An essential amino acid.

phosphagens Compounds such as ATP and phosphocreatine that serve as a source of high energy in the body cells.

phosphates Salts of phosphoric acid, purported to possess ergogenic qualities.

phosphocreatine *See* PC.

phospholipids A lipid containing phosphorus, which in hydrolysis yields fatty acids, glycerin, and a nitrogenous compound. Lecithin is an example.

phosphorus A nonmetallic element essential to human nutrition.

phosphorus-calcium ratio The ratio of calcium to phosphorus intake in the diet; the normal ratio is 1:1.

phylloquinone Vitamin K, essential in the blood clotting process.

physical conditioning Methods used to increase the efficiency or capacity of a given body system so as to improve physical or athletic performance.

phytates Salts of phytic acid; produced in the body during the digestion of certain grain products; can combine with some minerals such as iron and possibly decrease their absorption.

polypeptides A combination of a number of simple amino acids; *also see* peptide.

polysaccharide A carbohydrate that upon hydrolysis will yield more than ten monosaccharides.

polyunsaturated fatty acids Fats that contain two or more double bonds and thus are open to hydrogenation.

positive caloric balance A condition whereby caloric intake exceeds caloric output; the resultant effect is a weight gain.

postabsorptive state The period of time after a meal has been absorbed from the gastrointestinal tract; in BMR tests it is usually a period of approximately twelve hours.

potassium A metallic element essential in human nutrition; it is the principal cation present in the intracellular fluids.

power Work divided by time; the ability to produce work in a given period of time.

power-endurance continuum In relation to strength training, the concept that power or strength is developed by high resistance and few repetitions, while endurance is developed by low resistance and many repetitions.

PRE Progressive Resistive Exercise.

pre-event nutrition Dietary intake prior to athletic competition; may refer to a two to three day period prior to an event or the immediate pre-event meal.

Pritikin program A dietary program developed by Nathan Pritikin severely restricts the intake of certain foods like fats and cholesterol and greatly increases the consumption of complex carbohydrates.

progressive resistance principle A training technique, primarily with weights, whereby resistance is increased as the individual develops increased strength levels.

proline A nonessential amino acid.

proof Relative to alcohol content, proof is twice the percentage of alcohol in a solution; 80 proof whiskey is 40 percent alcohol.

protein Any one of a group of complex organic compounds containing nitrogen; formed from various combinations of amino acids.

protein-calorie insufficiency A major health problem in certain parts of the world where the population suffers from inadequate intake of protein and total calories.

protein complementarity The practice among vegetarians of eating foods together from two or more different food groups, usually legumes, nuts, or beans with grain products, in order to ensure a balanced intake of essential amino acids.

protein sparing effect An adequate intake of energy calories, as from carbohydrate, will decrease somewhat the rate of protein catabolism in the body and hence spare protein.

provitamin A Carotene, a substance in the diet from which the body may form vitamin A.

pyridoxal A component of the vitamin B_6 group.

pyridoxamine A part of the vitamin B_6 group; an analog of pyridoxine.

pyridoxine A component of the vitamin B complex, vitamin B_6.

pyruvate The end product of glycolysis. Under aerobic conditions it may be converted into acetyl CoA while under anaerobic conditions it is converted into lactic acid.

radiation Electromagnetic waves given off by an object; the body radiates heat to a cool environment.

ratings of perceived exertion *See* RPE.

RDA Recommended Dietary Allowances; the levels of intake of essential nutrients considered to be adequate to meet the known nutritional needs of practically all healthy persons.

RE A measure of vitamin A activity in food as measured by preformed vitamin A or carotene, provitamin A; 1 RE equals 5 IU.

recommended dietary allowances *See* RDA.

recommended dietary goals Dietary goals for Americans which have been established by a U.S. Senate subcommittee on nutrition; goals stress dietary reduction of fat, cholesterol, salt, and sugar and increase in complex carbohydrates.

relative humidity The percentage of moisture in the air compared to the amount of moisture needed to cause saturation, which is taken as 100.

repetitions In relation to weight training or interval training, the number of times that an exercise is done.

resting metabolic rate *See* RMR.

retinol Vitamin A.

retinol equivalent *See* RE.

riboflavin Vitamin B_2, a member of the B complex.

RMR Resting metabolic rate; the energy requirement to drive all physiological processes while in a state of rest; *also see* BMR and EMR.

RPE A subjective rating, on a numerical scale, used to express the perceived difficulty of a given work task.

running Although the distinction between running and jogging is relative to the individual involved, a common value used for running is 7 mph or faster.

saccharide A series of carbohydrates from simple sugars (monosaccharides) to complex carbohydrates (polysaccharides).

salt depletion heat exhaustion Weakness caused by excessive loss of electrolytes as in excessive sweating.

satiety center A group of nerve cells in the hypothalamus that responds to certain stimuli in the blood and provides a sensation of satiety.

saturated fatty acids Fats that have all chemical bonds filled.

SDA Specific dynamic action; often used to represent the increased energy cost observed during the metabolism of protein in the body.

selenium A nonmetallic element resembling sulfur; poisonous to some animals.

serum lipid level The concentration of lipids in the blood serum.

sets In weight training, a certain number of repetitions constitutes a set; for example, a lifter may do three sets of six repetitions in each set.

shell temperature The temperature of the skin; *also see* core temperature.

SI Le Systeme International d'Unite, or the International System of Units; a system of measurement based upon the metric system.

silicon A nonmetallic element.

simple carbohydrates Usually used to refer to table sugar, or sucrose, a disaccharide; may refer also to other disaccharides and the monosaccharides.

skinfold technique A technique utilized to compute an individual's percentage of body fat; various skinfolds are measured and a regression formula is used to compute the body fat.

sling psychrometer A device that incorporates both a dry bulb and wet bulb thermometer thus providing a heat stress index incorporating both temperature and relative humidity.

slow twitch fibers Red muscle fibers that have a slow contraction speed; designed for aerobic type activity.

sodium A soft metallic element; combines with chloride to form salt; the major extracellular cation in the human body.

specific dynamic action *See* SDA.

specific heat The amount of energy or heat needed to raise the temperature of a unit of mass, such as one kilogram of body tissue, one degree Celsius.

sports anemia A temporary condition of low hemoglobin levels often observed in athletes during the early stages of training.

spot reducing The theory that exercising a specific body part, such as the thighs, will facilitate the loss of body fat from that spot.

standardized exercise An exercise task that conforms to a specific standardized protocol.

steady state A level of metabolism, usually during exercise, when the oxygen consumption satisfies the energy expenditure and the individual is performing in an aerobic state.

sterols Substances similar to fats because of their solubility characteristics; most commonly known one is cholesterol.

stimulus period In exercise programs, the time period over which the stimulus is applied, such as a HR of 150 for fifteen minutes.

storage fat Fat that accumulates and is stored in the adipose tissue; *also see* essential fat.

sucrose Table sugar, a disaccharide; yields glucose and fructose upon hydrolysis.

sulfur A pale yellow nonmetallic element essential in human nutrition; component of the sulfur containing amino acids.

suma wrestling A form of wrestling in Japan.

target heart rate In an aerobic exercise program, the heart rate level that will provide the stimulus for a beneficial training effect.

thiamin Vitamin B_1.

threonine An essential amino acid.

thyroxine A hormone secreted by the thyroid gland that is involved in the control of the metabolic rate.

tin A white metallic element.

tocopherol Generic name for an alcohol that has the activity of vitamin E.

total body fat The sum total of the body's storage and essential fat stores.

trace elements Those minerals essential to human nutrition that have an RDA less than 100 mg daily.

triglycerides One of the many fats formed by the union of glycerol and fatty acids.

tryptophan An essential amino acid.

tyrosine A nonessential amino acid.

underwater weighing A technique for measuring the percentage of body fat in humans.

United States recommended daily allowances *See* U.S. RDA.

Universal gym A brand name for exercise equipment, particularly weights for strength development.

unsaturated fatty acids Fatty acids that contain double or triple bonds and hence can add hydrogen atoms.

urea The chief nitrogenous constituent of the urine and the final product of the decomposition of proteins in the body.

U.S. RDA The United States Recommended Daily Allowances; the RDA figures used on labels, representing the percentage of the RDA for a given nutrient contained in a serving of the food.

valine An essential amino acid.

vanadium A light gray metallic element.

vascular water The body water contained in the blood vessels; a part of the extracellular water.

vasodilation An increase in the size of the blood vessels, usually referring to the arterial system.

vegan An extreme vegetarian who eats no animal protein.

vegetarian One whose food is of vegetable or plant origin; *also see* lactovegetarian, ovovegetarian, ovolactovegetarian, and vegan.

very low density lipoprotein *See* VLDL.

vitamin, natural Often referred to as vitamins derived from natural sources; *i.e.*, foods in nature; contrast with vitamin, synthetic.

vitamin, synthetic A man-made vitamin commercially produced from the separate components of the vitamin.

vitamin A An unsaturated aliphatic alcohol; fat soluble.

vitamin B_1 Thiamin; the antineuritic vitamin.

vitamin B_2 Riboflavin.

vitamin B_6 Pyridoxine and related compounds.

vitamin B_{12} Cyanocobalamin.

vitamin B_{15} Not a vitamin but marketed as one; usual composition is calcium gluconate and dimethylglycine (DMG).

vitamin C Ascorbic acid; the antiscorbutic vitamin.

vitamin D Any one of related sterols that have antirachitic properties; fat soluble.

vitamin deficiency Subnormal body vitamin levels due to inadequate intake or absorption; specific disorders occur dependent upon the deficient vitamin.

vitamin E Alpha-tocopherol, one of three tocopherols; fat soluble.

vitamin K The antihemorrhagic, or clotting vitamin; fat soluble.

vitamins A general term for a number of substances deemed essential for the normal metabolic functioning of the body.

VLDL Very low density lipoproteins; a protein-lipid complex in the blood that transports triglycerides, cholesterol, and phospholipids; has a very low density; *also see* HDL and LDL cholesterol.

VO_2 max Maximal oxygen uptake; measured during exercise, the maximal amount of oxygen consumed reflects the body's ability to utilize oxygen as an energy source; equals the cardiac output times the arterio-venous oxygen difference.

warm-up Low level exercises used to increase the muscle temperature and/or stretch the muscles prior to a strenuous exercise bout.

water A tasteless, colorless, odorless fluid essential to life; composed of two parts hydrogen and one part oxygen (H_2O).

water depletion heat exhaustion Weakness caused by excessive loss of body fluids such as through exercise-induced dehydration in a hot or warm environment.

watt A unit of power in the SI.

WBGT index Wet bulb globe thermometer index; a heat stress index based upon four factors measured by the wet bulb globe thermometer.

wet bulb globe thermometer A device that takes into account the various factors determining heat stress: air temperature, air movement, radiation heat, and humidity.

work Effort expended to accomplish something; in terms of physics, force times distance.

zinc A blue-white crystalline metallic element essential to human nutrition.

Index

Acclimatization
    to heat   197–98
Acetyl CoA   48, 79
ACSM. *See* American College of Sports Medicine
Additives   221–22
Adenosinetriphosphate   108–18
Adipose tissue   44, 51
Adolescent nutrient needs   240–41
Age
    and exercise in the heat   196
Alanine   55
    use during exercise   64
Alcohol   205–13, 217
    and blood lipids   52
    in diets   165
    and fat synthesis   46
    and folacin   79
    and physical performance   209–12
    and vitamin B_{12} 80
    and vitamin supplements   74
Alcohol dehydrogenase   209
Alcoholic beverages
Aldosterone
    and sodium retention   89
Alpha tocopherol   82–83. *See also* Vitamin E
Amenorrhea   238
American College of Sports Medicine   152
    recommendation on hyperhydration   232, 248
American Council on Science and Health   233
American Dietetic Association   165
American Medical Association   247
Amino acids   55, 60
    essential   2, 56
    and fat synthesis   48
    glucogenic   60
    ketogenic   60
    nonessential   56
Aminostatic theory   154
Ammonia   61
Anabolic steroids   152
Anabolism   121. *See also* Metabolism
Anaerobic threshold   112, 120
Anemia
    and folacin   79
    iron deficiency   93
    sports. *See* Sports anemia
    and vitamin B_{12} 80
Antidiuretic hormone   100
Appetite
    effect of exercise on   173

Archery
    energy expenditure in   262
Ascorbic acid   80–81. *See also* Vitamin C
Atherosclerosis   50. *See also* Coronary heart disease
    and dietary fiber   24
Athletes
    pre-event nutrition   241–43
Athletic performance
    and ergogenic aids   230–33
ATP-PC energy system   110–13

Badminton
    energy expenditure in   262
BAL. *See* Blood alcohol level
Banister, R.   248
Basal metabolic rate   122–26, 141. *See also* Metabolism
    estimation of   122–24
Baseball
    energy expenditure in   262
Basic Four Food Groups   6, 155
    and balanced diets   10–13
    common foods in (table)   7
    and dieting   164–65
    in fast foods   228–29
    major nutrients in   8–9
    recommended minimum servings   10
    serving sizes   10
    and weight gaining   149
Basketball
    energy expenditure in   262
Bee pollen   232
Beer
    energy content   207
    food value   207
Behavioral strategies
    and dieting   161–63
BHA   223
BHT   223
Bicycling
    energy expenditure in   262
Biotin   114
    high content foods   80, 84
Blood alcohol level   209
Blood glucose   21–22, 26. *See also* Hypoglycemia
Blood lipids   51–52
    and alcohol   212–13
    effect of diet   51–53
    effect of exercise   53
Blood pressure
    in cardiac risk index   278
Blood sugar. *See* Blood glucose
BMR. *See* Basal metabolic rate

Body composition   133–42
    measurement of   137–39
Body fat
    Calories in pound of   140
    dietary losses   153
    effect on physical performance   139
    essential   139
    losses through exercise   171–86
    measurement of   137–39
    normal values   137–40
    safe losses   142
    storage   137
    total body   137
Body punch   201
Body temperature. *See* Temperature, body
Body water
    losses   158–59, 184–85
    replacement of   200
Body weight   133–42
    desirable. *See* Weights, body
    dietary losses   153–70
    gaining   143–52
    ideal   133–35
    metabolic control of   154
    prediction of losses   156–57
    slow versus fast losses   158
    water losses   158
Borenstein, B.   220
Bowling
    energy expenditure in   264
Brake Time®   201
Bread-Cereal Group
    cholesterol content   45
    common foods in   7, 20
    exchange lists   258, 289
    fat Calories   42
    nutrients in   9
    protein content   59
    recommended servings   10
    serving size   10
    vitamin content   84
Breakfast
    and physical performance   244–45

Caffeine   205, 213–17
    and FFA use during exercise   50
    physiological effects   214–16
Calcium   86–87
    food sources (table)   94
    and osteoporosis   241
    in sweat   198–99
Calcium-phosphorus ratio   88
Caloric concept of weight control   140–41

Calories
    in alcoholic beverages   207–8
    counting   155–56
    daily consumption   159–61
    daily expenditure (table)   126
    deficit in weight loss   156–57
    defined   106–7
    diet plans   282–91
    expenditure during exercise   130–32, 262–71
    in fast foods   276–77
    and METS   129
    and oxygen consumption   129
    percentage from fat   43
    RDA   251
    recording daily intake   160–61
    and weight maintenance   141–42
Calorimeter   106
Carbohydrate diets
    health implications   25–27
Carbohydrate loading   31–37
    different methods   33
    effects of   35
    examples of diets   34
    possible health problems   36–37
    protein phase   64
    protein sparing effect   64–65
Carbohydrates   19–37
    caloric equivalents   107–8
    complex   20, 34–35
    current dietary intake   14
    digestion of   21
    energy sources   22
    as energy source during exercise   118–20
    energy stores in body   110
    as ergogenic aid   232
    and exercise   27–37
    and fat synthesis   48
    food sources of   3, 20
    from protein and fat   23
    functions of   4
    metabolism in body   21–22
    and niacin   77
    in pre-game meal   242–43
    protein sparing effect   62
    and protein synthesis   61–62
    recommended dietary intake   14
    simple   19, 34–35
    and thiamine   76
    types and sources   19
Cardiac risk index   278–79
Carotene   71
Catabolism   121. See also Metabolism
CHD. See Coronary heart disease
Children
    and caffeine   216–17
    nutritional requirements   239–41
Chloride   91. See also electrolytes
Cholecalciferol   81–82

Cholesterol   12, 43–46
    blood, effect of diet   51–53
    and carbohydrate loading   36
    in cardiac risk index   278
    and coronary heart disease   46–47, 50–54
    current dietary intake   14
    diet, low in   280–81
    and dietary fiber   24
    dietary goals   14, 48
    effects of exercise   53–54
    HDL   47, 245
        and alcohol   212–13
    LDL   46
    and Lipoproteins   46–47
Choline   80
    high content foods   84
Chromium   95
Chylomicron   44
Cobalt   95
Coenzyme   70
Coffee
    caffeine in   213
Colas
    sugar content   30
Complex carbohydrates
    dietary goals   25
Conduction   188
Contraceptives, oral
    and folacin   79
    and nutrient requirements   238
    and vitamin B$_{12}$ 79–80
Convection   188
Cooper, K.   183
Copper   95
Coronary heart disease   240
    and alcohol   212–13
    and caffeine   216–17
    and carbohydrate loading   37
    and cholesterol   50–54
    and recommended dietary goals   14–15
    risk factors   51, 278–79
Costill, D.   34
Cramps, heat   194
Cyanocobalamin
    See also Vitamin B$_{12}$ 79–80

Dancing
    energy expenditure in   264
Dayton, S.   51
Dehydration   97, 184–85, 199
    and caffeine   214, 216
    effects of alcohol   212
    in wrestlers   246–48
Deutsch, R.   123
Dextrose   19
Diabetes
    and exercise   246
Diet
    balanced   9, 12
    development of personal   166–67

free foods   260, 287
high calorie   150
low calorie   165–69
low cholesterol   280–81
personal   165–69
plans   282–91
polyunsaturated fat   280–81
and your health   245–46
and weight gaining   143–52
for weight gains   149–52
Dietary goals   14
    carbohydrate   25
    cholesterol   48
    fat   48
    protein   63
Dietary intake
    current American   14
    proposed American   14
Disaccharides   19, 21
Diuretics   242, 247
    caffeine   214, 216
Durnin, J. V.   66, 219, 248

Electrolytes   29, 86, 99–100, 198–203
    RDA (table)   252
    See also individual electrolytes
Elements, trace   95–96
    RDA (table)   251–52
Endurance
    and iron   93
Energy   103–20
    Calorie concept   106–8
    during exercise   262–71
    expenditure, daily (table)   126
    human systems   110–14
    intake, RDA   251
    measures of   103–9
    metabolism   121–32
    sources, human   103–20
    stores in body (table)   110
    utilization
        during exercise   115–20
        during rest   114–15
English-Metric conversion   272–73
Ensure®   243
Ensure-Plus®   243
Environmental Effects
    on exercise   187–203
    heat stress   191–93
Enzymes   70
ERG®   201
Ergogenic Aids   230–33
Ethanol. See Alcohol
Ethyl Alcohol. See Alcohol
Evaporation   188
Exchange lists, food   166, 255–60
Exercise
    acute effects of   236
    aerobic   112, 171–86
    and blood cholesterol   53–54
    and blood lipids   53–54

calculation of energy expenditure 129, 262–71
and caloric expenditure 130–32, 262–71
and carbohydrates 27–37
in cardiac risk index 278–79
chronic effects of 236
cool down 176–77
duration concept in weight control 174
effect on appetite 173
effect on body temperature 189–93
energy requirements 121–32
energy sources during 115–20
fluid replacement 201–3
hazards in heat 193–98
heart rate as guide to 177–83
in heat 187–203
    dangers 185
heat, precautions in 176
and human energy systems 115–20
and hypoglycemia 26
intensity 21
    and caloric expenditure 174
    and energy systems 118–19
metabolic aftereffects of 127, 172
metabolic rate 124–32
muscle groups (table) 146–47
and nutritional requirements 235–41
and osteoporosis 87, 241
precautions 175–76
progressive resistance 145
and protein catabolism 65
self-initiated program 175–83
spot reducing 183
warm-up 176
and weight gaining 143–52
and weight loss 171–86
weight training 145–48
and your health 245–46
Extracellular water 98

Fast foods 228–29
    Calories in 276–77
Fasting 169–70. *See also* Starvation
Fat, Body. *See* Body fat
Fats 39–54
    animal 40
    caloric equivalents 107–8
    current dietary intake 14
    dietary goals 14, 48
    as energy source during exercise 49, 119–20
        effects of training 49–50
    energy stores in body (table) 110
    exchange list 259–60, 290
    in fast foods 229
    food energy (table) 41–42
    foods high in 41–42
    food sources 3
    health hazards 50–54
    hydrogenated 39
    metabolism in body 44–48
    monounsaturated 14

niacin 77–78
polyunsaturated 259–60
    dietary intake 14
    diet plan 282–86
    and protein synthesis 62
saturated 185, 260
    dietary intake 14
    as source of carbohydrate 23
    synthesis from protein 60
    types and sources 39
    vegetable 40
    and vitamins 48
Fatigue
    and carbohydrates 27–37
    and hypoglycemia 31
    and lactic acid 111–12
Fatty Acids
    essential 2, 40
    polyunsaturated 39
    saturated 39–40
    unsaturated 39–40
FDA. *See* Food and Drug Administration
Feeding center 154
Feingold hypothesis 222
Females
    exercise in the heat 195–96
    nutritional requirements of active 237–39
Ferritin 92
FFA. *See* Free fatty acids
Fiber 1, 20
    and cholesterol 24
Fluid
    replacement of body 200–203
Fluoride 95
Folacin 79, 114
    and alcohol 208
    high content foods 84
Folic acid. *See* folacin
Food
    cultism 229–30
    nutritional labeling of 226–29
    nutritional value of 220
    processing 220
Food and Drug Administration
    and food additives 222
    and pesticides 223–24
Food exchange lists 166, 255–60
    diet meal pattern 167
Food exchanges 287–91
    bread 289
    fat 290
    fruits 288
    meat 290
    milk 291
    vegetables 287
Food and Nutrition Board 248
Foods
    fast 228–29
        Calories in 276–77
    functions of 4
    natural and organic 224–25

Football
    energy expenditure in 264
Foot-pound 105
Fox, E. 110
Free fatty acids 109–10
    effects of caffeine 214–16
    as energy sources in exercise 49
        effects of training 49–50
    glycogen sparing effect during exercise 50
Fructose 19
    as energy source during exercise 31
Fruits
    exchange list 257, 288
Fruit-Vegetable Group
    common foods 7, 20
    and fat Calories 42
    nutrients in 8–9
    protein content 59
    recommended servings 10
    serving size 10
    vitamin content 84

Gatorade® 31, 201
GES. *See* Glucose-electrolyte solution
Gluconeogenesis 23, 60
    from protein during exercise 64–65
Glucose 19, 21
    and alcohol 211
    blood. *See* blood glucose
    and caffeine 215
    in electrolyte solutions 29–30
    in fat synthesis 46
    in GES solutions 201–2
    from protein 60–61
Glucose electrolyte solutions 29–30, 201–2
Glucose polymer 29
Glucostatic theory 154
Glycerol 39
Glycogen 21–24, 109, 118, 184
    and carbohydrate loading 34–35
    liver 21–22
    muscle 21–22, 24, 30–37
    and weight loss 158
Glycogen loading 31–37. *See also* Carbohydrate loading
Glycogen sparing effect
    caffeine 215
Glycolysis 112
Golf
    energy expenditure in 264
Grain products
    exchange list 289
GRAS 222
Growth and development
    nutrient needs 239–41

Handball
    energy expenditure in 264

Heart rate
  determination of 177
  exercise in the heat 197–98
  and exercise intensity 177–83
  maximal 179
  maximal reserve 179
  and oxygen consumption 128
  target 179
Heat 187–203
  acclimatization 197–98
  loss 188
  specific 189
  syncope 194
Heat balance equation 188
Heat illnesses 193–98
  prevention of 196–98
  table of 195
Height-weight charts 134–35
Hemoglobin 4–5, 92
Herbert, V. 75, 233
High density lipoproteins. See Cholesterol, HDL
Homeostasis 100
HR Max. See Heart rate, maximal
Human energy systems 110–20
  major characteristics (table) 116
Humidity, relative 191
Hypercholesteremia 51–52
Hyperglycemia 29–31
Hyperhydration 100, 203, 232
Hypertension 245
  and sodium 90
Hypertriglyceridemia 51–52
Hypervitaminosis 75, 82
Hypoglycemia 26, 29, 242
  and alcohol 211
  in exercising diabetics 246
  and fatigue 31
Hypohydration 100
Hypothalamus
  body temperature regulation 189
  and weight control 154

Index of Nutritional Quality 4, 225–26
Indicator Nutrients 227
Inositol 80
INQ. See Index of nutritional quality
Insulin 26
Intercellular water 98
International Olympic Committee 212, 215
Intracellular water 98
IOC. See International Olympic Committee
Iodine 95
Ions 86. See also Electrolytes
Iron 92–94, 114, 236
  and female athletes 237–39
  and fiber 24
  food sources (table) 94
  in sweat 198–99

Jogging 180–81. See also Running
  energy expenditure in 266–67
Joule 105

Kannel, W. B. 51
Ketones
  and alcohol 209
Kilogram-meter 105

Labeling, nutritional 222, 226–28
Lactate
  and alcohol 209
Lactic acid 112
Lactic acid energy system 111
Lactose 19
Lean body mass 137
  increases in 144–52
Lecithin 88–89
Legumes
  and fat Calories 41
  protein content 58
  vitamin content 84
Lipases 44
Lipids, serum 46
Lipoproteins 46–47. See also Cholesterol, HDL, LDL
  and coronary heart disease 53–54
Lipostatic theory 154
Liquid meals
  in pre-event nutrition 243–46
Liquid protein diets 64
Liver
  and alcohol metabolism 209–10
  and carbohydrate metabolism 21
  and fat metabolism 46
  and protein metabolism 60

Magnesium 91
  food sources (table) 94
  in sweat 198–99
Maltose 19
Manganese 95
Marathon running
  and carbohydrates 29–37
Maximal oxygen uptake 117
  See also VO$_2$ max
Mayer, J. 171, 248
Mayo Clinic 165–66
Measurements
  English-metric 272–73
  systems
    English 104–5
    international unit 105
    metric 104–5
Meat
  exchange list 259, 290
Meat Group
  cholesterol content 47
  common foods 7
  and fat Calories 41
  nutrients in 8–9

protein content 58–59
recommended servings 10
serving size 10
vitamin content 84
Metabolic aftereffects of exercise 127
Metabolism 121. See also Basal metabolic rate and exercise, metabolic rate
Metric-English conversion 272–73
METS 129
Milk
Milk Group
  cholesterol content 47
  common foods 7
  and fat Calories 41
  nutrients in 8–9
  protein content 58–59
  recommended servings 10
  serving size 10
  vitamin content 84
Minerals 85–96
  essential 1
  table 87
  food source 3
  major 86
  RDA 250–52
  roles in body 85
Molybdenum 95
Monosaccharides 19, 21, 24
Monosodium glutamate 223
Muscle fibers 31–32
  fast twitch 32, 118
  slow twitch 31, 118
Muscles
  major groups 146–47
Myoglobin 114

Natural foods 224–25
Nautilus 147
Niacin 77–78, 114
  equivalent 77
  and fat utilization during exercise 50
  high content foods 84
Nickel 95
Nicotinamide. See Niacin
Nicotinic acid. See Niacin
Nitrogen
  losses during exercise 63–64
  in protein 61
Normohydration 100
NPU. See Net protein utilization
Nutrament 243
Nutrient density 4, 225–26
Nutrients
  for active people 235–41
  caloric equivalents 107–8
  essential 1–15
  table 2–3
  and food processing 220
  indicator 227
  key food sources (table) 3
  and weight loss 158–59

Nuts
    and fat Calories 41
    nutritional value of 260

Obesity 13, 133–42
    in children 239–41
    and heat intolerance 196
Oral contraceptives. *See* Contraceptives, oral
Organic foods 224–25
Osteoporosis 86–87, 241
Overload principle 145
Oxygen
    caloric equivalent 107–8
Oxygen energy system 112–14
    nutrients used 115–17

PABA. *See* Para-aminobenzoic acid
Pangamic acid 232–33
Pantothenic acid 78–79, 114
    high content foods 84
Para-aminobenzoic acid 80
Peas, dried. *See* Legumes
Peptides 55
Perceptual-motor activities 210–11
Perspiration. *See also* Sweat
    insensible 97
Pesticides
    in food 223–24
Phosphates 88
Phosphocreatine 108–11
Phospholipids 44
Phosphorus 88
    food sources (table) 94
Phosphorus-calcium ratio 88
Phylloquinone 83
Polysaccharides 21
Polyunsaturated fat
    diet low in 282–83
Potassium 90. *See also* Electrolytes
    food sources (table) 94
    sweat losses 90
Power 104–5
Power-endurance continuum 116
Pre-event nutrition 241–43
Pre-game meals 241–43
Pregnancy
    nutrient requirements 238
Pritikin Program 25
Proof, alcohol 207
Protein
    animal 56–57
    breakdown during exercise 65
    caloric equivalent 107–8
    chemical structure 56
    current dietary intake 14
    dietary goals 14, 63
    as energy source 115
        during exercise 64, 236
    energy stores in body (table) 110
    as fat carrier 44

and fat synthesis 48
food sources 3, 58–60
functions of 4–5
liquid diets 64
losses in sweat 66
metabolism 60–62
    and exercise 64–66
nutritional labeling of 227
plant 56–57
in pre-game meal 242
RDA 57, 63–64
as source of carbohydrate 23
specific dynamic action of 155
and sports anemia 65–66
supplementation 151
    and athletes 65–66
    as ergogenic aids 232
synthesis 61
types and sources 55
vegetable 57
Protein-Calorie insufficiency 63
Protein diets
    health aspects 63–64
Protein sparing effect 62
Provitamin A 75
Pyridoxine 78, 114

Quackery 219
    nutritional in athletics 229–33
Quickick® 201

Radiation 188
Ratings of perceived exertion 178–83
RBC. *See* Red blood cells
RDA. *See* Recommended dietary allowances
Recommended dietary allowances 5–6
    minerals (table) 87
    protein 57–59
    table 250–52
    vitamins. *See* individual vitamins
Recommended dietary goals 14–15
Red blood cells 5
    and folacin 79
    and vitamin B_{12} 80
Relative humidity 191
Resting metabolic rate 122. *See also* Metabolism
Retinol 75
Retinol equivalent 75
Riboflavin 76–77, 114
RMR. *See* Resting metabolic rate
RPE. *See* Ratings of perceived exertion
Running
    caloric cost of 131–32, 266–67
    and carbohydrates 29–37
    and energy expenditure 174, 266–67

Saccharide 21

Saccharin 223
Salt
    current dietary intake 14
    dietary goals 14
    in diets 165
    tablets 200–201
Salt-depletion heat exhaustion 194–95
Satiety center 154
Saturated fats 12. *See also* Fats, saturated
    dietary reduction of 52
Sedentary activities
    energy expenditure in 262–63
Selenium 95
Senate Select Subcommittee on Nutrition 14
Shephard, R. 83
Silicon 96
Simonson, E. 248
Simple carbohydrates
    and blood lipids 52
    dietary goals 25–26
    and exercise 28–29
Skiing
    energy expenditure in 265–69
Skinfold technique 138
Smoking
    in cardiac risk index 278
Sodium 89–90. *See also* Electrolytes
    salt tablets 200–201
    sweat losses 90
Sodium chloride ?
    food sources (table) 94
Sodium nitrate 223
Sodium nitrite 223
Specific heat 189–91
Sports anemia 65–67
Squash
    energy expenditure in 268–69
Starvation 141, 169–70
Stroke, heat 194
Sucrose 19, 26–27
Sugar
    and pre-game meals 242
Sulfur 96
SustaCal 243
Sustagen 243
Sweat 97
    composition 198–99
Sweating 187–203
Swimming
    energy expenditure in 268–69

Tarahumara Indians 25
Tatkon, M. 69
Temperature, body 187–93
    effect of exercise on 189–93
    regulation 187–89
Thermometer 191–92
    wet bulb globe 191–92
Thiamin 76, 114. *See also* Vitamin B_1

Index   313

Thirst 101
Tin 96
Trace elements. *See* Elements, trace
Training
   effect on carbohydrate use 119–20
   effect on fat use 119–20
Triglyceride 39
   structure of 40
Tryptophan
   niacin equivalent 77–78

Underwater weighing 137–38
Underweight
   causes of 143
Universal Gym 147
United States Recommended Daily Allowances 6
   and indicator nutrients 227
Urea 61
U.S. RDA. *See* United States Recommended Daily Allowances

Vanadium 96
Vegetables
   exchange lists 256, 287
Vegetarians 13
Very low density lipoproteins. *See* Lipoproteins
Vitamin A 75–76
   high content foods 84
Vitamin B$_1$ 76
   and alcohol 208
   high content foods 84
Vitamin B$_2$ 76–77
   high content foods 84
Vitamin B$_6$ 76
   high content foods 84
Vitamin B$_{12}$ 79–80, 114
   and alcohol 208
   high content foods 84
Vitamin B$_{15}$ 232–33
Vitamin C 80–81
   high content foods 84
Vitamin D 81–82
Vitamin E 82–83

Vitamin K 83
Vitamins 69–84. *See also* individual vitamins
   and active females 237–39
   and athletic performance. *See* individual vitamins
   as coenzymes 70
   deficiency 72
   as ergogenic acids 232
   essential 2
   fat soluble 2, 71
   and food processing 220–21
   food sources 3
      high content (table) 84
   formation in body 71
   megadoses 74–75
   and mineral interactions 72
   natural 71–72
   and natural foods 224–25
   RDA 250–53
   supplements 72–74
      to athletes 74, 83
   synthetic 71–72
   table of 71
   water soluble 2, 71
VO$_2$ max 118–19

Walking
   energy expenditure in 270–71
Water. *See also* Body water
   body losses 158
   and exercise 102
   extracellular 98–99
   intercellular 98–99
   intracellular 98–99
   metabolism 97–98
   replenishment in exercise 29–30
   and salt tablets 200–201
   vascular 98–99
Water-depletion heat exhaustion 194
Watt 105
WBGT Index 191–92

Weight control 133–86. *See also* Weight loss
   behavioral patterns 161–62
   caloric concept 140–41
   dietary losses 153–70
   diet versus exercise 185–86
   long haul concept 171
Weight gaining
   nutritional principles 149–52
Weight-height charts 134–35
Weight loss
   rapid 184–85
   spot reducing 183
   through exercise 171–86
Weights, desirable (tables) 134–35
   boys 274
   girls 275
Weight training 145–48
   energy expenditure in 270–71
Williams, J. 248
Wine
   energy content 207
   food value 207
Women. *See also* Females
   and iron 92–93
   osteoporosis 87, 241
Work 104–6. *See also* Exercise
   caloric equivalents 107–8
Wrestling
   energy expenditure in 270–71
   and rapid weight loss 246–48

Zinc 96, 114